DATE DUE			

THE ENCYCLOPEDIA OF

MULTIPLE SCLEROSIS

THE ENCYCLOPEDIA OF

MULTIPLE SCLEROSIS

Carol Turkington and
Kaye D. Hooper, M.P.H., R.N., M.S.C.N.

in collaboration with

Rosalind C. Kalb, Ph.D., and
Nancy J. Holland, Ed.D., R.N., M.S.C.N.

☑®
Facts On File, Inc.

The Encyclopedia of Multiple Sclerosis

Facts On File, Inc.
132 West 31st Street
New York NY 10001

Library of Congress Cataloging-in-Publication Data

Turkington, Carol.
The encyclopedia of multiple sclerosis / Carol Turkington.
p. cm.
Includes bibliographical references and index.
ISBN 0-8160-5623-4 (hc: alk. paper)
1. Multiple sclerosis—Encyclopedias. 2. Multiple sclerosis—Popular works. I. Title.
RC377.T875 2005
616.8'34'003—dc22
2004022858

Facts On File books are available at special discounts when purchased in bulk quantities for businesses, associations, institutions, or sales promotions. Please call our Special Sales Department in New York at (212) 967-8800 or (800) 322-8755.

You can find Facts On File on the World Wide Web at http://www.factsonfile.com

Text and cover design by Cathy Rincon

Printed in the United States of America

VB Hermitage 10 9 8 7 6 5 4 3 2 1

This book is printed on acid-free paper.

For
Robert Dayton Turkington
1912–1975
—C.T.

To people with MS and all those who journey through life with them.
May we continue to learn from and support each other well.
With loving thanks to my husband, Bruce, for his support and encouragement.
—K.H.

CONTENTS

FOREWORD

Every hour, someone receives a diagnosis of multiple sclerosis (MS). There are thought to be 400,000 people with MS in the United States and as many as 2.5 million others around the world with the disease. While certainly not the most common disease or the most threatening to the population at large, its chronic, variable, and unpredictable course can have a devastating impact on all those who have it or care about someone who does.

Although it can occur in very young children and older adults, MS is usually diagnosed between the ages of 20 and 50, when people are beginning their careers and families or just beginning to enjoy the fruits of their labors. MS is more common in women than men by a ratio of 2–3:1, and occurs more commonly in Caucasians of northern European ancestry than in other racial groups. The cause of MS is still unknown, but it is thought to be triggered in genetically susceptible individuals by an as-yet-unidentified environmental agent, such as a virus or bacterium.

Multiple sclerosis is an immune-mediated disease that primarily affects the central nervous system (CNS)—the brain, spinal cord, and optic nerves. It is believed to be an autoimmune disease in which the immune system mistakenly attacks the myelin sheath, the protective coating surrounding the nerves in the CNS that speeds the conduction of nerve impulses. Irreversible damage to the nerves themselves can occur as well.

This damage to the myelin in the CNS can produce a remarkable array of symptoms, including fatigue; weakness; problems with coordination; spasticity (stiffness); sensory changes such as numbness, tingling, and pain; impaired vision; bladder and bowel problems; tremor; sexual dysfunction; emotional changes such as mood swings and depression; and problems with thinking and memory. While most people will experience only a few of these symptoms, some will grapple with many. While some will experience relatively mild symptoms that come and go, others will have to deal with symptoms that come and stay, gradually worsening over time.

There are thought to be four basic types, or courses, of MS. *Relapsing-remitting MS,* which is the most common, is characterized by clearly defined inflammatory attacks that last for days or weeks and then subside, with no disease progression in between. *Secondary progressive MS* begins with a relapsing-remitting course that gradually becomes more consistently progressive, with or without acute attacks. *Progressive-relapsing MS,* which is relatively rare, is characterized by clear progression from the onset of the disease, with acute attacks superimposed along the way. *Primary progressive MS* is characterized by steady progression of disability from onset, without any acute attacks.

For most individuals with MS and their loved ones, the greatest challenge to coping with this disease is its unpredictability; each person's MS is unique, and there is no roadmap to guide the way. People with MS report that they seldom know how they are going to feel later in the day, let alone next week or next year.

The range and complexity of symptoms caused by MS can significantly impact a person's activities at home and at work. Although 90 percent of people with MS have worked at some time in their life, and approximately two-thirds are employed at the time of diagnosis, only 25 to 40 percent of Americans with MS are presently employed. The symptoms thought to figure most prominently in this early departure from the workforce are fatigue and cognitive impairment. These same symptoms, along with the many others that can occur, can also interfere with the performance of roles at home, leading to feelings of grief and loss, frustration and anger. Thus, while the numbers of people with MS are fairly small relative to other diseases, the emotional, social and economic impact is significant. The total *direct* (i.e., outpatient and inpatient medical care and services) and *indirect* (i.e., lost wages) costs per person per year in the United States come to $57,000, for a total cost of $23 billion per year.

Fortunately, tremendous progress has been made in the management of MS; although we still do not have a cure, more new tools to diagnose and treat this disease have been developed in the last 20 years than in all the decades since Jean-Martin Charcot first described it in 1868. Gone are the days of "diagnose and adios," a phrase coined in the 1980s by Dr. Labe Scheinberg—recognized by many as the father of comprehensive care in MS—to describe the lack of treatment and support provided to most people with MS. Today, people with MS have a range of treatment options provided by health-care professionals in a variety of disciplines.

At present there are five medications approved by the U.S. Food and Drug Administration for the treatment of relapsing forms of MS. Unfortunately, we still do not have any medications to treat the primary progressive form of the disease. Regardless of their disease course, however, every person with MS now has at his or her disposal a range of tools to manage symptoms, including medications, rehabilitation interventions, and general wellness strategies. In partnership with their health-care providers, people with MS can learn to manage their disease, avoid unnecessary complications, and remain healthy and active. And, individuals with MS and their families can access a variety of educational and support services from the National Multiple Sclerosis Society and other voluntary health organizations, a growing library of MS publications, and the Internet. No one needs to go it alone any more.

Between us, we have spent 55 years in the care of people with MS and their families and in partnership with a dedicated array of health professionals in the United States and around the world. We feel strongly that accurate, up-to-date information is a critical tool for anyone living with, or affected by, this disease, and we believe that this volume provides readers with the kind of information and resources they need to make life with this complex disease more manageable.

—Rosalind Kalb, Ph.D.
Director, Professional Resource Center
Clinical Programs Department
National MS Society

—Nancy Holland, Ed.D.
Vice President
Clinical Programs
National MS Society

ACKNOWLEDGMENTS

As always, the creation of a detailed encyclopedia involves the help and guidance of a wide range of experts, without whom this book could not have been possible. First of all, thanks to the National Multiple Sclerosis Society, the staffs of the National Institute of Mental Health, the American Medical Association, the National Institutes of Health, the Food and Drug Administration, and the American Autoimmune Related Diseases Association.

Thanks also to the American Academy of Child and Adolescent Psychiatry, the National Pediatric MS Center at Stony Brook University Hospital, the North American Children With MS Family Support Network, and the National Institute of Neurological Disorders and Stroke.

Thanks as well to the Multiple Sclerosis Foundation, the American Academy of Neurology, the American Neurological Association, the International Organization of MS Nurses, the MS International Foundation, the Boston Cure Project, Inc., the Montel Williams MS Foundation, the Myelin Project, and the International Essential Tremor Foundation. Hats off as usual to the medical librarians at the Hershey Medical Center medical library, the National Library of Medicine, and the Pennsylvania State Library.

Finally, thanks to agents Gene Brissie, Ed Claflin, and Bert Holtje, to James Chambers and Vanessa Nittoli at Facts On File, and to Kara, Michael, and Summer.

—C.T.

Appreciation and thanks to the National Multiple Sclerosis Society and also to the many MS centers, MS organizations, and individuals around the world who have contributed to the knowledge bank of MS.

—K.H.

INTRODUCTION

I was five years old when my father was diagnosed with multiple sclerosis (MS) in 1957. Doctors did not know a lot about MS back then, and what little they did know was not too encouraging. Although our family dealt with the limits of this disease every day, the situation was never discussed. This was the late 1950s. MS was the elephant in our living room, present in every moment of our lives but never, ever mentioned.

At six foot five, my father towered over most people—an athlete who climbed mountains, rode horseback, and played football, basketball, tennis, and golf. He loved camping and hunting, swimming, boating, and fishing. One by one, MS took each of these activities away from him. Ultimately, the disease forced him to sell his beloved farm in Pennsylvania and then the summer home in Connecticut.

This was a time before handicapped spaces, wheelchair access, and disability rights made the lives of those with MS somewhat easier to manage. The only available drug for the condition was the then-experimental adrenocorticotropic hormone (ACTH), and a diagnosis of MS was a bleak pronouncement of increasing disability. Every autumn, as my father's condition relentlessly worsened, he was hospitalized for another round of ACTH treatments that briefly gave him energy and sharpened his mind. In the last years of his life, vitamin B shots were added, but the only thing that really seemed to help was the cold weather.

Today, the outlook for patients with MS is infinitely brighter. With the diagnostic advance of magnetic resonance imaging, patients are more likely to start off with an accurate diagnosis. A host of new medications provide relief for a great many patients—indeed, most patients need never follow my father's debilitating course. Each year, scientists learning more about this neurological disease that strikes people in their prime.

The Encyclopedia of Multiple Sclerosis is designed to answer many questions about this condition and includes the most up-to-date information on all major forms and treatments for this disease. It has been designed as a guide and reference to a wide range of subjects important to the understanding of MS. It includes contact information for organizations and governmental agencies affiliated with MS issues, including current Web site addresses and phone numbers.

However, this book is not designed as a substitute for prompt assessment and treatment by neurological experts in the diagnosis and treatment of MS.

In this encyclopedia, we have tried to present the latest information in the field based on the newest research. Although this information comes from the most up-to-date medical journals and research sources, readers should keep in mind that changes occur quickly in the field of neurology. A bibliography has been included for those who seek additional sources of information.

—Carol A. Turkington
Cymru, Pennsylvania

ENTRIES A–Z

abducens nerve Also known as the sixth cranial nerve, this nerve (together with the third and fourth cranial nerves) is responsible for certain eye movements. It supplies just one muscle of each eye, the one responsible for moving the eye outward. This nerve begins in the abducens nucleus in the brain stem and emerges from the brain right below it. The abducens nerve then extends through the skull, entering the back of the eye socket through a gap between the skull bones.

Damage to this nerve from lesions of multiple sclerosis can lead to DOUBLE VISION or other eye problems.

abductor muscle A muscle used to pull a body part away from the midline of the body. For example, the abductor leg muscles are used to spread the legs.

ABLEDATA A national database of ASSISTIVE DEVICES and rehabilitation equipment for people with disabilities, sponsored by the National Institute on Disability and Rehabilitation Research of the U.S. Department of Education.

Assistive devices are tools or implements, including anything from electric can openers to wheelchairs, that make a particular function easier to perform.

ABLEDATA provides a description of the product with price and company information. The database also can provide information on prototypes, one-of-a-kind or customized products, and do-it-yourself designs. Database searches are free, and help is available from information specialists via phone, fax, or mail.

ABLEDATA also provides an online listing of resources relating to accessible housing and design. For contact information, see Appendix I.

acetylcholine A chemical messenger that brain cells use to communicate with each other, especially in parts of the brain important for thought, memory, and judgment. It carries nerve impulses across the gaps between cells from one neuron to another. It also carries impulses from a neuron to a muscle cell, where it generates muscle contractions. Acetylcholine is important to proper nervous system and muscle functioning. Several drugs used to treat the symptoms of multiple sclerosis operate by modifying the functioning of acetylcholine; such drugs include tolterodine, selective serotonin reuptake inhibitors, and cannabinoids.

Acetylcholine is found at all nerve-muscle junctions as well as at many sites in the central nervous system. There are two types of acetylcholine receptors—nicotinic and muscarinic—which are found in different parts of the nervous system. Both of these receptors respond to acetylcholine.

The actions of acetylcholine are called cholinergic actions and are blocked by anticholinergic drugs.

acid reflux See GASTROESOPHAGEAL REFLUX.

ACTH See ADRENOCORTICOTROPIC HORMONE.

activities of daily living (ADLs) Personal care activities necessary for everyday living, such as eating, bathing, grooming, dressing, and using the toilet. People with multiple sclerosis (MS) may not be able to perform these functions without help; therefore, the ability to perform ADLs is often used as a measure of ability and disability in MS.

See also ASSISTIVE DEVICES; HOME ADAPTATIONS; OCCUPATIONAL THERAPIST.

acupuncture An ancient medical treatment, developed centuries ago in China, in which long, very fine needles are inserted at specific sites in the body believed to control certain functions. Acupuncture has been used for centuries to treat a variety of conditions, but it is only since the 1970s that it has gained popularity in North America. There is some evidence that the use of acupuncture among people with multiple sclerosis (MS) may be more common than in the general population. According to two recent surveys in the United States and Canada, approximately 20 to 25 percent of respondents with MS had tried acupuncture for the relief of PAIN, SPASTICITY, NUMBNESS and tingling, FATIGUE, DEPRESSION, anxiety, and bowel and bladder symptoms. Of those who had tried acupuncture for symptom relief, 10 percent to 15 percent indicated that they planned to continue using it. To date, however, there have been no controlled clinical trials to evaluate the safety and efficacy of acupuncture in people with MS.

acute disseminated encephalomyelitis (ADEM)
A neurological disorder characterized by inflammation of the brain and spinal cord caused by damage to the MYELIN sheath (the fatty covering of nerve fibers that acts as an insulator).

ADEM, which appears more often in children than in adults, typically follows vaccination or infection. However, the condition has been poorly understood, and a variety of terminologies are used to describe it (including postinfectious, parainfectious, or postvaccinial encephalomyelitis). It is often confused with multiple sclerosis (MS), especially in the early stages of the disease. In fact, distinguishing ADEM from MS in the initial phases can be difficult; MAGNETIC RESONANCE IMAGING (MRI) and a SPINAL TAP may help. Typically the lesions of ADEM are different than those of MS.

ADEM predominantly affects the white matter of the brain. Under the microscope an invasion of white blood cells around small veins can be seen. Where these cells accumulate, myelin is destroyed. The association of the disease with a prior infection or immunization suggests an immune system problem. Detailed research of these patients has found evidence that these patients' bodies have mounted an allergic response against their own brain constituents.

The viral agents most often linked to ADEM infections are the viruses that cause St. Louis encephalitis, western equine encephalomyelitis, and California encephalitis and the mumps virus, ECHO viruses, and Coxsackie virus. This illness was first described 250 years ago by an English physician who noted that it occurred occasionally in patients who had smallpox.

Symptoms and Diagnostic Path
Symptoms appear suddenly with fever, headache, stiff neck, vomiting, and appetite loss quickly followed by confusion, stupor, delirium, and occasionally coma. During this early period a neurological examination usually reveals optic neuritis (inflammation of the optic nerve), clumsiness, paralysis on one side, and seizures. Some symptoms may last a few weeks to a month; fatal cases may progress rapidly in a downward spiral over a matter of days. Typically, once the disease ends, further attacks rarely develop. Recent long-term studies of patients with ADEM have shown that a small number will later develop MS.

The spinal tap will often reveal abnormal cerebrospinal fluid with an increase in white blood cells and protein. An electroencephalogram is usually abnormal, showing diffuse slowing. MRI typically shows multiple areas of abnormality in the white matter of the brain.

Treatment Options and Outlook
No specific treatment is available for viral encephalomyelitis. However, high doses of corticosteroids can often quickly improve symptoms, resulting in an excellent prognosis.

Overall the prognosis for ADEM is good when the disorder is diagnosed early and treated promptly, but the prognosis for children with ADEM varies. Some youngsters experience a complete or nearly complete recovery. However, permanent complications are common in infants and children who survive the initial infection. Some severe cases of ADEM may be fatal.

Adderall   A stimulant drug (a mixture of amphetamine and dextroamphetamine) that is approved for the treatment of attention deficit hyperactivity disorder. Adderall stimulates the central nervous system and causes an increase in motor activity while easing FATIGUE and aiding concentration. Amphetamines have a high potential for abuse or dependency. Although this drug may possibly decrease fatigue associated with multiple sclerosis (MS), it has not been rigorously tested in MS patients.

adrenocorticotropic hormone (ACTH)   An anterior pituitary hormone approved in 1978 as a short-term treatment for acute exacerbations of multiple sclerosis (MS). ACTH stimulates the adrenal glands to produce corticosteroids that reduce inflammation and autoimmune effects.

ACTH is no longer the preferred method of treatment for acute exacerbations of MS, since subsequent clinical trials have shown that treatment with high-dose, intravenous corticosteroids such as methylprednisolone (Solu-Medrol) and dexamethasone (Decadron) produce a more rapid response and have fewer side effects. They are also more potent, cause less sodium retention and less potassium loss, and are longer acting than ACTH. Moreover, the strength of ACTH varies depending on the preparation, and several studies have shown that the individual response to ACTH can be highly variable.

Other high-dose, intravenous corticosteroids used to treat MS include cortisone, prednisone, prednisolone, and betamethasone.

advance directive   A written document, completed and signed when a person is legally competent, that explains what the person would or would not want if unable to make decisions about medical care. Common advance directives include:

- HEALTH CARE PROXY (or health care power of attorney) that gives another person the authority to make decisions for the patient when the person is unable to do so
- LIVING WILL, which directs a doctor to use, not start, or stop treatment that is keeping a dying patient alive when the patient cannot make those wishes known
- nonhospital do-not-resuscitate order (DNR) that directs emergency staff to not resuscitate a person at home or at a health care facility other than a hospital

A patient with multiple sclerosis (MS) should prepare and sign advance directives because such documents allow someone else to make treatment decisions on his or her behalf when the person is no longer capable of doing so. Patients should prepare and sign advance directives that comply with state law and give copies to family, friends, and doctors. The documents should reflect the patient's wishes and appoint someone to make decisions who is willing to carry out those wishes. Advance directive requirements vary from one state to another and should therefore be drawn up in consultation with an attorney who is familiar with the laws of the patient's state.

advanced multiple sclerosis   As multiple sclerosis (MS) progresses, its symptoms tend to become more severe and pronounced, and disability progresses. Advanced MS manifests itself differently in everyone, but even in the earliest stages of MS, damage occurs within the brain, optic nerves, and spinal cord. MYELIN (the fatty material that insulates nerve fibers called axons) is attacked and destroyed (a process called DEMYELINATION), and the axons are sometimes damaged. Areas of demyelination tend not to repair themselves sufficiently, and with each attack more lesions (or areas of damage) tend to occur.

Whether MS is secondary-progressive (following a period of relapsing-remitting MS) or primary-progressive (meaning it has been slowly progressive from the beginning), "progressive" does not necessarily mean severe disability. It does mean that there are few or no recovery or remission periods.

While there are still no effective medical treatments to repair nerves or reverse permanent losses of function, there are many useful strategies and treatments to improve symptoms. It is possible to alleviate many symptoms and improve some functions; there are ways to compensate for disabilities and thus lessen their impact on life.

Advanced MS is a complex and unpredictable condition that often requires the attention of many specialists. A multidisciplinary MS center provides care by an MS specialist team. However, if an MS Center is not available, a multidisciplinary team will need to be created by the patient, working with the primary care physician and within the limits of insurance coverage. In MS, effective health care is best achieved by coordinated input from a range of specialist providers. It is important to contact the relevant professional early and to put a plan into action, because prompt attention to a problem can often reduce the impact it might have on life. Coordination among the team members is critical.

Treatment Options and Outlook

There are some treatments for progressive MS that should be discussed with a knowledgeable MS specialist. Some treatments may not be an option for certain individuals. The physician may suggest starting or staying with one of the DISEASE-MODIFYING AGENTS used to treat MS.

Drug treatments Mitoxantrone (Novantrone), methotrexate, intravenous methylprednisolone, and cyclophosamide have all been used with varying degrees of success, but also with the risk of serious side effects. Avonex, Betaseron, and Rebif are approved for use in secondary-progressive MS with relapses. Novantrone is approved for secondary-progressive, progressive-relapsing, and worsening relapsing-remitting disease. Careful monitoring is required for Novantrone, as cardiac toxicity (heart damage) is known to occur.

Experimental treatments Treatments such as BONE MARROW TRANSPLANTATION and a procedure called PLASMAPHERESIS have had very mixed results. These approaches have many risks, and because they are experimental they may not be covered by most insurance policies. To date, primary-progressive MS has been the most resistant to these treatments. Among the therapies currently being studied include those using monoclonal antibodies. These include alemtuzumab (CamPath 1H), daclizumab (Zenapax), and others.

Spasticity treatments In advanced MS, SPASTICITY is managed with a combination of medications, physical therapy, exercise, stretching, and adaptive devices. Severe spasticity can cause serious problems with positioning, sitting or lying down, and may impede personal care. This in turn increases the risk of BEDSORES and other skin problems. Untreated spasticity also may cause permanent joint contractures (stiff or frozen joints). Baclofen is the most commonly used anti-spasticity medication, while others used include DIAZEPAM, DANTROLENE, tizanidine, and botulinum toxin (BOTOX). Spasticity or periodic leg movements at night should be discussed with an MS nurse. (A partner may be more aware of this than the person with MS, who wakes up tired but is not quite aware of how frequently deep sleep is being disrupted). Very rarely, surgery is recommended for painful spasticity that does not respond to other measures.

Bladder treatments Loss of bladder control can increase the risk of pressure sores and skin breakdown. A urologist or a continence specialist should be involved in ongoing management of bladder issues if they are severe or persistent. Depending on the individual, a combination of management strategies with prescription medication, such as propantheline bromide, imipramine, or oxybutynin is effective. Difficulties with hand function, weakness, or tremor, or problems transferring on and off a toilet may make INTERMITTENT SELF-CATHETERIZATION inappropriate for some people.

For those with more advanced MS bladder problems, a suprapubic catheter can be the answer, although this involves minor surgery. A flexible tube is inserted into the bladder through an incision in the lower abdomen. The bladder empties via this tube into a collection bag, which is usually fastened to the leg. This technique may be more appropriate for long-term management, since it is associated with fewer complications than an indwelling catheter in the urethra. A urologist will need to assess bladder problems and discuss the options and management strategies that would be best.

Self-care help Showers, bed baths, or sponge baths are essential to keep skin clean and healthy, as is daily dental hygiene, hair care, and toileting. Should MS compromise the strength and coordination skills needed to accomplish them, there are ASSISTIVE DEVICES that can help patients remain independent or ease the burden on caregivers.

OCCUPATIONAL THERAPISTS are the experts in the area of assistive devices for personal hygiene and bathroom adjustments that make toilet functions more effective and safe. They have extensive practical information on both devices and techniques. A person with MS and a caregiver can develop a hygiene system that works to maintain dignity.

Some people manage independent lives with major disabilities by hiring personal care attendants, housekeepers, and home health aides. Home adaptations offer safety, ease of movement, and comfort; an occupational therapist can assess what can be done to modify homes.

Bowel treatments CONSTIPATION and DIARRHEA are both reasonably common in advanced MS, caused by decreased intestinal movement, weakened abdominal muscles, limited physical activity, poor diet, and decreased fluid intake. Pelvic floor muscles weakened by MS make having a bowel movement more difficult.

Swallowing problem solutions SWALLOWING PROBLEMS can be a serious issue in advanced MS. Choking and coughing when eating or drinking can be dangerous as well as disturbing, so problems should be discussed with a SPEECH PATHOLOGIST, who can assess individual needs and advise on feeding options.

Communication solutions With professional help, people can learn how to use their existing communication abilities to the fullest. Voice amplifiers may be useful if a person's articulation of words is adequate. In addition, speech problems can improve if the patient can learn to speak more slowly, use shorter sentences, and to choose words that are easy to pronounce.

To express themselves more widely and to share complex information, people with speech limitations often need assistive communication devices such as paper and pen, magic slates, or laptop computers. People with disabilities can control computers using adapted keyboards, sticks held in the mouth, or wireless devices worn on the head or eyeglasses. There are even computer controls that operate by eye blink. Text telephone, or TTY, systems and free translation services enable telephone use for those who speak too softly or slowly for a regular telephone. Those with profound disabilities can use a communication board, communicating basic messages by gazing at alphabet letters, symbols, words, or phrases.

Bedsore treatments Bedsores (pressure sores) can occur if patients cannot move around easily. These sores appear as a redness or break in the skin caused by too much pressure for too long a period of time. The pressure prevents blood from getting to the skin, so the skin dies. Normally the nerves send messages of pain or discomfort to the brain to signal the need to change position, but damage from MS interrupts these signals. People with MS who are immobile most of the day (even if they are not in bed) are at risk for pressure sores, also known as decubitus ulcers.

Sexual problem solutions Even in early MS, there may be physical changes that make sexual activity difficult or uncomfortable. Worsening MS may aggravate SEXUAL PROBLEMS. When MS becomes more severe, caregivers who are also spouses or partners face more hurdles in their sexual relationship. The couple may need new "cues" to initiate intimacy and set the stage for romance. Psychological and social issues may make the person with MS feel inadequate and unlovable. Consulting a trained sexual counselor can help couples work through these problems.

affective release See PSEUDOBULBAR AFFECT.

afferent pupillary defect (APD) An abnormal reflex response to light in which the pupil does not react appropriately to the level of light reaching it. In patients with multiple sclerosis, this condition is usually associated with damage to the OPTIC NERVE caused by inflammation. APD will often cause one pupil to appear larger than the other (relative afferent pupillary defect). The person with APD is often unaware of the condition unless he or she looks in a mirror.

APD is most clearly demonstrated by the swinging flashlight test. When a flashlight is shined first into the abnormal eye, then into the healthy eye, and then again into the eye with the pupillary defect, the affected pupil becomes larger rather than smaller.

African Americans and MS Although research indicates that multiple sclerosis is more common among Caucasians than African Americans, the course of disease may be more aggressive among African Americans. According to some research, more African Americans than Caucasians experience greater disability at first. However, once patients have moderate difficulty walking, the rate of progression is the same for both groups, albeit occurring at a later age for Caucasians than for African Americans.

age Multiple sclerosis (MS) is primarily a disease of young adulthood; most people with MS are diagnosed between the ages of 20 and 50. Although MS is usually considered a disease diagnosed in adults, it is occasionally discovered in children. About 5 percent of individuals with MS are diagnosed before age 21.

Late-onset MS is diagnosed after age 50 and appears to be more common than experts had originally believed, affecting about 9.4 percent of those with MS. However, because of other medical problems that affect older people, MS may be overlooked or misdiagnosed. Whether the prognosis is different among patients who are diagnosed at different ages is still controversial.

See also CHILDHOOD MS.

ageusia The absence or impairment of the sense of taste. This is an occasional symptom of multiple sclerosis that can occur as a result of certain lesions on nerves affecting taste sensation.

alcohol Patients with multiple sclerosis (MS) may notice changes in their ability to tolerate alcohol. Some people report that some of their symptoms (especially imbalance and lack of coordination) temporarily worsen after even one drink. For this reason, doctors often advise patients to reassess their alcohol intake and often suggest that they avoid alcohol completely because of its effects on the nervous system. In particular, the cerebellum's balancing mechanism is vulnerable to alcohol, especially if the nerves have lost their protective sheath. Because chronic alcohol use damages the nerve cells in the cerebellum and in other parts of the brain, this disease can have a significant impact on a patient with MS, whose brain cells may already be compromised.

Drinking even a small amount of alcohol may cause significant coordination problems, even when intellectual impairment is minimal. This may make it unsafe for people with MS to drive after drinking even a small amount of alcohol, even if the person's thought processes are still clear. Since alcohol depresses the central nervous system, it may also have an additive effect with certain medications that are commonly prescribed for MS, including BACLOFEN, DIAZEPAM, CLONAZEPAM, and some ANTIDEPRESSANTS. For all of these reasons, people with MS should talk to their physician about how much alcohol is appropriate for them to drink and how often.

alemtuzumab (Campath-1H) The generic name for an experimental multiple sclerosis (MS) drug that works by destroying the body's T cells. Although T cells are important in maintaining a healthy immune system, they are also believed to be responsible for initiating the destructive process seen in MS. In one small trial of 27 people with SECONDARY PROGRESSIVE MS, the drug virtually eliminated the formation of new lesions and the inflammation associated with the disease for at least 18 months. These results were demonstrated by magnetic resonance imaging (MRI) scans. Campath-1H has already been approved by the U.S. Food and Drug Administration for the treatment of chronic lymphocytic leukemia.

For 14 of the volunteers in this study, the progress of their disease initially appeared to be completely halted. In the other 13 MS symptoms continued to worsen although no new lesions were seen. MRI studies have discovered that the trial subjects whose disease continued to progress were the ones who had the greatest amount of existing lesions and brain atrophy. Unfortunately as time goes on, even some of those people whose progression appeared to have been stopped by the drug are now apparently beginning to deteriorate.

These results have led researchers to make several important inferences. First, inflammation is apparently not the only mechanism causing the disease to progress. Instead, further progression may be caused by the earlier death of central nervous system maintenance cells called OLIGODENDROCYTES.

These oligodendrocytes normally feed the neurons certain neurotrophic factors (in particular a factor called insulin-like growth factor 1, or IGF-1). Without IGF-1, the cell's axons wither and die, which interferes with nerve communication. This axonal death seems to take place long after the oligodendrocytes have died.

Campath-1H therapy works best when given early in the disease. As a result, a new clinical trial of Campath-1H for people with early RELAPSING-REMITTING MS has begun. Experts hope that if inflammation can be stopped right from the start, the progressive phase of the disease might never begin. The trial compares Campath-1H with Rebif and is being tested on 180 people in the United States and Europe. Preliminary results from this trial should be available in 2006.

Side Effects

Campath-1H appears to be reasonably well tolerated despite the fact that it kills T cells, which should mean that the immune system becomes seriously weakened. However, during the study there were few serious infections and no deaths.

The drug did cause one serious side effect. One-third of the trial subjects developed autoimmune thyroid disease (Graves' disease). Despite the seriousness of this condition, it is relatively easily managed with thyroxine supplementation, and most people with MS would rather exchange MS for Graves' disease. In addition, most volunteers experienced a temporary worsening of their symptoms immediately after their first infusion of the drug.

allergies and MS No evidence suggests an allergic reaction to a specific environmental allergen triggers the onset of multiple sclerosis (MS). Therefore, most experts believe there is no scientific rationale for the antiallergy MS treatments offered by some alternative therapists. Some of these treatments involve avoiding certain food groups or taking medication aimed at combating a particular allergen, but research has not yet established that MS is linked to a particular food allergy.

MS is generally considered to be an AUTOIMMUNE DISEASE in which the body's immune system attacks itself. Just what part or parts of the central nervous system the immune cells attack has not yet been precisely identified nor has the trigger that sets off this autoimmune process.

alopecia Loss of hair. This may occur with chemotherapeutic agents such as cyclophosphamide (Cytoxan), sometimes used to treat symptoms of multiple sclerosis.

alpha interferon See DISEASE-MODIFYING AGENTS; INTERFERON.

alternative medicine See COMPLEMENTARY AND ALTERNATIVE MEDICINES.

amalgam A soft metal that results from mixing a metal with MERCURY. Amalgams are commonly used in dental fillings. Studies have not shown a link between multiple sclerosis and amalgams.

See also DENTAL AMALGAM AND MS.

amantadine (Symadine, Symmetrel) An antiviral medication used to alleviate the symptoms of FATIGUE in people with multiple sclerosis (MS), also used to prevent or treat certain flu infections and to treat Parkinson's disease. The effectiveness of amantadine in treating MS fatigue was discovered accidentally when a number of people with MS were being treated for flu and instead experienced lessening of fatigue. Experts do not know why amantadine is sometimes effective in relieving this fatigue.

Amantadine also improves muscle control and reduces muscle stiffness, although scientists do not know exactly how it works. The antiviral properties of the drug may confer other benefits as well, because viral infections have been shown to be significantly correlated with relapses.

The usual dosage for managing fatigue in MS is 100–200 mg daily, taken in the earlier part of the day in order to avoid sleep disturbance. Doses in excess of 300 mg daily usually cause livedo reticularis, a blotchy discoloration of the skin of the legs.

Side Effects

Amantadine is generally well tolerated by people with MS, although it can cause insomnia, nausea, and dizziness. Since distinguishing between certain common symptoms of MS and some side effects of amantadine may be hard, patients should consult a doctor if sudden side effects appear.

Other common side effects include loss of concentration, dizziness, headaches, irritability, loss of appetite, nervousness, rashes, constipation, dry mouth, and vomiting. More rarely, amantadine can cause blurred vision, confusion, urinary hesitation, fainting, hallucinations, convulsions, coordination problems, eye irritation and swelling, depression, swollen feet, and shortness of breath.

Drinking alcoholic beverages while taking this medication may cause increased side effects such as circulation problems, dizziness, light-headedness, fainting, or confusion.

Although amantadine passes into breast milk, studies of the effects of amantadine during pregnancy have not been conducted on humans. Additionally, the effect of amantadine on newborn babies and infants is not known. Animal studies, however, have shown that amantadine is harmful to the fetus and causes birth defects.

See also PREGNANCY AND MS.

ambulation index (AI) A rating scale developed in 1983 to assess a person's ability to walk, evaluating the time and degree of assistance required to walk 25 feet. The AI has been largely replaced by the TIMED 25-FOOT WALK (T25-FW). While the AI uses a clinical rating of a performance category, the T25-FW measures the actual time needed to complete the task.

Scores on the AI range from 0 (asymptomatic and fully active) to 10 (bedridden). People are allowed to use assistive devices such as canes, crutches, walkers. During the test, the person is asked to walk a marked 25-foot course as quickly and safely as possible. The examiner records the time and whether any type of assistance (such as cane, walker, crutches) is needed. The test should take between one to five minutes. The AI is administered in person by a trained examiner, who does not need to be a physician or nurse.

Although the person's walking is timed, the time is used together with other factors to rate the person on a scale with 11 gradations. Gait speed in general has been demonstrated to be a useful and reliable functional measure of walking ability. In addition the rating scale has categories for persons who are unable to walk at all.

American Indians and MS Multiple sclerosis is very rare among the Native American cultures of North America; it is almost unheard of among the Inuit.

Americans with Disabilities Act (ADA) The first comprehensive legislation passed by any country in the world that prohibits discrimination on the basis of disability, enacted in 1990. The ADA guarantees full participation in American society for all people with disabilities and covers almost everyone with multiple sclerosis (MS)—not just people who use wheelchairs but every person with an impairment that substantially limits one or more major life activities. Even people with MS who have never had any disabling symptoms can be protected if they are perceived as disabled or they have records of such impairments.

The ADA's guarantee of full participation in American society includes protection from discrimination on the job, in public accommodations, in transportation, in telecommunications, and in government agencies and facilities.

A patient with MS does not have to provide a diagnosis before being given a job offer. If the person needs accommodations for a job interview or to do the job if it is offered, that person will have to discuss personal limitations but not diagnosis. If, and only if, the employer requires a medical exam of everyone who fills the position for which the MS patient is applying would that person need to say he or she has MS.

Most employers are prohibited from asking job applicants about medical history or disability, and they cannot ask about a person's medical status when checking references. However, a potential employer may ask if the person can walk, for example, if walking is an essential function of the job. An employer may also make a job offer contingent on the results of a medical exam or inquiry if that exam is required for all candidates. If the results show a disability and the person with MS is denied the job, the employer's decision must be based on job-related factors and on the patient's specific, current impairments and not on a diagnosis or speculation about future impairments.

MS patients may have to take a medical examination to keep a job if the medical exam is job related. If the exam reveals a disability, the employer must make reasonable accommodations for the disability so the MS patient can perform essential job functions.

If There Is a Problem

If a person with MS believes he or she has been discriminated against, the first step is to call the local chapter of the NATIONAL MULTIPLE SCLEROSIS SOCIETY. Local chapters have information on the ADA, on local and state laws, and on enforcement. Acting quickly is wise if action is needed. In employment-related matters, for example, a person may have only 180 days from the time a discriminatory incident occurs to make a formal complaint.

The ADA has established Disability and Business Technical Assistance Centers to provide information and referrals, technical assistance, public awareness, and training on all aspects of the ADA. To contact the nearest center, a patient should call 800-949-4232 or visit http://www.adata.org.

The Job Accommodation Network is an international information and consulting resource. Both people with disabilities and employers can contact them for practical help in making accommodations at 800-526-7234 or http://www.jan.wvu.edu.

Any person with MS who believes an employer or potential employer is not living up to the obligations of the ADA should call the Equal Employment Opportunity Commission District Office or the National Office: 800-669-4000 (TTY 800-669-6820). Written information can be obtained by calling 800-669-EEOC (3362) or visiting http://www.eeoc.gov.

The Disability Rights Education and Defense Fund (DREDF), based in Berkeley, California, is a national law and policy center dedicated to protecting and advancing the civil rights of people with disabilities through legislation, litigation, advocacy, technical assistance, and other services. The DREDF can be reached at 510-644-2555 or at http://www.dredf.org.

For more information on the Air Carrier Access Act, patients can visit the U.S. Department of Transportation's Web site at http://www.dot.gov/airconsumer.

4-aminopyridine (4-AP, Fampridine-SR) A potassium-blocking compound that is being studied as an experimental treatment for multiple sclerosis (MS). It appears to work by improving the transmission of nerve impulses along damaged areas of nerves where the protective covering (MYELIN) has been destroyed by the disease process, but it does not actually replace damaged myelin.

In small, preliminary trials, 4-aminopyridine (4-AP) has been linked with mild-to-marked improvement in PARESTHESIA, vision, strength, and coordination. However, the beneficial effects lasted only a few hours.

A related compound (3,4-diaminopyridine, or DAP) also temporarily improved nerve conduction, without harmful side effects, for several weeks at a time. However, one study comparing the two drugs found that 4-AP was better at improving walking, fatigue, and overall function.

Side effects of 4-AP may include dizziness and confusion, whereas DAP may cause abdominal pain, numbness, or tingling. Agriculturally, 4-AP is used as an extremely effective poison that is highly toxic to all mammals (including humans) if dosages are exceeded. As an experimental drug, recommended dose data is unavailable, but there is a narrow safety margin. Overdose can occur at relatively low doses. Additionally, either drug may cause epileptic seizures.

A slow-release formulation of 4-aminopyridine is supplied by the Irish drug company Elan Corporation and is currently being tested by Acorda in two phase II trials in the United States. It is currently awaiting approval by the U.S. Food and Drug Agency.

Medicines for multiple sclerosis are divided into two classes: Symptomatic medications treat symptoms and improve function, while preventive medicines target the disease itself. Fampridine-SR is a symptomatic medication, which would best help a patient who has already been affected by MS and needs medication to improve function.

Experts hope the drug will improve walking speed for people using canes or walkers and also help these patients better handle ACTIVITIES OF

DAILY LIVING. Experts are also hoping the drug will improve FATIGUE, one of the primary disabling symptoms of MS.

This treatment would be best for patients who have had MS for some time and who have developed WEAKNESS (especially leg weakness). The drug, which is still in the experimental stages and is not yet available for the general public, is currently being studied in 20 medical centers around the country.

amitriptyline (Elavil)   A tricyclic ANTIDEPRESSANT that is also often used in multiple sclerosis to treat painful burning sensations (paresthesias) in the arms and legs caused by damage to the pain-regulating pathways of the brain and spinal cord. Other tricyclic antidepressants are also used to manage neurologic pain symptoms, including clomipramine (Anafranil), desipramine (Norpramin), doxepin (Sinequan), imipramine (Tofranil), nortriptyline (Pamelor), and trimipramine.

Side Effects

Amitriptyline adds to the effects of alcohol and other central nervous system depressants (such as antihistamines, sedatives, tranquilizers, prescription pain medications, seizure medications, muscle relaxants, and sleeping medications) and may cause drowsiness. This medication also may increase sensitivity to sunlight. As a result, even brief exposure to sunlight may cause severe sunburn or a skin rash, itching, redness, or other skin discoloration. Amitriptyline may affect blood sugar levels of diabetic individuals.

Side effects that do not require medical attention unless they continue for more than two weeks or are bothersome include

- dry mouth
- constipation or diarrhea
- increased appetite and weight gain
- dizziness
- drowsiness
- decreased sexual ability
- headache
- nausea and vomiting
- unpleasant taste

- heartburn
- increased sweating

Uncommon side effects that should be reported to a physician as soon as possible include

- blurred vision
- confusion or delirium
- difficulty speaking or swallowing
- eye pain
- fainting
- hallucinations
- loss of balance
- nervousness or restlessness
- urinary problems
- shakiness or trembling
- stiffness

Rare side effects that should be reported as soon as possible include

- anxiety
- breast enlargement
- hair loss
- inappropriate milk secretion in women
- increased sensitivity to sunlight
- irritability
- muscle twitching or weakness
- rash or itching
- buzzing or other unexplained sounds in the ear
- sore throat and fever
- swelling of face and tongue
- yellow skin

Symptoms of acute overdose include

- confusion, restlessness, or agitation
- convulsions
- severe drowsiness, unusual fatigue
- enlarged pupils
- unusual heartbeat or shortness of breath
- fever

- hallucinations
- vomiting

Amsler chart   A type of eye test featuring a colored grid with a red dot in the center. During a NEUROLOGICAL EXAMINATION, patients will be asked to focus on the dot; if they have trouble seeing the dot, this can indicate a potential visual problem in the OPTIC NERVE common in patients with multiple sclerosis (MS). (Seeing a dark hole in the center of vision is a possible indication of MS.)

See also VISUAL LOSS; VISUAL PROBLEMS.

amyotrophic lateral sclerosis (ALS) vs. multiple sclerosis   Amyotrophic lateral sclerosis (also known as Lou Gehrig's disease) is a disease of the central nervous system, just like multiple sclerosis (MS). However, unlike MS, it does not attack the MYELIN sheath that surrounds and protects the nerve fibers of the brain and spinal cord.

Instead, ALS is a motor neuron disease, which means that it destroys the motor neurons in the brainstem, motor cortex, and spinal cord that directly affect muscle control. As these nerve cells are gradually destroyed, muscles become weaker and lose their ability to control both voluntary movements, such as walking and eating, and involuntary actions, such as breathing.

anesthesia   There are two broad types of anesthesia. General anesthesia is given to put people to sleep during surgery. Local anesthesia is given to numb a small part of the body.

Although administering general anesthesia presents a very small health risk to any patient, no matter how healthy, the risks are about the same for people with multiple sclerosis (MS) as for others. However, a small percentage of people with MS with severe, advanced disease may be seriously weakened by MS or have respiratory problems that would put them at greater risk for anesthetic complications.

Local anesthesia poses no risk to a person with MS unless the person happens to be allergic to the commonly used local anesthetics (such as Novocaine). In one study that reviewed this risk, 98 patients who together had received more than 1,000 doses of local anesthetics produced only four instances when the dose was followed by a sudden worsening of an MS symptom.

A third type of anesthetic—commonly called an epidural—is often injected into a woman's spine during labor and delivery. A recent study of pregnant women with MS showed that women who had anesthesia injected directly into the epidural space of the spine during delivery did not have a higher number of relapses than those who did not receive an epidural. Epidural anesthesia appears to be well tolerated by most people with MS.

However, because some neurologists believe that there is a greater risk of complications with spinal anesthesia (a method related to but different than epidural anesthesia), spinal anesthesia is generally not recommended for people with MS.

ankle-foot orthosis   A brace, usually plastic, worn on the lower leg and foot to correct FOOT DROP. It holds the foot in the proper position for heel-toe walking.

See also GAIT; PHYSICAL THERAPIST.

antibodies   Proteins of the immune system that are dissolved in blood or other body fluids and that are produced in response to bacteria, viruses, and other types of foreign ANTIGENS.

anticholinergic drugs   Certain medications commonly used in the management of NEUROGENIC BLADDER dysfunction that interfere with the transmission of parasympathetic nerve impulses and thereby reduce spasms of smooth muscle in the bladder. Such bladder problems may be one symptom of multiple sclerosis.

anticonvulsants   Medications designed to prevent SEIZURES, which may occur in 3–5 percent of people with multiple sclerosis (MS). Seizures may occur as part of the disease or may be related to infection, fever, or the abrupt withdrawal of certain medications.

In addition to controlling seizures, several anticonvulsants may be used to treat some types of PAIN typical of MS. CARBAMAZEPINE (Tegretol), phenytoin (Dilantin), and GABAPENTIN (Neurontin) can help manage pain that occurs when nerve impulses cross from one fiber tract to another. TRIGEMINAL NEURALGIA (a stabbing facial pain that may occur in MS) is usually treated with carbamazepine.

Side Effects

These drugs may cause side effects including dizziness, loss of balance, nausea, excessive gum inflammation, and blood abnormalities.

antidepressants Medications used to treat depression, including tricyclics, monoamine oxidase inhibitors, and selective serotonin reuptake inhibitors (SSRIs). SSRIs include fluoxetine (Prozac), sertraline (Zoloft), citalopram (Celexa), and paroxetine (Paxil). Other related antidepressants include venlafaxine (Effexor), nefazodone (Serzone), and bupropion (Wellbutrin).

Some evidence suggests that Elavil may help prevent the uncontrollable laughing or crying that sometimes affects people with multiple sclerosis (MS). Because some tricyclic drugs act to retain urine, they are also used in low doses to help control bladder incontinence. Some antidepressants (such as Prozac) may also help reduce MS-related FATIGUE.

Side Effects

Side effects vary from one drug to the next and from one person to the next. In general, they may include dry mouth, blurry vision, constipation, excessive excitement or lethargy, and sexual dysfunction.

antigen Any substance that triggers the immune system to produce an ANTIBODY.

antioxidants Chemicals that oxygen finds more attractive than the structural components of cells. In a sense, antioxidants sacrifice themselves to preserve the body. The safety of taking antioxidants for people with multiple sclerosis (MS) has not been established. One small, five-week study indicates that antioxidants are safe for people with MS, but experts believe the study is too small and short to be conclusive.

In fact, MS experts believe there is limited evidence suggesting that antioxidants may be beneficial, and there is also some evidence suggesting

potential harm. Antioxidant vitamins stimulate the immune system in laboratory experiments and in some groups of people. In MS, where an overactive immune system appears to be part of the disease process, stimulation may be dangerous.

Instead, the most reasonable course for people to obtain antioxidants would be to eat two to four servings of fruits and three to four servings of vegetables every day. If antioxidant supplements are used, experts suggest it may be best to use them in moderation.

Although the immune system is complex, experts assume that immune stimulation might be dangerous for MS patients and that slowing down the immune system may be beneficial. Accordingly, supplements that are supposed to "boost" or "improve" immune function may be the worst choice for people with MS.

See also COMPLEMENTARY AND ALTERNATIVE MEDICINES.

antiviral drugs Drugs that target VIRUSES and, according to some researchers, may help fight multiple sclerosis (MS). The reason that these drugs may help fight MS has to do with MYELIN, the layer of fatty substances that normally insulates the nerves and gets damaged as a result of MS. Because several viruses have chemical structures similar to that of a major protein making up myelin, some experts believe that the body of patients with MS may be reacting to these constituents of myelin that look like viruses. However, studies have failed to link a variety of viruses, including herpes simplex types 1, 2, and 6, herpes zoster (shingles), measles, and EPSTEIN-BARR, to MS.

Nevertheless, some experts still suspect there is some type of viral link with MS and therefore study specific antiviral agents such as acyclovir as potential treatments.

See also HERPESVIRUS 6; VACCINES AND MS.

anxiety Feelings of anxiety may be experienced by a patient with multiple sclerosis for a variety of reasons. If anxiety continues, it may be successfully treated with a variety of antianxiety medications, such as lorazepam or buspirone; antidepressants also may help. Supportive psychotherapy in combination with medication may be recommended as well.

aphasia An acquired language disorder caused by damage to the left half of the brain, which affects speaking and understanding speech. Very rarely, people with multiple sclerosis (MS) may develop aphasia.

Aphasia is usually related to brain problems such as a stroke and is not expected in diseases such as MS. However, MS lesions that are anatomically connected to certain language centers in the brain may lead to aphasia.

People with aphasia may be affected in different ways in any or all four language areas: reading, writing, comprehension, and expression. Language is affected not only as talking and understanding but also in its written form of reading and writing. Typically people have much more problems with reading and writing than speaking. However, the nature of the problems varies from person to person depending on the amount and location of damage to the brain. The impairment can be so subtle that it appears only when a patient is in unfamiliar surroundings and the language includes unusual words. This is why aphasia is often called an "invisible" disorder.

aquatic exercise See WATER EXERCISE.

arthrogryposis Fixation of a joint in a straight or contracted position.

aseptic necrosis of the hip Massive deterioration of the hip joint that may occur in a person after repeated courses of steroids used to treat relapses of multiple sclerosis (MS). Pain and difficulty walking may thus be the result of steroids, rather than disease progression.

Ashworth Spasticity Scale A scale of tone density used to measure SPASTICITY in people with multiple sclerosis.

Asian Americans and MS Cases of multiple sclerosis are quite rare in Asia, but Asian Americans have a comparatively higher incidence rate. Still MS occurs most frequently among Caucasian Americans and is uncommon among Asian Americans. This fact points to the possibility of environmental factors behind the disease.

aspiration pneumonia An infection of the lungs and bronchial tubes that can be caused when patients with multiple sclerosis have SWALLOWING PROBLEMS and inhale food into their lungs. The aspirated material provides a breeding ground for infection, which leads to pneumonia in the lower part of one or both lungs.

Once food has been inhaled, the inflamed lungs can become infected with multiple species of bacteria, leading to an abscess. A protective membrane may form around the abscess. If acute respiratory failure develops, the patient may have a prolonged illness or die.

Symptoms and Diagnostic Path

Symptoms may include fever; fatigue; cough with foul-smelling, bloody, or greenish sputum; chest pain and shortness of breath; bluish skin discoloration caused by lack of oxygen; rapid pulse; and wheezing. Other symptoms may include excessive sweating, swallowing difficulty, choking when swallowing, and breath odor.

Complications may occur if the infection spreads into the bloodstream (bacteremia) or to other areas of the body, resulting in low blood pressure and shock.

Physical examination can reveal crackling sounds in the lungs. Other tests may include a chest X-ray, sputum culture to check for bacteria in lung material, complete blood count to measure white and red blood cells, blood culture to check for bacteria, arterial blood gasses to measure oxygen and carbon dioxide levels in the blood, and bronchoscopy to assess lung health.

Treatment Options and Outlook

Hospitalization may be required to manage this type of pneumonia. Intravenous antibiotics and a ventilator may be needed to keep an open airway and provide oxygen. The trachea may be suctioned to clear secretions and aspirated particles out of the airway.

A chest X-ray, sputum culture and blood tests may be ordered to make sure the aspiration pneumonia is clearing and responding to medication. A patient's prognosis depends on the severity of the pneumonia, the type of organism, and the extent of lung involvement. If acute respiratory failure develops, the condition may be fatal.

Once the patient is discharged from the hospital, special breathing treatments may be prescribed.

Risk Factors and Preventive Measures

A swallowing evaluation will generally help patients who repeatedly inhale food into their lungs. Following certain food safety rules may help those with swallowing problems avoid the risk of aspiration pneumonia. Patients with swallowing problems should

- sit upright or lean slightly forward when eating or drinking
- keep the chin parallel with the table or slightly tucked down
- first eat soft, moist foods and thick, cold liquids (such as a sherbet shake or a fruit or vegetable smoothie) since they are the easiest to swallow; dry solids and thin liquids are more difficult and require closer attention for safe swallowing
- take one small bite or sip at a time without consecutive swallowing
- never wash food down with a liquid; instead, moisture should be added to the food
- avoid thin liquids altogether when tired; a good rule is to consume thin things in the morning and thick things in the evening
- eat quietly during a calm and social meal, saving discussion of difficult or controversial topics for times when the patient is not trying to eat
- swallow at least two times per mouthful of solid (the first time to send the food down, followed by a dry swallow to catch any residual particles)
- swallow hot, thin liquids and then clear the throat and swallow again before taking more liquid
- sleep in a bed with the head elevated to a 30-degree angle

assisted living   A type of housing for people who need various levels of medical and personal care in a homelike atmosphere. The philosophy of assisted living is to provide supervision, assistance and individualized personal-care services to individuals with disabilities such as multiple sclerosis (MS). Assisted living offers a unique mix of security and independence, privacy and companionship, and physical and social well-being.

Assisted-living services include 24-hour protective oversight, food, shelter, and a range of services that promote the quality of life of the individual. Because there is no common definition for assisted-living facilities, it is difficult to pinpoint the exact number of facilities, but experts have estimated that there are 33,000 assisted-living residences nationwide.

Assisted-living services can be provided in freestanding residences, near or integrated with skilled nursing homes or hospitals, as components of continuing care retirement communities, or at independent housing complexes. Living spaces can be individual rooms, apartments, or shared quarters. The facilities generally provide a home-like setting and are physically designed to promote the resident's independence. The services offered by assisted-living communities vary from facility to facility. Services often include

- one to three meals a day
- monitoring of medication
- help with personal care, including dressing and bathing
- housekeeping and laundry
- 24-hour emergency care
- some medical services
- social and recreational activities

The philosophy of assisted living emphasizes the right of the individual to choose the setting for care and services. Assisted-living clients share the risks and responsibilities for their daily activities and well-being with a staff geared to helping them enjoy the freedom and independence of private living. Assisted-living residences have adopted the philosophy of allowing the person to remain at the residence as long as the care staff can properly provide for their health, safety, and well-being.

Assisted-living arrangements are licensed by state governments and may also be called by a variety of different names, including residential care, board and care, congregate care, and personal care. Assisted-living care is not a substitute for, but rather a complement to, nursing facility care.

Costs

Costs vary with the type of residence, room size, and the range of services the resident needs, but daily basic fees range from $15 to $200. Many facilities charge a basic fee that covers all services; some facilities add on additional charges for special services. In addition, most assisted living residences charge a monthly rate, and a few residences require long-term arrangements.

The costs of care at these facilities are usually paid by the families or residents themselves; about 90 percent of the country's assisted-living services are paid for with private funds, although some states have adopted Medicaid waiver programs. Costs may be reimbursed if they are covered under health insurance or long-term care insurance. Some facilities also offer financial assistance programs, since government coverage for assisted-living residences has been limited. Some state and local governments do offer subsidies for rent or services for low-income elders; others may provide subsidies in the form of an additional payment for those who receive Supplemental Security Income (SSI) or Medicaid. Some states also use Medicaid waiver programs to help pay for assisted-living services.

See also ASSISTIVE DEVICES.

assisted suicide The completion of suicide by a patient with a chronic or terminal illness, such as multiple sclerosis (MS), with the help of another person in such a way that the patient technically dies by his or her own hand. For example, a person who dies by swallowing pills supplied by a doctor for the purpose of causing death would be considered an assisted suicide. Oregon, Belgium, and the Netherlands are the only three places in the world where laws specifically permit assisted suicide.

Assisted suicide is different than euthanasia, in which another person intentionally causes a patient's death. Giving a lethal injection to a terminally ill patient or putting a plastic bag over the patient's head would be considered euthanasia. Assisted suicide indicates that the person who dies actually performs the final act and gets only "assistance" from the other person.

The National Multiple Sclerosis Society (NMSS) has been dedicated to improving the quality of life for people with MS and their families for more than 50 years. According to a statement, the society believes that suicide and assisted suicide are fundamentally inconsistent with this mission. Although acknowledging how difficult life with MS can be, the society notes that although MS is a chronic, incurable condition, it is not fatal. In 1936, only 8 percent of patients were reported to survive more than 20 years after onset of illness; in 1961, more than 80 percent of MS patients were surviving 20 years after onset of illness. By 2002, a patient with MS could expect to live only about seven years shorter than an average life expectancy.

People with MS may develop DEPRESSION, but this affective disorder can be effectively treated. People with certain types of MS now have a choice of treatments that can slow the progression of the disease. Symptom management, ASSISTIVE DEVICES, and supportive services also can enhance the quality of life for those who have MS.

While noting that the society respects autonomy and the right to self-determination, the NMSS nevertheless asserts that the society affirms life and offers programs and services that promote positive coping with multiple sclerosis.

Assisted suicide remains extremely controversial in the United States and in many countries around the world because it reverses the physician's usual approach to patient care. Some patients desire an assisted suicide if they believe adequate relief is not possible. Others may request earlier death to exercise autonomy and to end their lives on their own terms. Proponents argue that terminally ill patients should have the right to end their own suffering and that involving another person (such as a doctor) makes the suicide easier and less risky. Critics worry that assisted suicide might lead to abuse, exploitation, and erosion of care for vulnerable people.

Many other U.S. states have attempted to pass laws legalizing assisted suicide; all have failed. In November 1998, an initiative in Michigan that would have legalized assisted suicide was defeated by a vote of 71 percent. In January 2000, an attempt to legalize assisted suicide in California failed. In November 2000, voters in Maine rejected the proposed Maine Death With Dignity Act. This law was virtually identical to the assisted-suicide law that passed in Oregon in 1994.

Although assisted suicide is against the law in all states but Oregon, giving general information to people about ways to kill themselves is not against the law.

assistive devices Tools or implements that make a particular function easier or possible to perform. An assistive device may be as simple as an electric toothbrush or as elaborate as an environmental control system that can be operated with a mouth switch by someone who has lost the use of his or her arms or legs. For example, tub and wall grab bars can help people with multiple sclerosis (MS) get in and out of the bathtub and keep their balance while showering. Button and zipper hooks can be used to help fasten clothes, and Velcro on clothes can make getting dressed easier. Combs, brushes, and toothbrushes can be fitted with easier-to-hold handles. Electric can openers, rocker knives to minimize wrist motion, and cookware designed for those with limited hand, wrist, and forearm strength can make cooking manageable. The heavy lifting and bending often involved in housekeeping can be minimized by putting cleaning supplies and equipment on wheels and by using long-handled dusters, brooms, and sponges. Extendable reachers can help grasp objects on shelves or in closets.

Special grips can help a person with MS securely handle a pen or a drawing implement. Special lenses and magnifying devices may correct some visual problems associated with MS.

Braces, canes, or walkers can help those who have trouble walking, while wheelchairs and electric scooters can provide some measure of independence for those who can no longer walk. Transfer boards and lifts can be used to help people with MS get in and out of a bed, tub, automobile, or wheelchair and to help lift those who have fallen. People with MS may drive safely with the help of hand controls, low-energy steering wheels, and other aids.

Assistive devices are usually prescribed by an occupational, physical, or speech therapist following referral by a physician. Many catalogs, websites and surgical supply stores are excellent sources for assistive devices.

See also Appendix I.

astrocytes Neuroglial cells that form a scar after the layer of MYELIN that normally insulates nerve fibers is destroyed.

Atarax See HYDROXYZINE.

ataxia Problems with coordinating limb actions that result in shaky movements and unsteady gait, caused by the brain's failure to regulate the body's posture and the strength and direction of limb movements. These types of coordination problems are common among people with multiple sclerosis.

Damage to the cerebellum—the part of the brain responsible for posture—or to the spinal cord causes problems with directing individual limb movements and also coordinated limb movements. This means that a patient may be able to move one leg smoothly but not be able to walk using both legs without staggering.

In cerebral ataxia, a clumsiness occurs in intentional movements, including walking, speaking, and movements of the eye. Sensory ataxia causes unsteady movements that are exaggerated when a patient closes her eyes; it occurs from a lack of sensory feedback.

Cerebellar ataxia is caused by a lesion in the cerebellum. Vestibular ataxia is caused by a lesion in the brain stem or the vestibular nuclei. Sensory ataxia results from dysfunction of position-sensing nerves.

atrophy A wasting away or decrease in the size of a cell, tissue, or organ of the body because of disease or lack of use.

auditory agnosia The inability to hear because the auditory stimulus cannot be interpreted, in spite of the presence of a normal sense organ (can hear sounds but not interpret). This is sometimes a symptom of multiple sclerosis.

autoimmune disease A disease in which the body's immune system reacts against its own healthy cells, organs, or tissues in the body that are essential for good health. Most experts believe that multiple sclerosis (MS) is an autoimmune disease like other diseases such as systemic lupus erythematosus, rheumatoid arthritis, and scleroderma.

Many experts believe that in MS, the target of the immune attack is a component of MYELIN, the fatty sheath that surrounds and protects nerve fibers in the central nervous system (CNS). When this process occurs, certain white blood cells (called T cells) become sensitized to myelin and enter the CNS. These T cells then injure myelin and secrete chemicals that damage nerve fibers (axons), recruiting more damaging immune cells to the site of inflammation. Experts do not know what activates T cells in patients with MS but suspect that both genetic and environmental factors are important.

Scientists have begun to identify the receptors on the T cells that bind to the myelin, which may lead to the development of more specific treatments designed to suppress the immune activity. Much of the ongoing research in MS is directed toward finding answers to questions about the role of the immune system in the development of MS.

autoinjector A device that can be used to help administer injectable subcutaneous drug treatments.

autonomic nervous system The part of the nervous system that regulates involuntary vital functions, including the activity of the cardiac muscle, smooth muscles (such as of the gut), and glands. The autonomic nervous system has two divisions: the sympathetic nervous system accelerates heart rate, constricts blood vessels, and raises blood pressure; the parasympathetic nervous system slows heart rate, increases intestinal and gland activity, and relaxes sphincter muscles.

Avonex See DISEASE-MODIFYING AGENTS; INTERFERON.

axon The extension of a nerve cell (neuron) that conducts impulses to other nerve cells or muscles. Axons are generally smaller than 1 micron (1 micron = 1/1,000,000 of a meter) in diameter, but can be as much as a half-meter in length.

axonal damage Injury to the AXON in the nervous system that may involve temporary, reversible effects or permanent severing of the axon. Axonal damage usually results in short-term changes in nervous system activity or permanent inability of nerve fibers to send their signals from one part of the nervous system to another or from nerve fibers to muscles. The damage can thus result in a variety of symptoms relating to sensory or motor function.

The brain controls the functions of the body by sending out electrical signals along the nerves, which act like wires in an electrical circuit. A nerve has a central core called an axon, which is covered by a protective sheath made of a protein called MYELIN.

In multiple sclerosis, the axons and myelin get damaged so that the brain's electrical messages are disrupted. Experts used to think that damage to the myelin sheaths occurred first and that damage to axons occurred later in the disease progression, but recent evidence suggests that axonal damage occurs in the earliest stages of the disease. Unfortunately, the body has no way of efficiently replacing or renewing damaged axons.

Minor damage to the myelin can cause a mild symptom, such as numbness or a tingling sensation, but more extensive damage can cause more serious symptoms. For instance, when axons become damaged, electrical impulses from the brain are cut off completely, causing paralysis or loss of bodily functions.

azathioprine (Imuran) A controversial immune-modifying medication that may be used to suppress multiple sclerosis (MS). Azathioprine suppresses the immune system and so is commonly used to treat autoimmune diseases such as rheumatoid arthritis and as part of chemotherapy for some cancers.

Over the past 20 years, azathioprine has been studied around the world as a possible MS treatment. However, results—using different patient populations, different doses, and different protocols—have been mixed. Slowed progression or fewer relapses were reported in 60 percent of the trials, but no apparent benefit occurred in the rest.

Side Effects

Some patients have not been able to take azathioprine because of severe nausea. Other potential side effects include severe anemia (a drop in white blood cell count), liver damage, and a long-term increased risk of developing cancers such as leukemia or lymphoma. The decision to use azathioprine is a complicated one and should be made by the physician and the patient together after a discussion of the potential risks and benefits.

Babinski reflex Also called Babinski's sign, a reflex that extends the big toe upward and fans the other toes when the sole of the foot is stroked. This reflex occurs during infancy but is abnormal in children and adults. After infancy, the normal response to stroking the foot is a bunching downward movement of all the toes.

In anyone over age two, the appearance of the Babinski reflex may indicate multiple sclerosis, a brain injury, or other neurological conditions. The Babinski reflex can occur in just one foot or in both feet.

baclofen (Lioresal) Medication used to treat SPASTICITY in patients with multiple sclerosis (MS). Usually well tolerated, baclofen acts on the central nervous system, easing spasms, cramping, and tight muscles. It is most helpful in cases of severe spasticity with fairly good limb strength. On the other hand, if the arm or leg is weak and spastic, eliminating the spasticity may not help overall limb usefulness. In fact a weak leg kept straight by spasticity is probably easier to walk on than a weak leg with normal muscle tone. On the other hand, sometimes severe spasticity causes severe pain, so easing spasticity makes good sense.

Patients with MS usually begin taking a dose of 5 mg every six to eight hours, which can be increased by 5 mg per dose every five days until symptoms improve. The goal of treatment is to find a dosage level that relieves spasticity without causing excessive weakness or fatigue. After a few days or weeks at the lower dose, the patient can usually begin to tolerate a higher dose with little sedation. The effective dose may vary from 15–160 mg per day or more.

Physicians must check the blood level of patients who use this drug every few weeks or months because occasionally, the drug can alter kidney function in some people.

Patients taking more than 30 mg daily should not stop taking this medication suddenly. Doing so could cause convulsions, hallucinations, increases in muscle spasms or cramping, mental changes, or unusual nervousness or restlessness.

Side Effects

Side effects typically go away as the body adjusts to the medication and do not require medical attention unless they continue for several weeks. These side effects include drowsiness or unusual tiredness, increased weakness, dizziness or lightheadedness, confusion, unusual constipation, new or unusual bladder symptoms, trouble sleeping, and unusual unsteadiness or clumsiness.

Unusual side effects that require immediate medical attention include fainting, hallucinations, severe mood changes, skin rash, or itching.

Symptoms of overdose are sudden onset of blurred or double vision, convulsions, shortness of breath or troubled breathing, or vomiting.

Since distinguishing between certain common symptoms of MS and some side effects of baclofen may be difficult, patients should consult a doctor if abrupt symptoms occur.

balance The ability to remain upright and not fall over when walking is a complex process that depends on a continuing flow of information to the brain about the position of the body. The body maintains its balance due to a complex integration of this information combined with a constant flow of instructions from the brain to various parts of the body, performing the necessary changes to keep the body in balance.

The brain receives information about body position from many sources: eyes; sensory nerves in skin, muscles, and joints; and the three semicircular canals of the labyrinth in the inner ear that detect placement and speed of head movements. The cerebellum is the part of the brain mainly responsible for collecting and integrating this information and conveying data to other motor centers to coordinate body movement.

Because multiple sclerosis (MS) often affects the cerebellum, some of the most common symptoms of MS include clumsiness, speech disorders, and other features of impaired muscular coordination.

balance problems   The ability to stand upright is moderated by the cerebellum in the brain, although the eyes, ears, and spinal cord connections also are involved. Balance problems and incoordination are common problems in people with multiple sclerosis (MS). If MS lesions affect the cerebellum, they may adversely affect a person's sense of balance, making it difficult to stand upright.

Balance problems may also be affected by DIZZINESS or a spinning sensation called VERTIGO.

Cerebellar incoordination and tremor are some of the most difficult MS symptoms to treat and are often incapacitating. There are no effective medications that can improve balance. However, if the balance problem is related to an MS relapse, treatment with steroids may be helpful.

An aid to enhance ambulatory mobility becomes essential if balance and coordination are problems. A cane, crutch, or walker can be used, preferably ones that have been measured for correct size and model for the individual. Instruction should be given to the user by a skilled therapist. New large wheel walkers with hand controls, a seat, and a basket have improved activities of daily living for people with balance, tremor, and mobility problems.

No treatments are available for dizziness, but several drugs can help control vertigo, including dimenhydrinate, ondansetron, or prochlorperazine. These drugs, however, may cause sedation.

See also PHYSICAL THERAPIST.

Barthel index   A scale of function in 10 areas encompassing mobility, function of ACTIVITIES OF DAILY LIVING, and urinary control.

basal ganglia   A part of the brain deep within the CEREBRUM and the upper parts of the BRAIN STEM that play an important part in producing smooth, continuous muscular actions and in stopping and starting movement. Fibers pass from almost every region of the CEREBRAL CORTEX (especially the MOTOR CORTEX) to the basal ganglia. After processing in the basal ganglia, nerve signals are then transmitted back to the supplementary motor area and premotor cortex of the frontal lobe.

Diseases such as multiple sclerosis can affect the basal ganglia and their connections, leading to the appearance of involuntary movements, trembling, and WEAKNESS.

bathroom aids   Safety aids for use in toileting and grooming in the bathroom are important for people with multiple sclerosis. Safety rails and grab bars, nonskid rugs, plastic cups, and adhesive safety strips for the shower or tub floor are vital.

Electric shavers are safer and easier to use than the nonelectric type and are recommended if hand or arm tremor is a problem. Those with a weak grip may find that an electric toothbrush and toothpaste tube squeezers (or pump toothpaste containers) can be helpful. Long-handled grips that fit on shaving cream cans can also help people with weak grips. Other helpful products include wall-mounted nail clippers and nail files, a long-handled scrub brush for the shower, flexible mirrors that can be set at an angle, bath pillows to support the head while bathing, and extension combs and brushes. Special bath mitts with Velcro closures can help people who lack grip strength.

A variety of toilet devices can help people who have uncertain balance or who cannot easily bend over. High-back or raised toilet seats are available from a variety of dealers, and extensions for toilet handles are available. Toilet splash guards, step stools, and toilet safety handrails also are available.

Bathing can be difficult and sometimes dangerous for a person with uncertain balance or coordination problems. Because sitting down in the shower makes sense for these patients, bathtub seats are a good option and can be obtained at a drugstore or medical equipment supply house. These seats include either a four-legged stool placed in the middle of the tub or a flat variety that clamps across the tub sides. In addition, replacing standard shower controls with push button or easy on/off controls can help patients who lack hand strength.

B cell   A type of lymphocyte (white blood cell) manufactured in the bone marrow that makes antibodies.

bedding   Because heat can worsen the symptoms of multiple sclerosis, selecting the right bedding and equipment is vital. Bedcovers should provide warmth without weight. Woven knit sheets are easy to put on the mattress because the corners stretch easily. However, if turning over in bed is difficult, woven satin sheets will help the patient slide more easily, especially while wearing nylon or silk pajamas. If turning over or changing sleeping positions in bed is difficult, the patient might do better by pushing the side of the bed up against the bedroom wall and installing a railing or grab bar on the wall. The railing must be attached to a stud and installed at the right height to help the patient turn over easily.

To minimize the amount of walking involved, patients may want to make one side of a bed completely and then finish the other side. A two-foot stick or a dowel with a cup hook attached to one end can help the patient arrange the blanket and sheet. However, the stick cannot be used with an open-weave or thermal blanket because the hook will snag the threads.

bedsore   The common name for a decubitus ulcer—a sore spot on the skin caused by pressure and lack of movement, typically in wheelchair-users or people who spend a great deal of time in bed. This pressure cuts off the blood supply to the underlying skin, fat, and muscle.

The ulcers occur most often in areas where the bone lies directly under the skin, such as the elbow, the hip, or over the tailbone. However, pressure sores are not limited to these areas and can occur in other places as well. The skin is much more likely to break down if it is moist or infected, so incontinence can add to the problem. A decubitus ulcer may become painful, infected, and worsen a patient's health.

Symptoms and Diagnostic Path
Pressure sores begin innocently enough. If left untreated, however, they may progress to much more serious, advanced stages:

- *Stage 1*   In this early stage, the bedsore may simply look like a small area of warm, reddened or purpled skin that does not return to its natural color when pressed.
- *Stage 2*   Now the outer layer of skin breaks down, and blistering, swelling, warmth, and redness may appear.
- *Stage 3*   At this stage, live tissue begins to ulcerate and die; the ulcers now penetrate the deep skin layers and the fat and muscle immediately beneath the skin; this hole or crater has a foul smell.
- *Stage 4*   The sore or ulcer extends down into the deep muscle, possibly down to the bone; infection may occur and may tunnel under the skin, increasing the size of the sore.

Treatment Options and Outlook
Seeing a doctor for proper treatment of bedsores is very important. The treatment of pressure sores becomes more difficult as the wound becomes more severe. A stage 1 ulcer can usually be managed by simply eliminating the source of the pressure. Stage 2 sores can be treated by medication and protective coverings. The treatment for a stage 3 or stage 4 ulcer may involve long-term care, including surgery (debridement), dressings, a special bed, medications, and antibiotics.

Risk Factors and Preventive Measures
Several related risk factors have been identified in the development of pressure sores, including immobility or inactivity, decreased sensation, bowel or bladder incontinence, poor nutrition, and older age. In addition, obesity or being underweight can both lead to sores, as can too-dry or too-moist skin and smoking. Other health conditions, such as diabetes, anemia, or cardiovascular disorders, also can contribute to bedsores.

The best way to treat a pressure sore is to avoid developing one in the first place. Pressure sores can be prevented by maintaining mobility, drinking lots of fluids, and having a well-rounded diet. If the patient with multiple sclerosis is not able to get out of bed, the person's position must be changed at least every two hours. The bed should have a mattress or pad that is capable of alternating and distributing the pressure applied by the body. Padding or boots for pressure points such as heels should be worn. Patients who use a wheelchair should sit on a gel-filled seat cushion to distribute the weight.

bee sting therapy   Some people with multiple sclerosis insist that their condition has improved following multiple bee stings, but objective studies have not yet proven this technique. Proponents of this treatment believe that the bee venom triggers an immune response that can affect the course of the disease. Risks of this therapy are considerable, especially since some people have a fatal reaction to bee stings (especially multiple stings) because of the venom's effect on the immune system.

behavioral neurologist   A physician who specializes in the diagnosis and treatment of behavioral and memory disorders caused by brain disease. A typical neurological evaluation takes about one to two hours and involves testing for sensory and movement problems as well as a brief review of mental function. The neurologist may prescribe medications to treat memory disorders or troublesome behavioral symptoms.

Bell's palsy   A form of facial paralysis (usually on one side of the face) caused by damage to the seventh (facial) cranial nerve. Bell's palsy can occur as a consequence of a serious neurological condition such as multiple sclerosis (MS) or by a viral infection such as the common cold sore virus or herpes simplex. The condition begins suddenly and can be transient or permanent. Named for the 19th-century Scottish surgeon Sir Charles Bell who first described the condition, Bell's palsy is the most common cause of facial paralysis, affecting about 40,000 Americans each year. The incidence rate in the United States is about 20–30 cases per 100,000. Worldwide, Bell's palsy afflicts between 10 and 30 people per 100,000.

Bell's palsy occurs when the nerve that controls the facial muscles becomes swollen, inflamed, or compressed, resulting in facial weakness or paraly-

sis. The etiology of this form of facial palsy is unknown, and therefore exactly what causes this damage is also unknown.

The disorder is more commonly seen in young adults, diabetics, and also pregnant women. Unfortunately, it is possible to suffer from Bell's palsy on more than one occasion, although the recurrence rate is only about 7 percent.

Between 80 and 90 percent of those with the condition make a gradual but full recovery over a period of weeks or months, depending on the severity of the facial paralysis.

benign multiple sclerosis   About one out of five people with multiple sclerosis has a very mild form of the disease in which only a few episodes occur. These occasional flares fade away quickly and do not lead to permanent disability. However, it is not possible to identify those who will have a mild course.

Berg balance scale   A scale of BALANCE that is sensitive to change, sometimes used to assess people with multiple sclerosis.

Betaseron   See   DISEASE-MODIFYING   AGENTS; INTERFERON.

biofeedback   A type of therapy that translates skin temperature, muscle contractions, blood pressure, pulse, brain waves and other bodily functions into audio or video signals so that people can use these signals to modify symptoms. Biofeedback has been used to teach people to reduce muscle PAIN and tension headaches. It has been used to manage SPASTICITY in people with multiple sclerosis, although studies have not substantiated its effectiveness in this area.

biological markers   A component of a person's body, such as a protein or gene, that can be measured to determine whether the person has a particular disease. The search for biological markers in multiple sclerosis (MS) has been made difficult by the nature of the disease, which occurs in the brain and cannot be accessed by routine sampling.

If researchers could identify an accurate biological marker for MS, diagnosing the disease would be much simpler. In addition, an effective biomarker would help predict the onset of MS and monitor its progression and response to treatment. Because new and evolving therapies have the potential for slowing the progression of the disease, earlier treatments may mean better outcomes.

black holes Lesions in the brain that emit very low signals on a MAGNETIC RESONANCE IMAGING scan. Severe disease progression can be gauged by the presence of these black holes; some evidence suggests that they may represent iron deposits in the brain.

bladder dysfunction Urinary and bladder problems are common symptoms that appear in about 80 percent of people with multiple sclerosis (MS). This occurs because the disease blocks or delays transmission of nerve signals in areas of the central nervous system that control the bladder and urinary sphincter. (The sphincter is the muscle surrounding the opening of the bladder that either keeps urine in or allows it to flow out.)

Just like other MS symptoms, bladder problems may be an issue only occasionally—at least in the beginning. With severe forms of the disease, the bladder problems may progress to a chronic condition. If left untreated, bladder dysfunction may cause emotional and personal hygiene problems that can interfere with normal life.

The bladder is a muscular bag that slowly expands as urine collects; the muscular part of the bladder is called the detrusor muscle. At the point where the bladder meets the urethra is a muscle called the external sphincter that remains closed when the patient is not urinating. The bladder and sphincter are normally under voluntary control, which means that a person has conscious control over when and where to urinate. Voluntary control of urination is managed by the brain.

When the bladder is full, it signals the brain via impulses up the spinal cord; impulses needed for normal urination are transmitted from the brain back to the bladder. As one or two cups of urine collect in the bladder, it gradually stretches until it reaches peak capacity. At this point, the person will experience an urge to urinate. For urination to occur, two events must take place simultaneously.

The bladder detrusor muscle must contract to expel urine at the same time that the sphincter muscle relaxes and opens, permitting a free flow of urine out of the body. When the person decides the time and place are right, the bladder contracts to push out the urine, while the sphincter opens to allow urine to exit.

MS-related lesions (areas of inflammation, DEMYELINATION scarring, and/or neuronal damage) in the brain or spinal cord can disrupt this normal process by interfering with the transmission of signals between the brain, spinal cord, and urinary system. Three primary types of bladder dysfunction can result:

Storage problem If the patient has a storage problem, the bladder is unable to retain urine as it accumulates. In this case, the detrusor muscle of the bladder is overly active. Contractions of the bladder occur when only a small amount of urine has collected, and the sphincter opens in a normal way, resulting in frequent and urgent urination.

Emptying dysfunction If the patient has an emptying dysfunction, the bladder is unable to eliminate stored urine completely. In this case the urethra is blocked by a spastic or tight sphincter, which prevents the bladder from emptying completely. The urinary sphincter tightens instead of relaxing when the bladder's detrusor muscle contracts to push the urine out. Although some urine is usually eliminated, a significant amount remains in the bladder.

Another form of emptying dysfunction occurs when the detrusor muscle is too weak to expel all the urine. However, this occurs infrequently in patients with MS.

Combination storage emptying problems Failure to store in combination with failure to empty (medically known as DETRUSOR–EXTERNAL SPHINCTER DYSSYNERGIA) results from a lack of coordination between muscle groups. Instead of working in coordination with one another (with the detrusor contracting to expel urine while the external sphincter relaxes to release it), the detrusor and external sphincter contract simultaneously, trapping the urine in the bladder. The resulting symptoms can include: urgency, hesitancy, dribbling, incontinence.

Urinary tract infections In addition to these common types of bladder dysfunction, people with

MS are at increased risk of urinary tract infections. Although anyone can develop an infection in the urinary tract, they are more common in people who are unable to fully empty their bladder.

Urine that remains in the bladder over a prolonged period of time breeds excessive bacteria, eventually leading to infection. Storage of urine also allows mineral deposits to settle and form stones that promote infection and irritate bladder tissues. The symptoms of a urinary tract infection can include urgency, frequency, a burning sensation, abdominal and or lower back pain, elevated body temperature, increased spasticity, dark-colored and foul-smelling urine.

Symptoms and Diagnostic Path

MS can disrupt the urinary system because of MS lesions in the brain and spinal cord that interrupt the transmission of signals to and from the brain. This in turn can result in problems storing urine to normal capacity or problems emptying the bladder completely. Many patients with MS have at least some—but not enough—control over emptying the bladder. They may have a sudden urge to urinate, which is followed very quickly by involuntary urination.

Any of these symptoms may occur, regardless of the underlying problem:

- urgency
- incontinence
- overflow incontinence—loss of urinary control due to a very full bladder, causing dribbling or leaking
- urinating several times during the night (NOCTURIA)
- trouble starting the flow of urine
- sensation of incomplete emptying, causing a feeling that some urine remains in the bladder after voiding
- urine flow that is thin and slow

Getting a proper diagnosis is an essential first step, so people must inform their doctor as soon as any problems occur for an accurate bladder diagnosis. The symptoms alone cannot reveal whether the basic problem involves storage, emptying, or another medical problem. Virtually all these symptoms could signal a urinary tract infection (UTI), which might not be related to MS but which must be promptly treated with an appropriate antibiotic. However, UTIs are often associated with an increase in other MS symptoms, such as spasticity and fatigue.

If a urine culture rules out a UTI, one or more other bladder function tests will be needed to help identify the problem and determine the treatment. Tests of bladder function include

- *Urinalysis and urine culture*   These lab tests of a fresh urine sample determine if infection is present and which antibiotic is appropriate if infection is detected.

- *Post-void residual urine*   After the patient urinates, a catheter is inserted to determine how much urine has remained in the bladder; this is the simplest test to determine bladder function, but the bladder sonogram (see below) is a non-invasive alternative that may be an option.

- *Bladder sonogram*   An ultrasonic scan that evaluates the urinary system.

- *Intravenous urogram (IVP)*   An X-ray with contrast dye of the entire urinary system that provides information about the kidneys as well as the bladder.

- *Radioisotope renal/residual urine scan*   A variation of the IVP in which radiation-emitting radioisotope is injected and traced on its path through the body to provide details on the kidneys and bladder.

- *Urodynamics*   A test in which a doctor or nurse uses a urinary catheter and rectal probe to determine the storage capacity of the bladder and function of the urinary tract.

Since bladder and sphincter function may vary over time, repeating diagnostic tests and varying the strategies over time may be necessary.

Treatment Options and Outlook

Patients can do some things themselves to help their bladder problems. Drinking at least eight glasses of fluid every day is recommended for general health and the health of the urinary system.

This often requires learning how to spread fluid intake over the course of the day and perhaps drinking less at night if awakening to urinate is a problem. Restricting fluids is not recommended for managing bladder problems.

Although fluids are important, patients should avoid consuming beverages containing caffeine, which is a bladder irritant that can make some symptoms worse. On the other hand, drinking cranberry juice daily can help reduce the risk of urinary infections because it contains a chemical that prevents bacteria from sticking to the bladder wall. Cranberry tablets are a useful alternative. Health care professionals can offer other possible diet changes and adaptations that may ease bladder problems since what a patient eats and drinks can contribute to good management.

Some people also use absorbent pads to provide security; many pads contain a powder that turns to a gel when wet, guarding against leaks. Although pads should not be used as the sole solution to bladder problems, they can help patients feel more comfortable. The ideal outcome is to eliminate leaking or loss of control so that pads are not needed.

In addition to self-help strategies such as dietary and fluid management, medical treatments for bladder problems may include medications and intermittent catheterization (inserting a thin tube into the bladder to remove urine) or an INDWELLING CATHETER.

Storage dysfunction   Treatment for the most common type of storage dysfunction is aimed at relaxing the bladder detrusor muscle so that a normal amount of urine may build up before the patient feels the urge to urinate. This may include medications such as Pro-banthine (propantheline bromide), Tofranil (imipramine), or Ditropan (oxybutynin), all of which relieve spasms of the bladder. Ditropan XL delivers oxybutynin, the most common drug for calming the bladder, packaged as a controlled-release, one-a-day tablet that maintains a steady level of medication in the body. Detrol (tolterodine) works by reducing bladder muscle contractions.

Alternatively, the nasal spray DDAVP (desmopressin acetate) is a different kind of medication that increases urine concentration and decreases urine production.

All of these medications also reduce the frequency of bathroom trips by increasing the volume of urine passed each time.

Emptying dysfunction   Some people with a mild emptying problem in which a small amount of urine is retained may respond well to the drug BACLOFEN (Lioresal). However, most people with emptying problems will need to use intermittent catheterization (IC), which is the most successful way to manage emptying dysfunction. In this method, urine is periodically drained by inserting a thin tube into the bladder through the urinary opening. This painless procedure is generally much easier to do than it sounds, with a little instruction and a few practice sessions with a nurse. Women are often more receptive than men to IC. Once men overcome their resistance and realize the benefits, they have an easier time than women since the male urinary opening is more accessible.

If symptoms are not controlled by IC alone, medications such as Ditropan XL or Detrol may be added to the routine in order to relax the bladder. The sometimes dramatic relief of symptoms and the prospect of avoiding serious complications over the long term usually encourage people to continue IC.

Some patients need to perform IC for only a few weeks or months since the bladder often returns to normal or near-normal function in time.

On the other hand, some people experience more complex bladder problems that resist other strategies. Options are available. Some individuals may ultimately need a catheter permanently inserted into the bladder. In other rare situations, surgery is required for an improved quality of life and better health.

Risk Factors and Preventive Measures

Serious complications can usually be prevented with good care and follow-up. Since emptying dysfunction leads to urinary retention, bacteria may multiply freely in the stagnant urine. This postvoid residual urine may predispose a person to frequent urinary tract infections. Kidney damage can occur if infected urine backs up through the ureters into the kidneys due to an exit that is blocked by a contracted or tight sphincter. Bladder or kidney stones are other potential complications of incomplete emptying since minute mineral particles normally expelled in urine may clump together to form stones that cannot be passed through urination. Stones can further complicate normal voiding.

Frequent UTIs, kidney or bladder stones, and kidney damage all suggest a problem with chronic urinary retention.

In the past, people with retention problems were taught "credé," in which the patient pushed down on the lower abdomen while voiding. This is now considered harmful since the pressure of credé may often move the urine up, not down. It is no longer recommended.

A person who has a urinary tract infection may also experience a pseudo-exacerbation. The infection and accompanying elevation in body temperature may cause other MS symptoms to flare temporarily, mimicking a true exacerbation, even though there is no underlying disease activity. Once the infection has been treated, these MS symptoms resolve and return to the person's pre-infection baseline. Thus health care providers look for bladder symptoms or other evidence of infection when trying to determine if a person is having an exacerbation.

bladder incontinence See BLADDER DYSFUNCTION.

blood-brain barrier A protective, semipermeable layer of cells lining the blood vessels in the brain and spinal cord that lets oxygen, essential nutrients, carbon dioxide, and other waste materials move between the blood and the central nervous system (CNS). This same barrier also prevents large molecules, immune cells, and potentially damaging substances and germs from moving out of the bloodstream into the CNS. However, immune system cells are somehow capable of crossing into the brains of people with multiple sclerosis (MS) but not into the brains of people without the disease. Some scientists think this implies that the blood-brain barrier of patients with MS has become damaged and that this breach may underlie the disease process.

Preventing these immune system cells from entering the brain and spinal cord had been the aim of a medication for MS called natalizumab (Tysabri), which was recently pulled from the market.

blood test for MS Although no blood test is currently available to diagnose multiple sclerosis (MS), preliminary research suggests that antimyelin antibodies may be a tool to an MS diagnosis, and may be used to predict future MS attacks.

Researchers in Austria have studied a simple blood test that identifies antibodies in the blood produced to fight off substances that are damaged during MS disease activity (myelin OLIGODENDRO-CYTE glycoprotein [MOG] and MYELIN BASIC PROTEIN [MBP]). In the Austrian study, of 103 participants with a clinically isolated syndrome and positive results with magnetic resonance imaging (MRI) and cerebrospinal fluid analysis, 22 individuals had antibodies against both MOG and MBP. Of these 22, 21 participants (or 95 percent) experienced a relapse eight months later. Of the 39 who did not have either antibody, only nine (23 percent) had a relapse, and on average, this occurred almost four years later. The third group of 42 people had positive readings for the MOG antibody only, and 35 of them (83 percent) had a relapse after a little more than a year on average.

According to researchers, this blood test could thus provide a rapid, inexpensive, and precise method for predicting early conversion to clinically definite MS. The advantage of such a method would be to allow doctors to identify better those patients who should begin treatment immediately in order to delay the occurrence of a second attack and a definite MS diagnosis. Theoretically, such a test may even hold the potential of one day predicting upcoming disease activity in those already diagnosed, allowing for steroidal treatment or other proactive strategies for individuals prior to the onset of an exacerbation. This would be an important development. MS has always been associated with a variety of symptoms that may occur unpredictably and mimic other conditions. In most cases, patients visit a neurologist after the first flare-up of neurological symptoms, which is labeled as a "clinically isolated syndrome." Up to 80 percent of those who experience a clinically isolated syndrome will eventually develop MS, but predicting who will be among this 80 percent is difficult. To diagnose MS, the physician must confirm that two MS-like events have occurred and/or lesions have appeared in more than one location and at two different times. This process may be both expensive and time-consuming, involving continued evaluation and repeated MRI scans. The development of a reliable blood test, however, could save patients from uncertainty as well as saving them time and money.

board-and-care homes   A type of residential health care, suitable for patients with advanced multiple sclerosis, that involves more care than ASSISTED LIVING but less than would be available in a nursing home. Also called personal-care homes or residential-care facilities, board-and-care homes are often single-family houses serving fewer than 10 residents in quiet, residential neighborhoods.

The caregivers (usually two per home) are health care aides, not registered nurses. Some board-and-care facilities provide 24-hour care for frail patients who do not need ongoing medical attention but might otherwise have to go to a nursing home. In the best situations, residents of board-and-care homes feel part of a family, eating in a dining room and enjoying social activities in the home.

bone marrow transplantation   An experimental treatment (also called hemopoietic stem cell transplantation) used for severe forms of multiple sclerosis (MS). The long-term benefits of this experimental procedure have not yet been established.

In this procedure, the individual receives grafts, often of his or her own blood stem cells. Stem cells are produced in the bone marrow and are the early forms for all blood cells in the body (including red, white, and immune cells). Early studies indicate that bone marrow transplantation may slow progression of MS, although at this point it is not a cure.

botulinum toxin (Botox, Myobloc)   A toxin derived from the bacterium *Clostridium botulinum*, used in a class of drugs called neurotoxins. Although not currently approved for the treatment of patients with multiple sclerosis (MS), a growing number of health care providers now consider the use of botulinum toxin as an effective short-term treatment option for certain types of MS-related problems,

such as muscle stiffness and urinary problems, when first-line treatment is ineffective. Although experts believe that Botox will probably not be resubmitted for specific approval to relieve MS-related SPASTICITY or BLADDER DYSFUNCTION, some doctors treating MS have begun to prescribe it.

The brain should send electrical messages to muscles so that they can contract and move. This message is transmitted to the muscle by a substance called acetylcholine. Botulinum toxin blocks acetylcholine, so the muscle does not receive the message to contract. Because Botox selectively paralyzes nerves, it appears to be partly effective in treating spasticity, a nerve-driven condition common among people with MS. A study published in 1990 revealed marked improvement and no adverse effects after Botox injections to 10 nonambulatory people with MS who had spastic contraction of the thigh muscles.

SPASTICITY refers to a wide range of involuntary muscle contractions that result in muscle spasms or stiffness, interfering with voluntary muscle movement and usually involving the muscles of the legs and/or arms. Spasticity may vary based on many factors, including infections, stress, pain, temperature, position, and time of the day. Over time, severe spasticity may cause decreased range of motion in the affected limbs. Some doctors believe that an increased sensitivity in the parts of the muscles that are responsible for contracting, relaxing, and stretching contributes to spasticity.

Botox also has been studied as a possible treatment for a bladder problem called DETRUSOR–EXTERNAL SPHINCTER DYSSYNERGIA (DESD), which causes urinary urgency, frequency, incontinence, difficulties emptying the bladder, and urinary infections in people with MS. DESD is a serious problem that can sometimes lead to damage of the kidneys and ureters (the tubes connecting the kidneys with the bladder). In two case studies, each involving someone with MS who had DESD, Botox relieved symptoms for about three months after injection. A 2003 study by University of Pittsburgh researchers showed that 41 of 50 people with a variety of bladder problems, including MS-related difficulties, reported a decrease or absence of incontinence after a Botox injection. Symptom relief came within seven days of the injection and lasted for as long as six months. No long-term complications occurred.

Two types of botulinum toxin are available for therapeutic use: botulinum toxin type A (Botox) and botulinum toxin type B (Myobloc). The patient's doctor will decide which type of botulinum toxin is more appropriate. Although many other types of botulinum toxin have been identified, they are not used to treat MS symptoms. Botulinum toxin is given as an injection into the affected muscles.

The effects of the medication begin to appear from one to two weeks after the injection and remain effective for two to six months, depending on the individual. Injections are not repeated more often than every three months to minimize the risk of developing antibodies to the botulinum toxin. If the muscles to be injected are small or hard to reach, recording electric signals from the muscles may be necessary to make sure the right ones are receiving the injected medication. A very fine needle is used for the injection, but some people report minor, temporary discomfort from the injection. The medication itself does not sting or cause irritation after it has been injected.

The benefit of botulinum toxin is limited to the injected muscles. This treatment may not be a good choice when many muscles are involved.

Side Effects

Side effects may include temporary weakness of the injected muscle, temporary weakness in some nearby muscles, and brief flu-like symptoms that may appear one week after the injections and last for about a day. In addition, patients may have a slight chance of developing antibodies to the botulinum toxin, which would make it less effective. If this occurs, switching to the other type of toxin (for example, from type A to type B) may be helpful. To minimize the risk of developing antibodies, specific guidelines are followed to restrict the frequency of injections and the dose of medication that is injected.

Botox   See BOTULINUM TOXIN.

bovine myelin   A highly experimental treatment for multiple sclerosis (MS) in which the insulating material of a cow's central nervous system is fed to the patient. Some people insist they find some benefit from this treatment. However, the risks of this treatment are considerable in the wake of mad cow disease (bovine spongiform encephalopathy), which may be transmitted by ingesting central nervous system material from infected cows.

Adequate human studies of this treatment have not yet been conducted, and positive results have been elusive.

bowel dysfunction   The bowel (also known as the colon or large intestine) is the lower portion of the digestive system. Major digestive action starts in the stomach and is continued in the small or upper intestine. Food is moved through the digestive system by a propulsive action and becomes mainly waste and water by the time it enters the bowel. When the stool reaches the final section of the bowel, it has lost much of the water that was present in the upper part of the digestive system. The stool is eliminated from the body with a bowel movement through the anal canal.

Normal bowel functioning can range from three bowel movements a day to three a week. The rectum (the last four to six inches of the digestive tract) signals when a bowel movement is needed. It remains empty until just before a bowel movement. The filling of the rectum sends messages to the brain via nerves in the rectal wall that a bowel movement is needed.

From the rectum, the stool passes into the anal canal, guarded by ring-shaped internal and external sphincter muscles. The stool is admitted to the anal canal by the internal sphincter muscle, which opens automatically when the rectal wall is stretched by a mass of stool. The external sphincter is opened by a conscious decision of the brain so that bowel movements occur only at appropriate times.

Constipation and Diarrhea

If the contents of the bowel move too fast, not enough water is removed and the stool reaches the rectum in a soft or liquid state called diarrhea. If movement of the stool is slow, too much water may be absorbed by the body, making the stool hard and difficult to pass—a problem called CON-STIPATION. Constipation can prevent any of the stool from being eliminated, or it can result in a partial bowel movement, with part of the waste retained in the bowel or rectum.

Constipation and MS

Constipation is the most common bowel complaint in multiple sclerosis (MS) and is often caused by poor dietary habits or limited physical activity. MS can lead to loss of MYELIN in the brain or spinal cord, a short-circuiting process that may prevent or interfere with the signals from the bowel to the brain indicating the need for a bowel movement, and/or the responding signals from the brain to the bowel that maintain normal functioning. Common MS symptoms such as difficulty in walking and FATIGUE can lead to slow movement of waste material through the colon. Weakened abdominal muscles can also make the actual process of having a bowel movement more difficult.

People with MS often have problems with SPAS-TICITY. If the pelvic floor muscles are spastic and unable to relax, normal bowel functioning will be affected. Some people with MS also tend not to have the usual increase in activity in the colon following meals that propels waste toward the rectum.

Constipation can be made worse when some people with MS try to solve another common problem—BLADDER DYSFUNCTION—by reducing their fluid intake. The first step for a person with MS may be to get medical help for bladder problems so that adequate fluid intake, which is critical to bowel functions, will be possible.

A long-term delay in dealing with bowel problems is not an option. Besides the obvious discomfort of constipation, complications can develop. Stool that builds up in the rectum can put pressure on parts of the urinary system, increasing some bladder problems. A stretched rectum can send messages to the spinal cord that further interrupt bladder function. Constipation aggravates spasticity, and constipation can be the root cause of the most distressing bowel symptom: incontinence.

Diarrhea and MS

In general, diarrhea is less of a problem for people with MS than is constipation. Reduced sensation in the rectal area can allow the rectum to stretch beyond its normal range, triggering an unexpected, involuntary relaxation of the external anal sphincter, releasing the loose stool. MS sometimes causes overactive bowel functioning, leading to diarrhea or sphincter abnormalities that can cause incontinence. The condition can be treated with prescription medications such as Pro-Banthine or Ditropan.

Bulk-formers can be used to treat diarrhea instead of constipation, when taken without any additional fluid. If bulk-formers do not relieve diarrhea, medications that slow the bowel muscles, such as Lomotil, may be useful. These remedies are for short-term use only.

Maintaining a Healthy Bowel System

After age 40, all people should have periodic examinations of the lower digestive system. The methods include a rectal exam or a sigmoidoscopy or colonoscopy. These last two tests, in which the bowel is viewed directly with a flexible lighted tube, are used increasingly as early diagnostic exams. They do not require a hospital stay. The colonoscopy, which examines the entire large intestine, is widely considered the better choice. Drinking adequate fluids, adding dietary fiber, exercising, and a regular timed bowel-elimination program are integral to good bowel management.

Fluid intake of two to three quarts of fluid (8–12 cups) daily, including water, juices, and other beverages, is recommended. Fiber intake is also important, since it helps keep the stool moving by adding bulk and by softening the stool with water. Fiber is plant material that holds water and is resistant to digestion. It is found in whole-grain breads and cereals as well as in raw fruits and vegetables. Incorporating high-fiber foods into the diet will help lessen the chances of gas, bloating, or diarrhea.

If limited mobility is a problem, as it is with many people with MS, as much as 30 grams of fiber a day may be required to prevent constipation. Regular exercise, such as walking, swimming, or chair exercises, is important to encourage bowel activity.

Although the emptying reflex is strongest after breakfast, MS can decrease the sensation in the rectal area, and the urge to eliminate may not be present.

Stool softeners, bulk-forming supplements, suppositories, enemas, or manual stimulation may be necessary to treat and maintain good bowel habits on the advice of health professionals. These techniques may need several weeks before it is clear how well they are working.

Impaction and Incontinence

Impaction refers to a hard mass of stool that is lodged in the rectum and cannot be eliminated; it is a problem that requires immediate attention. Impaction can usually be diagnosed through a rectal examination, but symptoms may be confusing because impaction may cause diarrhea, bowel incontinence, or rectal bleeding. Impaction leads to incontinence when the stool mass presses on the internal sphincter, triggering a relaxation response. The external sphincter, although under voluntary control, is frequently weakened by MS and may not be able to remain closed. Watery stool behind the impaction thus leaks out uncontrollably. Loose stool as a side effect of constipation is not uncommon in MS.

Total loss of bowel control happens only rarely in people with MS, but it usually can be managed effectively. Some people with MS report that a sensation of abdominal gas warns them of impending incontinence.

People with the problem should work closely with a doctor and nurse for a solution; a regular schedule of elimination may be the key. When the bowel becomes used to emptying at specific intervals, accidents are less likely. Dietary irritants, such as caffeine and alcohol, should be considered contributing factors and be reduced or eliminated. In addition, medications that reduce spasticity in striated muscle may contribute to the problem. Dosage adjustment may be required.

Drugs prescribed for bladder spasms can be helpful when a hyperactive bowel is the underlying cause of incontinence. Since these drugs also affect bladder function, starting on a low dose and slowly increasing may obtain the best results.

Protective underwear can be used to provide peace of mind. An absorbent lining helps protect the skin, and a plastic outer lining contains odors and keeps clothing from becoming soiled. If bowel problems persist or worsen, a gastroenterologist should be consulted for specialized investigation of bowel and digestive problems.

brain   Part of the central nervous system, along with the spinal cord and optic nerve. It functions as a primary receiver, organizer and distributor of information for the body. The brain houses a complex network of nerve cells and fibers that is responsible for controlling all the processes in the body and orchestrating all thought, speech, emotion, and memory. Messages along the nerves extending from the central nervous system to every other part of the body are received, sorted, and interpreted by the brain.

Physical symptoms such as NUMBNESS, SPASTICITY, or VISUAL PROBLEMS are common in MS. They are usually the result of damage to specific areas in the brain and spinal cord. On the other hand, what causes problems in thinking (also called COGNITIVE DYSFUNCTION) is not always obvious. The ability to think is sensitive to many disruptive influences ranging from normal aging to disease or injury. Cognition also can be temporarily affected by stress, depression, sleep disturbances, hormones, fatigue, or nutritional factors such as low blood sugar (hypoglycemia). Prescription drugs or substance abuse also can influence the ability to think clearly.

Brain Hemispheres

The brain is split into two halves—the left and the right hemisphere. They are separated by a groove, called the CORPUS CALLOSUM, that helps each half of the brain communicate with the other. Although the two halves look identical, they control different parts of the body.

The left side of the brain controls the right side of the body, and the right brain controls the left side. This is because the nerves to each side of the body cross over at the top of the spinal cord. Although the two hemispheres are linked by the corpus callosum and share information, one-half of the brain is always considered dominant. Right-handed people almost always have a dominant left hemisphere. Left-handed people probably have a dominant right hemisphere.

In addition, each half of the brain specializes in certain areas. The right hemisphere controls painting, music, and creative activities; recognizing faces, shapes, and patterns; and judging size and distance. It is also the seat of imagination, emotion, and insight.

The left hemisphere is the center of speech, reading and understanding language, understanding mathematics and performing calculations, and writing and language. It is the logical, problem-solving side of the brain.

On each side of the brain are three main areas: the CEREBELLUM, the CEREBRUM, and the extension of the spinal cord deep within the brain called the BRAIN STEM.

The brain stem controls basic body functions, such as heart rate and breathing, that are responsible for life, and it typically operates without any conscious control. It is made up of the midbrain, the MEDULLA, and the pons. Right behind the brain stem is a small apricot-sized cerebellum, responsible for controlling coordination and balance. The largest area of the brain is the cerebrum, whose four sections completely wrap around the midbrain. It is this area that handles conscious and complicated jobs like thinking, speaking, and reading. The cerebral cortex is the gray outer surface of the cerebrum, as wrinkled as a walnut, where sensory messages are received and interpreted. Although its wrinkled surface does not take up much space within the skull, if it was flattened out, the cerebral cortex would cover an average office desk.

Deep within the brain, in front of the brain stem, are a variety of structures of crucial importance in maintaining body functions, including the thalamus, hypothalamus, BASAL GANGLIA, and pituitary gland.

The four lobes of the brain are broad surface regions in each hemisphere that are named for the bones of the skull lying above them: the frontal, parietal, temporal, and occipital lobes. The frontal lobe is the seat of a person's personality and the critical area for thought. Within the parietal lobe are areas that control pain and sensations of itching, heat, and cold. The occipital lobe's job is to interpret what a person sees.

MS scarring occurs with roughly equal frequency in the right and left halves of the brain and in those areas of the brain called white matter, where a lot of myelin is present. MS lesions are particularly common near the inner cavities of the brain (ventricles) through which the cerebrospinal fluid flows.

More recent studies using MAGNETIC RESONANCE IMAGING have shown a definite relationship between the lesions and intellectual problems, leaving no doubt that MS is the cause. Damage to the structures that join the left and right halves of the brain are particularly serious.

Thinking Problems in MS

Problems with short-term MEMORY are the brain problems most often reported by patients with MS. For example, a person may have trouble remembering an important phone number but usually has no trouble recalling details from the distant past, such as definitions learned in childhood.

Several studies suggest that although most people with MS are able to remember or store information, they may have difficulty recalling it quickly and effectively. A few people with MS may take longer to learn new information. This may mean that poor recall may be the result of not having adequately learned something. Not everyone who experiences a few memory lapses needs counseling. However, therapy can help people deal with the impact intellectual problems have both on self-esteem and on practical everyday living. A therapist can also address depression or anxiety, which can adversely affect intellectual function.

Other patients report problems with abstract reasoning and problem-solving skills, affecting their capacity to analyze a situation, identify the important points, plan a course of action, and carry it out. Occasionally people with MS report that their judgment is sometimes poor. More often family members or employers notice changes in problem solving or reasoning.

MS also can affect visual-spatial abilities, including the ability to recognize objects accurately and to draw or assemble items. Patients use these abilities in many everyday tasks such as driving, following a map, or packing a suitcase.

Verbal fluency is still another area affected in MS. Fluency problems are usually experienced as having a word "on the tip of the tongue." These are a different type of problem than speech problems, which slow down speech or change voice quality.

Both recall and fluency skills require rapid processing of information. Researchers at the Medical College of Wisconsin have found that people with MS performed as well as healthy volunteers on a specialized memory task—but at a significantly slower speed. This supports the belief by many people with MS who feel that their thinking is slowed.

Brain, W. Russell (1895–1966) A British neurologist who published a major review of "disseminating sclerosis" in 1930, more than 60 years after the seminal work of Dr. Jean-Marie CHARCOT. In 1933, Dr. Brain went on to publish *Diseases of the Nervous System,* which contained a section on multiple sclerosis (MS), regularly revising it until his death in 1966.

Dr. Brain was the first to collect statistical data on the incidence and course of MS. His accounts of the underlying pathology of the disease were so accurate that they remain almost unchanged today. Because his understanding of MS was profound, Dr. Brain's books have helped guide neurologists throughout the 20th century and up through today, and many of his opinions and predictions have since been proved correct.

brain atrophy Shrinkage of the brain. As MYELIN, axons, myelin-producing cells (OLIGODENDRO-CYTES), and NEURONS are destroyed, the brain begins to shrink. Processing MAGNETIC RESONANCE IMAGING (MRI) images to determine brain volume may help monitor progression of the disease and treatment effects. MRI also can detect shrinkage in the spinal cord, which is a very strong marker of disease progression.

brain cells There are two kinds of brain cells—neurons and glia. Although most brain cells are glial, the remaining 15 percent—the neurons—make the brain the most important organ in the body. Glial cells play a supportive role in brain function, helping to remove waste products, supplying nutrients, maintaining electrical balance, and guiding the brain's development. The neurons control all the brain's activities and emotions.

Neurons in the brain are structurally the same as nerve cells throughout the body, with a main cell body composed of a nucleus and cytoplasm. The nucleus contains the genetic material that allows a cell to reproduce; the cytoplasm provides energy for the cell. Neurons have very long extensions called axons that allow neurons to communicate with each other. At the end of each axon are many branches or dendrites that reach out toward a neighboring neuron. One neuron has more than 10,000 dendrites, which receive impulses from the axons of other neurons. The human brain has more than 15 billion neurons.

As multiple sclerosis destroys the nerve covering (MYELIN), it disrupts the ability of nerve cells to send messages. Unlike nerve cells in the limbs or trunk, nerve cells and tracts in the brain and spinal cord do not recover their function if they have been destroyed.

brain scans An important group of diagnostic tests increasingly used as a tool to detect changes in brain anatomy and function in patients with multiple sclerosis (MS). Brain scans can be used to rule out physical causes of MS symptoms such as a brain tumor.

Brain scans are generally divided into those that measure brain structure (such as computed tomography [CT] scans) and those that measure brain function (such as positron emission tomography [PET] scans).

Functional Tests

Two main types of brain scans used to measure brain function are PET and single photon emission computed tomography (SPECT). By using these tools, researchers can "see" which areas of the brain are most active after injecting a substance into the bloodstream. Many scientists are using PET, SPECT, and some newer functional imaging methods to study how brain activity changes during disease. PET and SPECT are available at any hospital with a nuclear medicine division.

PET scan PET SCANS provide information about how the brain functions (instead of how it looks) by measuring the rate of sugar metabolism or blood flow in the brain. PET scans are designed to show the activity of brain cells in different regions of the brain by appearing as differently colored areas. PET scans can also be used with magnetic resonance imaging (MRI) to create three-dimensional images of the brain so that scientists can measure the rate at which various regions of the brain use, deposit, or metabolize certain chemicals.

SPECT scan This procedure measures blood flow in different areas of the brain. SPECT is less expensive and more widely available than PET and is used more often in clinical settings.

Structural Tests

Scans designed to reveal brain structure include CT or CAT scans and MRI.

CT scan A CT SCAN provides a three-dimensional picture of the anatomy of the brain by taking multiple X-rays and reconstructing the image of the brain with a computer. CT scans are used in patients with symptoms of stroke, tumor, or hydrocephalus to rule out these conditions. Sometimes a contrast agent or dye is injected into a vein in the arm before the CT scan to obtain a more detailed picture of the brain's anatomy.

MRI scan MRI scans use a strong magnetic field and radio frequency waves, rather than X-rays, to provide pictures of the structure of the brain. As a result, MRIs are radiation free and can also provide a more detailed picture of brain structures than do CT scans. MRIs are better than CT scans in diagnosing MS.

The CT or MRI may be normal in patients with probable MS, especially in the early stages. However, a normal scan in this case only means that there is no evidence of a tumor, stroke, or other structural abnormality that could cause MS symptoms—it does not mean that the brain is normal.

brain stem The part of the BRAIN located at the top of the spinal cord, connecting the forebrain and the midbrain to the spinal cord. It controls functions such as heartbeat and breathing and is the source for the cranial nerve serving the eyes, ears, mouth, and other areas of the face and throat. The brain stem is one of three major divisions of the brain responsible for monitoring muscular movement and also for receiving nerve impulses through the cranial nerves.

From the spinal cord upward, the brain stem includes the MEDULLA, the pons, and the midbrain. The medulla contains the nuclei of the ninth, 10th, 11th, and 12th cranial nerves. The pons is much wider than the medulla and contains bundles of nerves connecting with the CEREBELLUM, lying just behind the brain stem. The pons receives information from the ear, face, and teeth in addition to signals controlling the jaw, facial expression, and eye movement. The midbrain is the smallest part of the brain stem, containing the nuclei of the third and fourth cranial nerves, which control eye movement and pupil size.

The cerebellum is a separate brain organ that is directly attached to the back of the brain stem and is concerned mostly with balance and coordinated movement. Running through the middle of the brain stem is a canal that widens into the fourth ventricle of the brain, home of the circulating cerebrospinal fluid.

Multiple sclerosis damage to certain areas of the brain stem will result in different problems; damage to a specific cranial nerve can have particular effects. For example, damage to the seventh (facial) nerve will cause facial palsy.

brain stem auditory evoked response See EVOKED POTENTIALS.

breast-feeding A woman with multiple sclerosis (MS) can safely breast-feed her baby since there is no danger of transmitting the disease via breast milk. Most women with MS can physically breast-feed, although the disrupted evening and night-time schedules may worsen her fatigue.

Although the relapse rate drops during the second and third trimesters of pregnancy, it rises significantly in the six months after delivery. Research shows that because the relapse rate is temporary for women with very active disease, many MS experts favor restarting disease-modifying medication quickly to keep the disease controlled. Since no studies have been conducted to determine if these drugs pass into breast milk, medications are not approved for use in nursing women. A woman who chooses to nurse should not take any of the disease-modifying drugs until she stops nursing.

Thus experts believe that the only truly safe course for the baby is to avoid disease-modifying drugs during breast-feeding even though doing so means the mother is giving up the protection of medication at a time when the danger of relapse is heightened. Many women prefer to breast-feed in any case because breast milk is highly recommended for infants, and the experience of nursing a baby is treasured by many women. A woman who wishes to breast-feed should consult with her doctor.

Although experts generally do not recommend that nursing mothers use medications to treat fatigue, a woman could stop breast-feeding temporarily and simply use steroids for a couple of days. In addition, the antidepressant sertraline (Zoloft) is known to be safe for nursing mothers, and the implication is that other antidepressants in this class also can be used.

Other new research suggests that intravenous immunoglobulin in the postpartum period may help prevent relapses for women who do not take disease-modifying drugs while breast-feeding.

breathing problems and MS Multiple sclerosis (MS) rarely directly affects breathing. Breathing is controlled by the autonomic nervous system (the part of the central nervous system that controls vital functions, such as heartbeat, without conscious thought), and MS does not usually affect this system. However, the few people with MS who are very severely disabled may develop breathing problems as a result of weakened chest muscles.

Treatment Options and Outlook

If people with MS do develop breathing problems, they may try using breathing exercises and devices to encourage deep breathing (incentive spirometers). Patients may also find that sitting upright rather than lying flat can be helpful. Chest percussion, which involves tapping lightly on the chest to loosen secretions, may also be beneficial.

Patients with SWALLOWING PROBLEMS may require a feeding tube to avoid continued risk of ASPIRATION PNEUMONIA.

If breathing problems occur abruptly, a patient with MS must see a health care provider immediately or go to the emergency room.

Risk Factors and Preventive Measures

Breathing problems also may be caused by aspiration pneumonia, which is linked to the inability to clear secretions from the nose and throat, or from swallowing problems causing food to be inhaled. A swallowing evaluation may help patients who repeatedly take food into their lungs.

Because some medications (such as tranquilizers or muscle relaxants) can also depress breathing, their use should be carefully monitored in anyone with a history of respiratory distress.

calcium ethylamino-phosphate (calcium EAP)
A type of treatment for multiple sclerosis (MS) whose usefulness is based only on anecdotal evidence. No objective evidence suggests that calcium EAP is an effective treatment for MS.

In fact, treatment with the calcium EAP protocol has been classified as unsafe and unapproved for use by the U.S. Food and Drug Administration. The calcium EAP protocol is likewise not recommended by the Medical Advisory Board of the National MS Society.

Because the treatment protocol includes many different agents and may include a powerful drug that suppresses the immune system, the proposed therapy is not without serious risk. The major proponent of the calcium EAP protocol was the late physician Hans Neiper in Germany.

Campath-1H   See ALEMTUZUMAB.

Canada   Canada has one of the highest rates of multiple sclerosis (MS) in the world; 50,000 Canadians have the disease, which means it affects 100 out of every 100,000 Canadians. Every day, three more Canadians are diagnosed. MS is the most common neurological disease affecting young adults in Canada.

MS is at least twice as prevalent in the prairie provinces as it is on the island of Newfoundland. It is also much higher in Pincher Creek, Alberta, for unknown reasons. Saskatchewan has the highest rate on the prairies.

Canadian Occupational Performance Measure (COPM)   A test designed for use by OCCUPATIONAL THERAPISTS to detect change in a client's self-perception of occupational performance over time, as a result of multiple sclerosis. The COPM is designed for use with clients with a variety of disabilities and across all developmental stages. Any change in scores between assessment and reassessment are the most meaningful way to detect change in occupational performance.

canes   Many patients with multiple sclerosis use one or two canes to help compensate for unsteadiness or staggering. A cane is usually used on the opposite side of a weak leg, preceding or accompanying it. Two canes may be needed if weakness is severe, although a walker may be more helpful in this case.

See also OCCUPATIONAL THERAPIST.

cannabinoids   These are compounds in MARIJUANA (cannabis) that may help protect nerve cells and that, therefore, may have a role in easing some symptoms of multiple sclerosis (MS). Some recent studies have suggested that cannabis may improve PAIN, spasms, tremor, mood, appetite, FATIGUE, vision, sexual and urinary function, and MEMORY. However, not all persons with MS respond to these substances, which may worsen balance and posture in persons who struggle with SPASTICITY.

cannabis   See MARIJUANA.

carbamazepine (Tegretol)   An antiepilepsy medication used to treat the tingling pain that may occur in patients with multiple sclerosis.

This drug must be taken regularly if it is to be effective; the physician should check the patient's blood level of medication every few months to prevent an overdose. The doctor also should periodically check the patient's white blood cell count, which may drop in response to this drug. However, in most cases the white blood cell level should not drop low enough to cause problems.

The drug is usually given in doses of 200 mg to 400 mg three or four times a day. Skin rashes may also occur.

Side Effects

A smaller initial dose is prescribed at first to prevent nausea or fatigue that may be caused by a large initial dose of this drug.

Carbamazepine increases the effects of alcohol and other central nervous system depressants that may cause drowsiness (such as antihistamines, sedatives, tranquilizers, prescription medications for pain or seizures, and muscle relaxants). Some people who take carbamazepine may become more sensitive to sunlight, experiencing a severe sunburn or skin rash, itching, redness, or other discoloration.

Because birth control pills containing estrogen may not work properly while taking carbamazepine, women should use an additional or alternative form of birth control while taking this drug. Carbamazepine also affects the urine sugar levels of diabetic patients.

Symptoms of overdose that require immediate attention include

- severe clumsiness or unsteadiness
- severe dizziness or fainting
- fast or irregular heartbeat
- unusually high or low blood pressure
- irregular or shallow breathing
- severe nausea or vomiting
- trembling, twitching, and/or abnormal body movements

Patients should check with a physician immediately if any of the following side effects occur

- blurred or double vision, hallucinations
- confusion or agitation
- skin rash or hives
- speech problems
- changes in frequency or color of urine; painful urination, bloody urine

- depression or other mood/emotional changes
- unusual numbness, tingling, pain, bluish color or weakness in hands or feet
- ringing or buzzing in ears
- swelling of face, hands, feet, or lower legs
- trembling, uncontrolled body movements
- pale or black tarry stools, or blood in stools
- bone or joint pain
- nosebleeds or other unusual bleeding or bruising
- wheezing, chest pain or tightness, shortness of breath, hoarseness, or coughing
- sores, ulcers, or white spots on lips or mouth
- sore throat, chills, and/or fever
- swollen glands
- unusual fatigue or weakness
- jaundice

Side effects that typically go away and do not require medical attention unless they continue for several weeks or are bothersome include

- mild clumsiness or unsteadiness
- mild dizziness, drowsiness, or lightheadedness
- mild nausea or vomiting
- aching joints or muscles
- constipation or diarrhea
- dry or irritated mouth or tongue
- sensitivity to sunlight
- appetite loss
- hair loss
- muscle or abdominal cramps
- male sexual problems

caregiver   The primary person in charge of caring for an individual with severe multiple sclerosis (MS). A caregiver is most often a partner or spouse, but can also be a child, parent, or friend.

Caregiving can be physically and emotionally exhausting, especially for the person who is the primary caregiver, in part because MS is extremely changeable and unpredictable; one day a person with MS can dress alone, the next day the person cannot. Caregiving can involve anything from helping with injections to assistance with toileting, dressing, transferring, and feeding, as well as administering medical treatments. Although the person with disabilities may need a great deal of assistance, the needs and concerns of both partners must be addressed if the relationship is to remain healthy.

Most people with MS do not develop such severe disability that they require full-time long-term care; however, it is impossible to predict who will develop severe disability. This is why it is a good idea to investigate the kinds and costs of local long-term options before a crisis occurs. This should include an early start to long-term planning, which will help the caregiver and patient feel more secure. Life planning includes an investigation of income-tax issues, protecting existing assets, saving for future financial needs, end-of-life planning, insurance, employment rights, and state assistance. Caregivers and patients need to understand the coverage and policies of their medical insurance, including Medicare, Social Security benefits, and available private disability insurance. Some people may qualify for state assistance programs, such as welfare, food stamps, or Medicaid. Hospital or clinic social workers are good sources of information regarding these programs. It is also a good idea for caregivers and patients to understand the Americans with Disabilities Act (ADA) and other laws that provide protections related to housing, transportation, recreation, and employment.

A medical team should be involved to assess treatments, adaptations, and to provide training for caregivers in administering medical treatments, advice on coping with FATIGUE and occasional relapses, and some long-range financial planning. Home-care, nursing home or assisted living center are choices that may need to be made. All these decisions should be made in consultation with a therapist or counselor.

At-Home Care

People with severe levels of disability can live at home successfully by addressing practical problems, such as transferring from wheelchair to bed or bath using the proper kind of lift, ensuring a home has wide doorways and grab bars, and having options for adult day care.

Adapting homes for safety, accessibility, and comfort makes caring at home possible. An OCCUPATIONAL THERAPIST (OT) can suggest ways to keep the person with MS as independent as possible, ensure safety, and reduce the physical strain on the caregiver. OTs also know tips and techniques for bathing, dressing, toileting, and safe transfers. Ramps, widened doorways, and renovations in the kitchen and bath can often solve accessibility problems. Sometimes the best choice involves moving to more accessible housing that is near public transportation, stores, and other public facilities.

A Child as a Caregiver

Sometimes children assume major household and personal-care responsibilities when a parent has disability due to MS, especially in single-parent households. When children take on household responsibilities, their needs must be carefully balanced with the amount and level of caregiving they are expected to do.

Children are not equipped to handle the stress of being a primary caregiver, so they should never be responsible for a parent's medical treatments or daily functions, such as toileting. Children under 10 can certainly handle some household chores, and young teenagers can take on more responsibility, but they also need to spend some time with their peers. Older teenagers and young adults may be competent carers, but they should not be expected to undertake long-term primary care.

A Parent as a Caregiver

The return of an adult child to the home can be stressful for both the parents and the adult child. Providing care will become more difficult as parents age. In time, one or both parents may become ill and require care themselves. Alternative care plans and living arrangements should be discussed with the adult child well before such a crisis occurs.

Family, Friends, and Hired Help

Friends usually want to help and need to be affirmed in their offers. Having a list of things to do or some tasks that are time limited and specific are good ways to participate in the ongoing friendship. If paid care is possible and necessary, the person with MS should always be part of the interview process.

Safety and Security

One of the major concerns in caregiving is safety and security. Advance planning and adaptation of the home means that compromising situations can be avoided for the most part. Accessible peepholes, portable telephones with speed dial, automatic door openers, and "life-net" call systems that summon help in an emergency may provide security. A person with severe disability should not be left at home alone.

Managing Symptoms

Many MS symptoms can be controlled by medications, management techniques, and rehabilitative therapies. The health care team can advise caregivers about diet and routines that will support regular toileting and sleep habits.

For some people, the most frightening aspect of giving care to someone with a chronic disease is being responsible for medical and symptom-management treatments. This may involve keeping track of medications, administering injectable drugs, or performing intermittent urinary catheterization. Caregivers can and should make appointments with health care professionals to get information, advice, and training. With proper training and a little experience, most caregivers feel confident about this part of their role.

Caregivers should get training in necessary medical techniques from a health professional. Treatment plans can fail if the caregiver does not know the medical staff, does not understand why and how a procedure is done, or gets instructions that are impossible to carry out. If there are problems with carrying out a medical or treatment procedure, contact the health care team and arrange for a follow-up training session.

Stress and Burnout

Providing emotional support and physical care to someone with MS is often deeply satisfying, but it is sometimes distressing or simply overwhelming. The strain of balancing a job, raising a family, increased responsibilities in the home, and the care of the ill person may lead to feelings of martyrdom, anger, and guilt. One of the biggest mistakes caregivers make is thinking that they can handle everything alone.

The best way to avoid burnout is to have the practical and emotional support of other people, which can not only relieve stress but can give new perspectives on problems. Caregivers also need to take care of themselves and not neglect their own health. If sleep is regularly disrupted because the person with MS wakes in the night needing help with toileting or physical problems, the problems should be discussed with a health-care professional.

Successful caregivers should not give up enjoyable activities. Many organizations have respite-care programs; it may be possible to arrange respite care on a regular basis.

Caregivers need an outlet to discuss concerns and fears openly; the person receiving care is not the only one who needs emotional support. Anger, grief, and fear can lead to guilt and resentment. Caregivers can have a fear of dependency and isolation and may not ask others for help.

It is important that caregivers and patients have personal and social support networks, because working out an outlet for angry feelings is important to avoid physical or emotional abuse.

Abuse

Abuse is never acceptable. Caregivers may be too rough during dressing or grooming, or the person with MS might scratch a caregiver during a transfer. Once anger and frustration reach this level, abuse by either person may become frequent.

Emotional abuse seen in humiliation, harsh criticism, or manipulative behaviors can undermine the self-esteem of either partner. Help can be provided by family and social groups, therapists and counselors, or support groups. Although most caregivers never experience such levels of distress or become abusive, separation—temporary or permanent—or a nursing home are healthier options than a corrosive relationship.

Sex and Intimacy

Caregivers who are also spouses or partners usually face changes in their sexual relationship that can have physical or emotional causes. Caregivers feel that they are performing a parental role rather than being a lover or spouse, and this can interfere with sexual intimacy. MS also can interfere with both sex drive and function.

Open and honest communication about sexual needs and pleasures without fear of ridicule or embarrassment is the crucial first step. Counseling by a sex therapist can be helpful in this process. Support groups can play a role in providing an outlet for emotions and a source of practical information.

See also ASSISTIVE DEVICES; HOME ADAPTATIONS; SAFETY ISSUES; SEXUAL PROBLEMS; Appendix I.

Carswell, Robert (1793–1857) A mid-19th-century pathologist who took the first important step toward recognizing the pathology of multiple sclerosis (MS) when he found strange lesions in the spinal cord of a patient during an autopsy. Unaware of their cause, he meticulously recorded their appearance. His hand-painted illustration of the lesions appeared, together with descriptive text, in his *Atlas of Pathology* published in 1838. Within the text, Carswell described the pathology as "a peculiar diseased state of the chord and pons Varolii, accompanied with atrophy of the discolored portions."

Despite his major contribution in describing the pathology of MS lesions, Carswell did not record any clinical associations with his observations. Clinical symptoms were not linked to the internal symptoms that Carswell described until much later, when Jean-Marie CHARCOT made further discoveries into the symptoms of the disease.

catheter A hollow, flexible tube inserted into the urethra of a patient with multiple sclerosis (MS) who is unable to control BLADDER DYSFUNCTION with medication. Two types of catheters are typically used for this condition—intermittent and indwelling catheters, although an external catheter also can be used.

Intermittent Catheter

An intermittent catheter is used on an as-needed basis, inserted whenever patients have an urge to urinate—attached, used, and then removed. This type of catheter is usually preferred by patients and is safe and effective. It can typically be used at any time in any place by an individual who has been trained to insert it. The catheter is a plastic or rubber tube much like a long straw with a plastic bag attached to one end. Before insertion, the end of the tube is washed, lubricated with a water-based gel, and then carefully inserted, usually while the patient is sitting or squatting. Once inserted into the penis or urethral opening, it is gently pushed into the bladder. Some women find that using a small mirror can help make insertion easier. Once in place, the urine will flow down the tube and into the attached bag. Once the bladder is completely emptied, the catheter is removed, washed, and returned to its carrying case until the urge to urinate recurs (usually within four to six hours).

Learning how to use this type of catheter can take some time because of the psychological stress it may cause. Actual physical insertion of the catheter is not particularly difficult. During the first few weeks, patients should record the times a catheter is used, the amount of urine, and the amount and types of liquid consumed during the day. After a few weeks, patients will clearly be able to see their urinary pattern and establish a catheterization routine. Once a schedule has been set up, a catheterization should never be missed; this could lead to infection.

When using an intermittent catheter, patients should be careful to remove all of the urine, never retaining more than 16 ounces in their bladder at any time. Patients are also advised to use the catheter right before having sex to prevent accidents.

Indwelling Catheter

An indwelling catheter—also called a Foley catheter—is inserted into either a penis or urethral opening by a health care professional and left in place permanently. It is used when patients cannot insert an intermittent catheter. These devices resemble the intermittent catheter. However, the Foley also has an inflation device attached to the insertion end of the tube that can expand inside the bladder, where it is anchored until it is removed for cleaning or replacement.

An indwelling catheter is much more difficult to insert and should be placed the first time by a health care professional under sterile conditions. Once in place, the catheter should be cleaned near the insertion site with soap and water at least daily. The bag should be emptied before it fills up and then rinsed with a water and alcohol solution. This bag should always hang below the patient's groin so that gravity can help remove the urine.

Unlike patients with an intermittent catheter, patients with an indwelling catheter should drink as much as possible, especially acidic fruit juices such as cranberry or orange juice. Doing so can help prevent calcium salts from building up in the tube and can discourage the growth of bacteria.

External Catheter

A third type of catheter is fitted over the urethral opening instead of inside of it. This device is an alternative to an intermittent catheter for those who do not want to insert a device or who have infections or malformations of the urinary tract. The male or female patient would urinate into the catheter and then empty the attached bag.

Several styles and shapes are available. The most popular is the condom catheter that surrounds the penis in a sheath much like a condom, with the other end attached to a bag strapped to the leg. Women add a silicone device, held in place by a special bonding cement.

External catheters are available at pharmacies and medical supply houses.

Caucasians and MS   Although multiple sclerosis (MS) occurs in all racial groups, it is far more common among Caucasians—especially those from northern Europe and in those countries populated by Caucasians of northern European descent. On the other hand, MS is fairly uncommon among Caucasians in South Africa, the southern United States, and Australia—areas of southern latitude.

MS is uncommon among AFRICAN AMERICANS and ASIAN AMERICANS. Interestingly, although AMERICAN INDIANS, the Inuit, and Laplanders all live in northern latitudes, MS is also very uncommon in these groups. This suggests they are genetically protected from the disease.

causes of MS   Experts still do not know exactly what causes multiple sclerosis (MS), but they suspect that the condition is triggered by a combination of immunologic, genetic, and environmental factors.

Immune-Related Causes

It is now generally accepted that MS involves an autoimmune process—an abnormal immune response directed against the central nervous sys-tem. The exact antigen (target) that the immune cells are sensitized to attack remains unknown. In recent years, however, researchers have been able to identify which immune cells are mounting the attack, some of the factors that cause them to attack, and some of the sites (receptors), on the attacking cells that appear to be attracted to the MYELIN and begin the destructive process. The destruction of myelin—the fatty sheath that surrounds and insulates the nerve fibers—as well as damage to the nerve fibers themselves slows or halts nerve impulses, producing MS symptoms. Researchers are looking for highly specific immune-modulating therapies to stop this abnormal immune response without harming normal immune functions.

Environmental Causes

Migration patterns and epidemiological studies have shown that people who are born in a part of the world where people are at low risk for MS and then move to an area with a higher risk before the age of 15 acquire the risk of their new home. Such data suggest that exposure to some environmental agent that occurs before puberty may predispose a person to develop MS later in life.

Infections

Since all children are exposed to numerous viruses and bacteria and since viruses are known to cause demyelination and inflammation, some experts believe that a virus or other infectious agent may trigger MS. Although many infectious microorganisms have been investigated, no one agent has emerged as a proven trigger. However, there are a number of reasons for the persistent belief in a link between viruses and MS.

First, the disease has a distinct geographical distribution, which suggests the condition could have a contagious aspect. The number of MS cases increases the farther away a person travels from the equator in either direction. Second, MS clusters also occur in certain areas, such as the clusters that occurred between 1943 and 1989 in the FAEROE ISLANDS, which lie northwest of Scotland. During World War II, this region was occupied by British troops, and the incidence of MS rose each year for 20 years after the war. This lead some researchers to think that the troops might have brought with them some disease-causing agent.

The third reason to suspect a viral basis to MS is that some viruses are strikingly similar to the myelin protein and may therefore cause confusion in the immune system, causing the T cells to continue to attack their own protein rather than the viral antigen. More than one antigen may be involved. Some may trigger the disease, and others may keep the process going.

People with MS may be affected by different organisms and infections may cause some, but not all, cases of MS. Organisms at the top of the suspect list are those that can affect the central nervous system. More than a dozen viruses and bacteria, including measles, hepatitis B, and canine distemper, are being investigated to determine if they are involved in the development of MS. The top three suspects are HERPESVIRUS 6, *CHLAMYDIA PNEUMONIAE*, and EPSTEIN-BARR VIRUS. So far, however, no germ has been definitively linked to MS.

Genetic Causes

Although MS is not hereditary in a strict sense, having a parent or sibling with the condition increases an individual's risk of developing the disease. The average person in the United States has about a one in 750 chance of developing MS. Children or siblings of a person with MS, however, have two to five in 1,000 chance of developing the disease.

Some studies suggest that certain genes have a higher prevalence in populations with higher rates of MS. Common genetic factors have also been found in some families where more than one person has the condition.

Some researchers theorize that MS develops because a person is born with a genetic predisposition to react to some environmental agent that, upon exposure, triggers an autoimmune response. Sophisticated new techniques for identifying genes may help answer questions about the role of genes in the development of MS.

cecocentral scotoma   A horizontal oval defect in the field of vision that causes a blind spot, interfering with central vision. In people with multiple sclerosis, this eye problem is caused by the loss of the fatty nerve sheath (DEMYELINATION) that protects the OPTIC NERVE.

See also VISUAL PROBLEMS.

Centers for Independent Living   Community-based organizations that exist in every state, and that are supported by state funds through the Department of Human Services. They are not-for-profit, nonresidential organizations that serve people with disabilities, providing programs and services that promote independent living, although there is variability in the specific programs offered at individual centers.

central nervous system   The collective term for the BRAIN, OPTIC NERVE, and SPINAL CORD, which is the two-way highway for messages between the brain and the rest of the body. It is this body system that is affected by the lesions of multiple sclerosis.

The central nervous system (CNS) is responsible for integrating all nervous activities and works with the peripheral nervous system, which consists of all the nerves that carry signals between the CNS and the rest of the body. The CNS receives sensory information from all sensory organs in the body, analyzes this information, and triggers appropriate motor responses.

cerebellum   An apricot-sized structure located above and right behind the BRAIN STEM, responsible for controlling coordination and balance. The cerebellum controls movement by collecting information about limb position, balance information, and vision, and it synthesizes the information to control movement by triggering nerve transmissions. Some evidence indicates that mental activities are also coordinated in the cerebellum, which could explain why COGNITIVE DYSFUNCTION is sometimes associated with damage to the cerebellum. Damage to the cerebellum is very common in multiple sclerosis, and is permanent. The severity of symptoms is directly proportional to how much the cerebellum has been damaged.

Mild damage in this area might mean a patient cannot judge the range of limb movements without watching them. Damage in this area could also affect the speed and cadence of speech, tremors, and certain eye movement abnormalities, such as

NYSTAGMUS. Severe damage could mean a person would be unable to move the arms or legs smoothly and efficiently. The most common symptoms that indicate the cerebellum has been damaged include

- a lack of muscular strength (asthenia)
- uncoordinated muscular activity with tremors and a swaying, unsteady, and wide-based gait (ATAXIA)
- the inability to stop a motion at the intended point (DYSMETRIA)
- slowed movements on one side
- flabby muscles (hypotonia)

cerebral cortex   The wrinkly gray outer layer of the BRAIN in which thought processes take place. The gray covering that makes up the cerebral cortex actually consists of the cell bodies of nerve cells (NEURONS); underneath lies the WHITE MATTER formed from the AXONS of these neurons. The surface of the cortex is wrinkled because the brain has grown at a faster rate than the skull, and so the surface of the brain must fold to fit inside the skull.

The cerebral cortex is divided into right and left halves that are mirror images of each other. In most cases, structures that appear on the left side have a matching structure on the right. In general, sensory and movement information from the left side of the body is processed in the right hemisphere and vice versa.

The cortex is divided into large regions, called lobes, based on function and anatomical structure. These include the frontal lobes, the parietal lobes, the occipital lobes, and the temporal lobes.

cerebrospinal fluid (CSF)   A watery, colorless, clear liquid that circulates through the ventricles of the brain and through the cavity of the spinal cord, helping to cushion these important areas and establishing uniform pressure. The composition of this fluid can be altered by a variety of diseases. Certain changes in CSF that are characteristic of multiple sclerosis (MS) can be detected with a lumbar puncture (SPINAL TAP), a test sometimes used to help make the MS diagnosis.

cerebrum   The largest, most highly developed section of the BRAIN. This area is the site of most conscious and intellectual activities. It can be affected by any of the DEMYELINATING DISEASES, including multiple sclerosis.

The cerebrum is made up of billions of nerve cells and is divided into two hemispheres, each containing a central cavity (ventricle) filled with cerebrospinal fluid. These two hemispheres are called the right and left cerebral hemispheres. These halves are the part of the brain is responsible for higher-order thinking and decision making.

Long ago the cerebrum functioned as part of the olfactory lobes. Over time it has grown over the rest of the brain, forming a wrinkly top layer. Because of its sophistication and size, the human cerebrum is unusual in the animal kingdom.

The outer layer of the cerebrum is called the cortex. Indentations (called fissures) divided each central hemisphere into four lobes. Although scientists have gained a general understanding of the cerebrum's function, the details of its mechanism remain a mystery, its complexity undeciphered.

Chaddock's sign   A reflex test that is one indication of multiple sclerosis (MS). In this test, a NEUROLOGIST touches a patient's skin at the outside of the ankle. Normally no response would occur. A patient with MS or other types of brain damage would reveal an upward fanning of the big toe. This abnormal reflex is similar to Babinski's sign (an extension of the big toe and fanning of other toes when the sole of the foot is stroked), which is also common in people with MS. Chaddock's sign is a signal that lesions are in the corticospinal tract.

See also BABINSKI REFLEX.

Charcot, Jean-Marie (1825–1893)   French pathologist who in 1869 was the first person to describe multiple sclerosis (MS) scientifically. Born in Paris, he was a founder of the field of neurology. He worked at the Salpêtrière and taught Sigmund Freud. He is best known for his contributions to the knowledge of chronic and nervous diseases, and for making hypnotism a scientific study.

Charcot also was the first to make definite links between the mysterious symptoms and the pathological changes seen in postmortem samples from patients with MS. Almost 40 years after the discovery of MS lesions by Robert CARSWELL, Charcot described MS as *sclerose en plaques,* and recognized the condition as a distinct disease. Charcot also helped to develop diagnostic criteria, which included the now-famous Charcot's triad of DOUBLE VISION (diplopia), disturbances of balance or coordination (ATAXIA), and difficulties with, or slurred, speech (DYSARTHRIA) that he observed in his own housekeeper.

Charcot also gave the first complete histological account of MS lesions. He described many important features, including loss of myelin and proliferation of glial fibers and nuclei.

chemotherapy The use of potent cell-killing drugs that are prescribed for some forms of cancer and that may also be used to treat multiple sclerosis (MS). These drugs kill both tumor cells and also normal cells, which is why most chemotherapy drugs cause a range of side effects. Cells that are most vulnerable to chemotherapy drugs are those that grow and divide rapidly, including cancer cells, hair and intestinal cells, red blood cells, and white blood cells.

Many experts believe that MS is an autoimmune disease and that it is caused by the abnormal action of certain white blood cells that attack the fatty covering (MYELIN) of nerves. Destruction of myelin slows or halts nerve impulses, producing the symptoms of MS. Since chemotherapeutic drugs diminish the numbers of white blood cells, using them should theoretically slow down or halt this autoimmune destruction.

MITOXANTRONE (Novantrone) was approved in 2000 for reducing neurologic disability and/or the frequency of clinical relapses in patients with secondary progressive, progressive-relapsing, or worsening relapsing-remitting MS. In addition to being the first drug approved in the United States for SECONDARY PROGRESSIVE MS, it offered new treatment options for others experiencing worsening of the disease.

Many other chemotherapeutic drugs have been used to treat MS, but the results of many studies have not conclusively shown them to be of definite value. Their use in treating MS remains controversial.

Azathioprine (Imuran)

This drug as a treatment for MS remains controversial. A drug that suppresses the immune system, azathioprine is commonly used to treat autoimmune diseases such as rheumatoid arthritis and as part of chemotherapy for some cancers. Over the past 20 years AZATHIOPRINE has been and continues to be widely studied both in the United States and abroad to see if it is useful as a treatment for MS. The results have been mixed. Some patients experienced slowed progression or fewer relapses (in 60 percent of the trials); no apparent benefit occurred in the other trials.

However, some patients have not been able to take azathioprine because of severe nausea. Other potential side effects of azathioprine include severe anemia or or leukopenia (shortage of white blood cells), liver damage, and a long-term increased risk of developing cancers such as leukemia or lymphoma.

The decision to use azathioprine is a complicated one. It should be made by the physician and the patient together after discussing the potential risks and benefits.

Cladribine (Leustatin)

Recent studies of CLADRIBINE have shown no benefit in MS. Side effects have included infections and bone marrow suppression with reduced platelet counts.

Cyclophosphamide (Cytoxan)

This potent immunosuppressive drug is usually given to treat cancer, but it has also been used to treat MS for many years in uncontrolled studies where it was often (but not always) reported to improve the condition of people with primary or secondary progressive MS. More recent studies have shown that at best CYCLOPHOSPHAMIDE provides only a modest benefit.

A study in people with rapidly progressive disease was under way as of 2004, but the drug is currently used only in selected situations. Its use should be discussed with a neurologist and decisions reached on an individual basis. Side effects of short-term treatment with high doses are hair loss, nausea, occasional bladder injury, and risk of infection. Long-term side effects include sterility, mutations, and the increased risk of cancer.

Cyclosporin A

This drug first received attention when it was shown to reduce rejection rates significantly in organ transplantation. Unlike most immune-suppressing drugs, it appears to have a specific action primarily against one type of white blood cell (helper T cells). Since some evidence suggests that these cells are abnormally active during acute exacerbations of MS and since it has been shown to be effective in treating other autoimmune diseases in humans and the animal model of MS, CYCLOSPORIN A (cyclosporine) was tried in a study with patients with progressive MS. The study enrolled almost 600 men and women and followed them for two years. Those who received cyclosporine had a slightly slower worsening of the disease. However, no significant differences were noted in patients' abilities to perform ACTIVITIES OF DAILY LIVING, and no change in brain scans or spinal fluid test results occurred. On the other hand, serious side effects are associated with cyclosporin A use, namely kidney damage and high blood pressure.

A German study compared cyclosporin A to azathioprine, but no significant differences between the two groups were apparent at the end of the study. However, cyclosporin A caused twice as many side effects as azathioprine. Therefore, experts believe that the risks of cyclosporine outweigh the benefits for treatment of MS and do not justify its use under most circumstances. It is rarely used today.

Methotrexate

METHOTREXATE is a synthetic immunosuppressive drug that is highly effective in the short term against rheumatoid arthritis, an autoimmune disease. It also effectively prevents the animal model for MS.

Although a clinical trial of methotrexate in the 1970s did not show any benefit to people with MS, a recent study showed the drug had modest benefit. In this trial, the drug slowed the deterioration of arm function but did not affect the worsening of leg function or overall disability.

child death and MS Parents who have a child who dies have up to a 50 percent higher risk of developing multiple sclerosis (MS), according to a Danish study published in the March 9, 2004 issue of *Neurology*. These results show that psychological stress may play a role in the development of MS. Researchers have long believed that stress plays a role in the onset of MS, but this is the first study to follow a large group of people before they developed MS.

Scientists have suspected that if stress causes MS, only severe stresses are likely candidates, because MS is not that common. The death of a child is one of the most serious stressors that occurs in a society with low infant mortality, so it was used as an objective indicator for severe stress.

The study found that the risk of developing MS was even greater for parents whose child died unexpectedly—they were more than twice as likely to develop MS as were parents who did not lose a child. This provides more evidence that stress plays a role in the disease, because losing a child unexpectedly is considered to be even more stressful for parents, experts noted.

Results could help researchers determine what processes in the body are affected by stress that could lead to MS.

Researchers, working in Denmark over a 16-year period, identified parents of children under 18 who died. They also identified 15 times as many parents who did not lose a child, randomly selected from the general population and with the same number of children in the family and of the same ages as the families who lost a child. The study involved 21,062 parents who lost a child and 293,745 parents who did not lose a child. People who had MS or suspected MS at the start of the study were not included. Parents were followed for an average of 9.5 years. Over that time, 28 of the parents who had not lost a child developed MS; 230 of the parents who had lost a child developed MS.

The risk of developing MS was the same regardless of the age or sex of the child who died. The risk was also the same regardless of the age or sex of the parent, which is of particular significance, as the risk in the general population is usually twice as high in women.

childhood (pediatric) MS Although multiple sclerosis (MS) was once thought to strike only adults, MAGNETIC RESONANCE IMAGING has made it possible to diagnose MS earlier and more accurately than ever before. Experts now acknowledge that, while still rare, MS can occur in children of all ages. (A diagnosis before the age of 10 is rare, although there have been reports of infants as young as 18 months diagnosed with MS.) Experts estimate that onset before 18 years of age has been reported to occur in between 3–5 percent of cases; as many as 20,000 U.S. children may have the disease yet remain undiagnosed.

New medical evidence suggests that the number of pediatric patients is rising, probably because more doctors are considering the diagnosis when they see a child suffering from telltale symptoms such as a sudden loss of vision.

Most studies of early-onset MS have reported a higher girl-to-boy ratio than is typically seen in adults with MS. Although the woman-to-man ratio in adults is approximately two to one, some studies of children with MS have reported ratios that are closer to three to one. In one study of 125 subjects, the overrepresentation of girls was even greater in certain subgroups.

Girls are also more likely to exhibit initial symptoms that are purely sensory (such as NUMBNESS or tingling), complete recovery from the initial episode, a nonprogressive type of MS, and less disability. Boys were more likely not to recover from the initial episode and were more likely to have progressive disease.

In a 1997 study of 149 children with MS, boys slightly outnumbered girls before age 12. After age 12, the number of girls steadily increased until the age of 15, when the ratio became four to one. The ratio for girls to boys between the ages of 12 and 15 was found to be three to one, echoing other studies. No evidence was found in this study to confirm prior reports of male sex and older age at onset being unfavorable prognostic indicators.

MS occurs when the body's immune cells mistakenly attack the thick sheath (myelin) covering the nerve fibers of the brain and spinal cord. When the myelin is destroyed, the underlying nerve can be damaged, triggering a range of symptoms such as tremors or slurred speech. However, no one knows what pattern of disease will occur in children.

A very small correlation occurs between parents with MS and their children who subsequently develop MS. The vast majority of individuals with MS have neither a parent nor a child affected with the disorder. Studies to date do suggest that genetic factors may make certain individuals more susceptible to the disease than others, but environmental factors may also be important.

Symptoms and Diagnostic Path
As with adults, most children are diagnosed with RELAPSING-REMITTING MS. Although most children with MS have mild cases, a small group of children have aggressive symptoms. Instead of one or two attacks a year, these children must deal with five or more. No one knows whether these children will go on to suffer from progressively worsening disease as they get older.

Children with MS generally experience the same types of symptoms as adults, including possible cognitive dysfunction that may affect school performance. Researchers worry that repeated attacks can leave a child with memory and learning problems. One study found that about 30 percent of the children tested had trouble with cognitive skills, such as remembering information for a test. Children with MS have not yet completed developing important intellectual and social skills or crystallizing their personalities; they are still in the process of acquiring new knowledge in every area of their lives. If MS interferes with this learning process by some combination of physical, social, or psychological changes caused by the disease, these children may have trouble acquiring the knowledge and skills needed in adult life.

The symptoms of MS can affect every aspect of a child's daily life, which can have important consequences for the development of self-confidence and self-esteem.

The lack of knowledge about pediatric MS means many children may not get a diagnosis right away. Only a few neurologists at urban centers in the United States and Canada specialize in pediatric MS.

Treatment Options and Outlook
When a childhood diagnosis is made, doctors, parents, and children are faced with a number of

unanswered questions. Researchers do not know whether the drugs used to treat adults will work for children nor do they know how quickly the disease will progress. The drugs that have fueled a revolution among adults with MS have not been tested in children. However, the drugs currently available to treat MS, including the beta interferons and GLATIRAMER ACETATE, have all been used in children with no obvious negative effects and essentially the same benefits as seen in adults.

The outcome for children diagnosed with MS seems to vary as much as it does for adults. Some children do quite well, with a significant period of time passing between relapses; others seem to have a more rapidly progressive course. Because MS does not significantly shorten a person's life expectancy, children with MS and their families will be living with the consequences of the illness for decades.

See also FAMILY SUPPORT NETWORK; INTERFERON.

chiropractic A type of treatment that involves manipulation of the spinal column, based on the theory that the state of a person's health is determined by the condition of the muscles, skeleton, and nervous system. Chiropractic therapy does not use drugs or surgery. The name "chiropractic" comes from the Greek *cheiro* meaning "hand" and *prakto* meaning "to use." The basic assumption of chiropractic is that misaligned vertebrae apply pressure to nearby nerves, which can cause pain or dysfunction in the organs or muscles served by those nerves. The goal of chiropractic therapy is to restore normal function to joints and their supporting structure—especially the vertebral column and pelvis.

Chiropractic was developed in the 19th century by Daniel David Palmer as a way of restoring hearing for one patient. Palmer believed that a displaced vertebra was applying extra pressure on a nerve in the man's ear, causing hearing loss.

After a complete examination that often includes X-rays, the chiropractic practitioner applies precise adjustments to the vertebral column in order to bring structures back into alignment and eliminate the nerve irritation, restoring normal function.

Although there is little to no incontrovertible evidence that chiropractic therapy works, according to the National Multiple Sclerosis Society, there is ample anecdotal testimony that such therapy is indeed effective. According to an editorial in a 1998 issue of *The New England Journal of Medicine,* treatment may be most effective in the case of lower back pain.

Nothing that a chiropractor can offer will affect the course of multiple sclerosis (MS) or the level of disability. On the other hand, if the individual with MS has lower back pain or certain other aches that may or may not be related to MS, a chiropractor may be able to ease some symptoms.

Chlamydia pneumoniae An atypical bacterium that has been associated with persistent inflammation in small vessels. A few studies have reported significantly higher rates of previous *Chlamydia pneumoniae* infection in patients with multiple sclerosis (MS). However, an analysis of many studies has reported no connection at all between *C. pneumoniae* and MS, and many experts now believe there is no strong evidence linking the germ to MS. It is still possible, however, that an infection—which can cause widespread inflammation—may play a role early in the course of the disease in some individuals.

chronic pain Any PAIN that persists for longer than one month. In multiple sclerosis, chronic pain may occur and persist independent of disease duration or disability. Chronic pain includes dysesthetic extremity pain, back pain, and painful leg spasms.

chronic-progressive multiple sclerosis A former catchall term for progressive forms of multiple sclerosis (MS), now categorized as two separate forms of disease: PRIMARY PROGRESSIVE and PROGRESSIVE-RELAPSING. The clinical course of MS usually falls within one of the following categories: primary progressive, progressive-relapsing, RELAPSING-REMITTING, and SECONDARY PROGRESSIVE.

ciliary neurotrophic factor (CNTF) A substance that promotes the survival of the MYELIN-producing cell called an OLIGODENDROCYTE. Some experts believe it may be this cell, and not the myelin sheath itself, that is the target of the agent causing multiple sclerosis (MS).

CNTF, a substance that normally occurs in a healthy nervous system, also helps oligodendrocytes survive. How CNTF does this is not known, although scientists do know that CNTF helps the cell resist the toxic activities of tumor necrosis factor. High concentrations of this factor are also found in areas of demyelination. However, scientists do not yet know whether CNTF will be helpful in patients with MS.

cladribine (Leustatin) An immune-modifying medication that has shown no benefit in multiple sclerosis. Side effects have included infections and bone marrow suppression with reduced platelet counts. However, cladribine's manufacturers planned to begin new tests by the end of 2004.

classifications of multiple sclerosis See TYPES OF MS.

climate Many people with multiple sclerosis (MS) experience a temporary worsening of their symptoms when the weather is very hot or humid. A few notice problems, such as increased SPASTICITY, in very cold climates. In general, experts recommend that people with MS who are sensitive to temperature try to avoid extremes of either hot or cold.

When they get overheated, some people with MS notice, for example, that their vision becomes blurred (a phenomenon known as UHTHOFF'S SIGN). These temporary changes can result from even a very slight elevation in core body temperature (less than half a degree) because a higher temperature further impairs the ability of exposed nerves, which are characteristic of MS, to conduct electrical impulses.

Typically, heat only temporarily worsens symptoms and does not cause actual damage to the tissue. Symptoms are usually quickly reversed when the source of the higher temperature is removed. People with MS who are planning to move to a very warm climate should therefore visit the area first to check if the hot weather seriously worsens their MS symptoms.

Of course the adverse effects of heat may be eased if the person with MS remains in air-conditioned surroundings as much as possible during periods of extreme heat. If an air conditioner is needed to help minimize the symptoms of MS, the cost of this equipment may be tax deductible as long as there is a prescription from a physician.

Some people with MS also notice a worsening of spasticity in cold weather.

clinically isolated syndrome (CIS) A single symptom typical of multiple sclerosis (MS), such as an attack of optic neuritis in one eye or an episode of NUMBNESS on one side, unaccompanied by any other symptom that indicates a loss of nerve fiber insulation (DEMYELINATION). Individuals who experience a clinically isolated syndrome may or may not go on to develop MS.

Studies have shown that when the CIS is accompanied by brain lesions that are consistent with those seen in MS, there is a high risk of a second episode within several years. Individuals who experience CIS with no evidence of lesions are at relatively low risk of developing MS over the same time period.

An MS diagnosis requires evidence of inflammation and demyelination that have occurred in different parts of the central nervous system. In addition, there must be no other explanation for these lesions. A clinically definite diagnosis of MS is made when the inflammation and demyelination is demonstrated by two separate attacks. In the event of a CIS, the physician must wait for the second attack to occur in order to make a diagnosis of clinically definite MS; this may take anywhere from months to years. A laboratory-supported diagnosis is made when other diagnostic tools (such as MAGNETIC RESONANCE IMAGING [MRI], a SPINAL TAP, and visual EVOKED POTENTIALS) are used to provide evidence of the second demyelinating attack even though the person may not have experienced any additional symptoms.

By using these tests, the physician can confirm a laboratory-supported diagnosis of MS without having to wait for a second clinical event or attack to occur.

In a 2003 study scientists found that individuals who had antibodies against two major proteins in myelin tended to experience a second clinical event significantly earlier than people without those antibodies. These findings could improve the quality of diagnostic information used to guide treatment decisions for MS in the future. However, the lab test used to detect the antibodies is not yet commercially available.

Studies suggest that INTERFERON beta-1a significantly delays the onset of clinically definite MS, as indicated by a delay in a second attack. In addition, MRI findings showed that the patient receiving interferon beta-1a had a significantly smaller increase in the volume of brain lesions as well as fewer new lesions.

clinical trial   A formal test of a medical procedure or medication, conducted by scientists. In the United States there are three major steps in the life cycle of a drug before it is ever approved: preclinical research, clinical studies, and Food and Drug Administration (FDA) review. Once scientists believe they have an idea for a new drug that they think will be effective and safe to use, they put this idea to the test with five or more years of preclinical research. This is the phase in which new compounds are discovered and initially tested, both in the laboratory and in the first phases of animal testing. Animal testing is a required phase before the FDA will give a compound consideration as a new drug.

Any new drug that is proposed for the treatment of multiple sclerosis (MS) in the United States must be approved by the FDA. Once significant research has been accumulated and proposals have been written, what is called an Investigational New Drug application, or IND, is filed with the FDA. The IND lets the government know what compound is being tested, describes what early results have shown, and asks permission to proceed to the second phase of the drug life cycle. This process typically takes several months.

If the application is approved, the company embarks on seven years of clinical studies in humans. The clinical trial phase is the longest and most expensive part of the process. To make it worth the time and money invested, it is absolutely critical that the trials are carefully planned, because the results of the trial will determine what claims a drug can make.

Before trials begin, researchers are required to identify what results, or outcomes, they intend to measure. The goals of different trials and whether or not these are achieved determine what indication, or particular use, the drug will be allowed to claim if it becomes approved by the FDA.

However, being indicated for something does not mean that the drug is useful for only this one thing. The indication is merely the use for which the drug received formal scrutiny. For example, if the researchers set out to prove that a particular drug can safely and effectively reduce the number of relapses in MS and that is the sole intention of the study, the FDA grants permission for the drug to be indicated for the reduction of relapses, assuming the trials show positive results. Sometimes, however, researchers discovered that the drug also prevents fatigue, a common problem in patients with MS. When this occurs, doctors are allowed to prescribe this medication for fatigue in MS patients, but the drug company cannot actively promote it as a fatigue-stopping drug or tell doctors this is an antifatigue medication—unless they do more clinical studies to test whether the drug is safe and effective for stopping fatigue. If possible, they may submit another IND using the same data to apply for a second indication. Either way could take years.

The FDA must carefully review each drug in a standardized set of trials before they allow it to be marketed for any purpose other than the one they have already approved. For people waiting for a treatment, this seems like an excruciatingly long process. The goal is not to deny treatment to the people who need it—rather, it is meant to ensure that the outcome is indeed the result of the treatment and not a matter of chance.

Phase 1: Safety

The first phase of a clinical trial typically lasts about five years and costs about $10 million. Often referred to as the safety study, this research involves testing compounds in the lab and in animals to find the maximum safe dose. Safety studies are also conducted in smaller groups of people. Because several side effects may still be unknown at this early stage, precautionary exams such as blood pressure, weight measurement, urinalysis, health questionnaires, or blood tests are usually done on a regular basis.

Phase 2: Endpoints

In the second phase of a clinical trial, researchers determine how the final and most important phase should be designed and what endpoints will be established. This helps ensure that the final and most expensive phase will be as efficient and as valuable as possible, which is one reason why this second phase takes a few years to complete. The cost for this phase is typically about $20 million.

Phase 3: Proving It Works

By the time a drug has made it to the third phase, researchers have a better idea of how promising the treatment looks. The ultimate goal of this phase is to prove a drug works. This is typically when researchers also try to establish the ideal dosage and dosage schedule and determine which patients will be most likely to benefit.

With the endpoints defined in the previous phase and the groups of patients most likely to benefit from this drug already defined, the final three to four years of testing can begin.

Double-Blind Studies

In order to find out if a drug is actually working, it is usually tested at the same time as a placebo (or dummy pill). Usually this is called a double-blind trial, where neither the researchers nor the patients know which patients are taking what. If the researcher knows but the patient does not, this is called single blinded. If both the patient and the researcher know whether they are taking an active drug or a placebo, this is called an "open-label study." Although a double-blind trial is the gold standard in clinical trials, sometimes running a double-blind trial is next to impossible.

Because the medications used to treat MS are so different and easy to spot (some are injected differently, others cause unique side effects), most of the head-to-head trials comparing the three main MS therapies are open label. This means that both the researchers and the patients are aware of which therapy they are taking.

Just because a drug has been on the market for a while does not automatically mean that it has been clinically proven to work long term. A drug's ability to continue to do its job over a number of years is arguably one of the most important outcomes researchers can set out to prove. In MS, there are occasionally reports of a loss of effectiveness after a period of time with some medications.

Clinical Trial Participation

Many people with MS want to participate in clinical trials for new or experimental forms of therapy. Clinical trials must be carefully controlled to make sure that the results are valid and not due to factors other then the drug or therapy being tested. This means that clinical trials must have strict criteria for participation. Not everyone who wants to participate in a particular study may be eligible to do so.

Most well-controlled clinical trials involve two groups: one that receives the experimental treatment and another that receives either a placebo (inactive substance) or a previously-approved treatment. People in these studies should realize that there is a 50/50 chance that they will not receive the treatment under study.

Other trial designs involve a "crossover" of treatment, generally meaning that the type of treatment given to each group is switched during the course of the trial. In these types of trials, all groups eventually receive the active treatment under study. The actual design and circumstances of the trial are explained by the investigators before being asked to give consent to participate.

General eligibility guidelines Requirements that must often be met for participation in a clinical trial include the following:

- The person should reside close to the research facility (usually within a radius of 150 miles).
- The person must have a specific type of MS. Often trials specify which clinical type of MS is under study (relapsing-remitting, secondary progressive, primary progressive, or progressive-relapsing).
- The person must fall within the study guidelines relating to age, sex, level of disability, and duration of disease.
- Previous or current treatment with certain drugs (such as drugs that suppress the immune system) may exclude a person from a study.

Potential risks and benefits   Persons who are eligible and who choose to enter clinical trials should be fully aware of the potential risks and benefits of the study. All aspects of a clinical trial should be discussed with the person's neurologist, so that a well-informed decision may be made. Physicians may also be able to help persons locate appropriate clinical research programs.

Before participating in a clinical trial, people must sign consent forms stating they know the purpose of the trial and how it will be conducted. People are also free to leave a clinical trial at any time, for any reason.

Placebo   The "placebo response" occurs when a person who is ill perceives an improvement or actually experiences an improvement in symptoms or overall health from the psychological effect of receiving treatment rather than from the treatment itself. Many factors influence the generation of a placebo response. Some scientists believe that certain psychological factors actually cause the body to produce hormones called endorphins, which act as the body's own painkillers, resulting in reduced levels of pain or discomfort. The placebo response may be due to a person's profound desire to get better, increased medical attention as result of being in an experimental study of a new treatment, or even an unconscious wish by the person to please the physician by getting better.

Some improvements triggered by the placebo effect can be measured objectively, but studies have demonstrated that placebo effects are rarely as strong as the effects of a medically valuable treatment. Moreover, placebo effects diminish over time, even if the individual continues with the treatment that elicited them. The widespread existence of the placebo response reinforces the need to build adequate controls for this response into the design of clinical trials of any new treatment or therapy, so that the actual therapeutic response to a treatment being tested can be separated from responses resulting from the placebo effect. In some trials, up to 70 percent of patients with MS have demonstrated a placebo response. Therefore, in order to be considered as an effective treatment, a drug must be demonstrated to have produced statistically significant benefit in the persons who received it, over and above the benefit experienced by a similar group of persons who received a placebo.

clinical signs and symptoms   Problems that may appear as the result of a disease. A *sign* in multiple sclerosis (MS) is an objective physical problem or abnormality identified by a physician during a NEUROLOGICAL EXAMINATION. Neurologic signs may differ significantly from the symptoms reported by the person because they are identifiable only with specific tests and may cause no obvious symptoms. Common neurologic signs in MS include altered eye movements and other changes in the appearance or function of the visual system, altered reflexes, WEAKNESS, SPASTICITY, and circumscribed sensory changes.

A *clinical symptom* is a subjectively perceived problem or complaint reported by the person. In MS, common symptoms include visual problems, FATIGUE, sensory changes, weakness or paralysis, tremor, lack of coordination, poor balance, bladder or bowel changes, and psychological changes.

The clinical symptoms and deficits are quite varied among persons with MS, and they typically change and worsen as the disease evolves. The most frequent include

- *Fatigue*   This has been reported in up to 90 percent of cases

- *Motor involvement*   This may occur quite early in the disease course of MS, especially in those who have multiple symptoms. Symptoms can include weakness in an affected limb, progressing to spasticity, hyper-reflexia, clonus, extensor plantar responses, and muscle contractures.

- *Visual involvement*   OPTIC NEURITIS is a common problem, especially double vision, blurring or haziness, and visual loss.

- *Sensory symptoms*   Vague and poorly characterized sensory symptoms may include tight and burning sensations, or numbness and paresthesias. Such symptoms are often transient, but some can progress and remain a problem.

- *Tonic spasms*   These are brief increases in muscle tone in one or more limbs, often associated with pain.

- *Brain stem symptoms*   Most common symptoms include ophthalmoplegia and NYSTAGMUS. Vertigo occurs as an initial symptom in about 5 percent of people but becomes more common as disease progresses. Facial numbness, weakness, and pain are less common but do occur (especially TRIGEMINAL NEURALGIA).

- *Cerebellar involvement* This may involve disabling intention tremor, ATAXIA, or DYSARTHRIA.
- *Genitourinary symptoms* At any time during the course of MS, urinary urgency, frequency, incontinence, hesitancy and retention, and urinary tract infections may occur. Bowel dysfunction (especially constipation) is also common.
- *Cognitive deficits* To some degree, these appear in about 40 to 60 percent of patients, especially short-term memory dysfunction, difficulty managing complex tasks, and confusion.
- *Depression* The second most common symptom in MS, which is not linked to how severe the disease may be. The incidence of suicide in people with MS is 7.5 times higher than in the general population.

clonazepam (Klonopin) A benzodiazepine that belongs to a group of medications called central nervous system (CNS) depressants. Although clonazepam is used for many different medical conditions, it is used in multiple sclerosis (MS) primarily for the treatment of tremor, PAIN, and SPASTICITY.

Side Effects
Side effects that may go away during treatment, and do not require medical attention unless they continue for several weeks or are bothersome, include:

- drowsiness or fatigue
- clumsiness or unsteadiness
- dizziness or lightheadedness
- slurred speech
- abdominal cramps or pain
- blurred vision or visual changes
- changes in sexual drive or performance
- gastrointestinal changes, including constipation or diarrhea
- dry mouth
- fast or pounding heartbeat

- muscle spasm
- urinary problems
- trembling

Since distinguishing between certain common symptoms of MS and some side effects of clonazepam may be difficult, patients should consult their doctor if an abrupt, serious symptom develops. Unusual side effects that should be discussed as soon as possible with a physician include:

- behavior problems, including difficulty concentrating and angry outbursts
- confusion or mental depression
- convulsions
- hallucinations
- low blood pressure
- muscle weakness
- skin rash or itching
- sore throat
- fever or chills
- bleeding or bruising
- excitement or irritability

Symptoms of overdose that require immediate emergency help include:

- continuing confusion
- severe drowsiness
- shakiness
- slow heartbeat or reflexes
- shortness of breath
- continuing slurred speech
- staggering
- unusual severe weakness

Clonazepam adds to the effects of alcohol and other CNS depressants (such as antihistamines, sedatives, muscle relaxants, tranquilizers, and prescription medications to treat pain, seizures, or sleeping problems). Taking an overdose of this medication or taking it with alcohol or other CNS depressants can be fatal. Because stopping this medication suddenly may cause withdrawal side effects, the dosage should be gradually reduced before stopping.

clonus   A sign of SPASTICITY, characterized by involuntary shaking or jerking of the leg, that occurs when the toe is placed on the floor with the knee slightly bent. The shaking is caused by repeated, rhythmic, reflex muscle contractions.

clusters of MS   An unusually large group of cases of multiple sclerosis (MS) that occurs over a specific time period and/or in a certain area. Such clusters of MS are of interest because they may provide clues to environmental or genetic factors that might trigger the disease. To date, cluster studies have not produced clear evidence for the existence of any triggering factor in MS.

Although MS is known to occur in people with a genetically determined predisposition for the disease, a great deal of evidence suggests that most people who are genetically susceptible must still be exposed to some other factor in order for MS to develop. These triggering factors might include infectious agents, environmental and industrial toxins, diet, trace metal exposures, and certain climatic elements such as varying amounts of sunlight. None has been proven to be causally linked to MS, and exactly what factors may be involved remains unknown. More than one factor may be capable of triggering MS in susceptible individuals.

Many problems arise when investigating clusters of MS. First, determining what constitutes a cluster is difficult. To do this, one needs to calculate the number of new cases of MS that would be expected to occur in a given area over a given period of time, based on the total population at risk in the area. The expected incidence can then be compared with the reported incidence. Since MS is not considered to be infectious and is therefore not a reportable disease according to the standards of the U.S. Centers for Disease Control (CDC) and because no nationwide MS registry exists, documented incidence rates may not exist for an area where a cluster has been reported. The problem then becomes one of finding a suitable comparison population where the incidence of MS is known. This figure can help to determine the expected incidence of MS in the area where the cluster has been reported.

MS rates also are known to vary by latitude. Additionally, MS occurs more often in women than men and more often in individuals of northern European ancestry than in others. Therefore, the expected incidence in an area must take into consideration not only the geographical location of that area but also the age, sex distribution, and ethnic makeup. In addition, MS is more common in families in which the disease already exists—an indication of the genetic susceptibility for the disease. Therefore, issues such as family relations within a reported cluster must also be taken into consideration.

A true cluster of MS means that there is a significantly higher incidence of definite MS in an area than expected. Surprising as it might seem, what may appear to be an extraordinary number of MS cases in one neighborhood or county may actually be no more than might be expected within that area.

Some of the other problems that make MS clusters hard to investigate include an uncertainty of the diagnosis of MS and a significant lag time between symptom onset and diagnosis.

One of the earliest and most famous groups of clusters known to MS investigators are a series of alleged epidemics that occurred on the Faeroe Islands, a Danish possession lying in the North Atlantic between Norway and Iceland. Although the inhabitants are Nordic and are considered a high-risk group for the disease, there were no known reports of MS prior to 1943 among native-born residents. That year, suddenly about 25 cases of MS in the Faeroes were diagnosed. The disease had apparently been brought into the Faeroes since it had not been reported there before.

The cases were linked to the British occupation during World War II shortly before 1943. When researchers later grouped the cases of MS with clinical onset from 1943–73 by puberty status at the time of the British occupation, they found three distinct peaks of MS incidence, corresponding to the three alleged epidemics. The first consisted of 18 cases, all of whom were past puberty at the time of the occupation. The second alleged epidemic consisted of nine cases who were not yet teens during the occupation but who reached age 11 between 1941 and 1951, with onset of MS from

1948–60. The third alleged epidemic included five cases who had reached age 11 between 1949 and 1963, with onset of MS from 1965–73.

Many of the occupation soldiers were from the Scottish Highlands, where the MS prevalence is quite high (90 cases per 100,000, comparable to rates in the northern United States).

Experts believe that if MS is somehow triggered by a virus, the disease may have been brought to the Faeroes by the occupying forces. Unfortunately, no factor has yet been identified that can definitively account for the alleged epidemics.

MS clusters may sometimes crop up in occupational settings as well. An industry-based MS cluster was reported in DePue, Illinois, in the late 1990s after residents of this small town (population 1,800) had been exposed to trace metals in water and soil from a zinc smelter plant that closed in the early 1980s. In conjunction with the Illinois Department of Public Health, the investigators confirmed the diagnoses of nine people with MS, all of whom had developed symptoms between 1971–90. Based on expected incidence rates, the investigators determined that the nine cases far exceeded the number expected to occur over a two-decade time period in a town of this size. The authors concluded that exposure to zinc or other trace metals could have been a factor in the occurrence of this MS cluster, although they had no direct evidence that zinc or any other metal is in fact related to MS.

Zinc was also identified as a possible exposure factor in an earlier report among employees at a manufacturing plant in Rochester, New York. When investigators checked workers' records, they found that 11 had developed MS during a 10-year period between 1970 and 1979, when two to four cases would have been expected. Even though the investigators concluded that this was a significant excess of MS cases, they could find no differences in exposure to zinc between the workers who had developed MS and those who had not. However, genetic susceptibility to MS was not taken into account in the investigation.

How to Report a Cluster

The major resource for individuals with concerns or questions about an MS cluster in their commu-

nity is the local public health department, whose job is to investigate suspected clusters. The health department also may refer such cases to the federal CDC Agency for Toxic Substances and Disease Registry. For contact information, see Appendix I.

cognitive abilities High-level functions carried out by the human brain, including comprehension and use of speech, visual perception and construction, calculation ability, attention (information processing), MEMORY, and executive functions, such as planning, problem solving, and self-monitoring. Multiple sclerosis can interfere with some cognitive abilities.

See also COGNITIVE DYSFUNCTION.

cognitive dysfunction Impairments in thought function caused by the disease process of multiple sclerosis (MS). MS has the potential to affect these brain functions, either directly or indirectly. Cognitive dysfunction is not correlated with duration or level of physical impairment but may be linked to the number of lesions as identified on MAGNETIC RESONANCE IMAGING (MRI) scans. Between 50 and 60 percent of all patients with MS will develop some degree of slowed ability to think, reason, concentrate, or remember, but only 5–10 percent develop problems that are severe enough to interfere in a significant way with everyday activities. Although cognitive dysfunction occurs more commonly among people who have had the disease for a long time, it can be seen early in the disease, even presenting as the first symptom.

Several reasons may cause MS to affect a person's ability to think clearly. First, MS damages both myelin and the nerve cells within the brain, which interferes with a variety of neural functions. In fact, magnetic resonance imaging studies have indicated that the extent of demyelination in the brain is directly related to the severity of cognitive dysfunction.

However, MS is also associated with DEPRESSION, ANXIETY, STRESS, and FATIGUE, all of which may slow down cognitive function. Just as the physical symptoms of MS can vary considerably from person to person, cognitive changes can vary in the same way. Moreover, it is common for certain functions to be largely intact while others are more severely affected.

Symptoms and Diagnostic Path

Impaired working memory is the most common cognitive problem experienced by patients with MS. Other cognitive functions frequently affected in MS include the speed of information processing, planning, and prioritizing, impairment in visual perception and constructional abilities, word-finding ability, abstract reasoning and problem solving, and attention and concentration. Sustained attention and the ability to divide attention between separate tasks are especially affected.

The first signs of cognitive dysfunction may be subtle. The patient may have trouble finding the right words or remembering what to do on the job or during daily routines at home. Decisions that once were easy now become more difficult. The patient may demonstrate poor judgment. Often the person's family becomes aware of the problem first, noticing changes in behavior or personal habits.

People with MS should seek medical help if they are concerned about cognitive dysfunction. Even early in the disease, disordered thinking can have an impact on daily life. In fact research has shown that cognitive symptoms and fatigue are the two primary reasons for leaving the workforce. Since cognitive function can also be affected by aging or medications, a careful evaluation is necessary to determine the cause of these mental changes.

A professional evaluation may be a good idea if the patient (or the patient's family or friends) notices a change for the worse in cognitive functions. An evaluation is a good idea if any of these changes interfere with work, school, or social life or if they distress the patient. People who are affected by cognitive problems are not always the ones who think they have a problem; some patients who think they have cognitive problems are in fact simply depressed. Others who are severely impaired are unaware that any changes have taken place.

Other causes for intellectual problems should be carefully ruled out and preliminary, less expensive testing considered before a formal neuropsychological evaluation is scheduled. This type of formal testing may require several hours, is expensive, and may not be covered by insurance.

Assessing intellectual function should be done by a qualified neuropsychologist, a specialist in the behavioral changes caused by brain disease or trauma—preferably a person who has had experience with people who have MS. A psychologist without this training may have difficulty selecting the proper tests and interpreting the results. A psychiatrist or neurologist can perform briefer evaluations, but these usually identify only the more severe forms of cognitive dysfunction. (In one University of Vermont study, almost half the patients whom neurologists considered to be without intellectual problems were found to have problems when tested by a neuropsychologist.) OCCUPATIONAL THERAPISTS and SPEECH-LANGUAGE PATHOLOGISTS also can perform cognitive assessments.

Treatment Options and Outlook

Cognitive rehabilitation is often recommended to patients with cognitive dysfunction, administered by a neuropsychologist, a speech pathologist, or an occupational therapist. This type of treatment involves a variety of strategies ranging from computer-mediated memory exercises to training people in using aids such as notebooks. Thus far, studies suggest that the greatest promise seems to be with straightforward compensatory techniques, such as organization strategies, notebooks, computers, and filing systems, to compensate for memory deficits and other changes.

Common memory aids include writing things down in notebooks, posting notes on the refrigerator, or carrying a pocket calendar. Time management methods may include special filing systems, checklists for complex tasks, reading comprehension strategies, and special-purpose diaries. Although compensatory strategies do not address the underlying problem of cognitive dysfunction, they offer an alternative way to perform a task that has become difficult.

Ordinarily, cognitive rehab involves one or more one-hour sessions a week over several weeks or months. In many instances, the cognitive rehab program may include meetings with family members to help them understand the nature of specific problems and how they can help. Stress management, counseling, or psychotherapy may round out the treatment plan if these seem to be warranted.

A comprehensive program of cognitive rehabilitation is likely to use a mixture of retraining and compensatory strategies. For example, supervised programs of graded practice can improve attention and concentration levels. This sets the stage for more effective use of compensatory strategies in everyday situations.

At present, not many medications can boost memory. A drug called Aricept (DONEPEZIL) is approved for the treatment of memory problems in patients with Alzheimer's disease, and MS experts have hoped it might help MS patients as well. A recent clinical trial of 69 patients with MS found that Aricept improved performance on memory tasks, but larger clinical trials are needed to confirm these findings.

A few studies have looked at the effects of three other MS disease-modifying agents (Avonex, Betaseron, and Copaxone) on cognitive function. One large clinical trial with Avonex showed modest benefits for a variety of cognitive functions, while two others using Betaseron had mixed results. A large clinical trial of Copaxone reported no benefits for cognitive function.

However, disease-modifying agents reduce the number and severity of MS attacks, reduce signs of damage to brain tissue, and delay the progression of disability, they may all also have beneficial effects on cognitive function. However, no studies are in progress of these disease-modifying agents specifically regarding cognitive function in MS.

cognitive rehabilitation   Techniques designed to improve the function of individuals with multiple sclerosis whose ability to think (cognition) is impaired disease. Rehabilitation strategies are designed to improve the impaired function via repetitive drills or practice or to compensate for impaired functions that are not likely to improve.

Psychologists, neuropsychologists, speech/language pathologists, and occupational therapists all can provide cognitive rehabilitation. Although these three types of specialists use different assessment tools and treatment strategies, they share the common goal of improving the individual's ability to function as independently and safely as possible in the home and work environment.

Cohen, Richard (1948–)   Journalist and former TV producer first diagnosed with multiple sclerosis (MS) in 1973, when he was 25. His book

Blindsided: Lifting a Life Above Illness: A Reluctant Memoir describes his battle with MS along with two bouts of colon cancer and blindness. Cohen's father, a physician, also had MS.

The first sign of MS occurred when he dropped a coffee pot while working on a PBS documentary about disability. He married actress Meredith Viera in 1986, and they now have three children.

Cohen, whose book was a *New York Times* bestseller, is unsparing about the difficulties that come from living with chronic illness. Yet he said he never considered suicide and has never been clinically depressed. Cohen is now working on a book proposal to examine how other people deal with chronic illness.

cold feet   The sensation of having very cold feet is related to NUMBNESS in patients with multiple sclerosis. This uncomfortable sensation is most likely related to the changes that the disease causes in the diameter of blood vessels. The disease creates the sensation of coldness in the feet because of nerve damage, but the feet are not really physically cold.

community resources   Many resources are available to help health professionals and the patient with multiple sclerosis (MS) obtain the most current information about MS and community resources. For more information, see Appendix I.

complementary and alternative medicines (CAMs)   Types of treatments beyond traditional medicine, including everything from exercise and diet to food supplements, stress management strategies, and lifestyle changes. These therapies come from many different disciplines and traditions—yoga, hypnosis, guided imagery, relaxation techniques, traditional herbal healing, Chinese medicine, macrobiotics, naturopathy, and many others. They are referred to as *complementary* when they are used in conjunction with conventional medical interventions, and *alternative* when they are used instead of conventional treatments.

As a result, there is little published documentation to substantiate claims made about most CAMs, and what is available may not be reliable. Even when conventional medical practices have never undergone clinical trials, health professionals are aware of clinical experience and health risks and communicate this information to people using that particular treatment. Most people, however, have little or no idea of the risks they are taking when they use a complementary or alternative therapy. Despite this lack of scientific rationale, CAMs appeal to a growing number of Americans. Recent studies indicate that about 75 percent of people with multiple sclerosis (MS) use some form of CAM. Alternative medicine is now a 15-billion-dollar-a-year industry.

Food supplements and other forms of CAMs are not regulated in the United States in the same way as prescription medications. Therefore, there is no way to know that the products being sold are safe or effective, or, in the case of supplements, that they are even accurately labeled. In fact, some alternative therapies are painful and produce serious side effects. In recent years, a number of food supplements proved so harmful that they had to be taken off the market. People who are considering using an alternative therapy should ask the following questions:

- What does the treatment involve?
- How and why is it supposed to work?
- How effective is it?
- What are the risks?
- How much does it cost?

The answers to these questions can help a person considering an alternative therapy to weigh the risks against the benefits. As well as seeking answers to these questions the person using CAMs should keep the physician informed and maintain conventional therapy. Some examples of CAMs used in MS include ACUPUNCTURE; herbal medicines; echinacea; vitamins A, C, and D; evening primrose oil (LINOLEIC ACID); ginkgo biloba; ginseng; grape seed; homeotherapy; St. John's wort; selenium; and valerian.

comprehensive care centers Centers established by neurologists to address the whole spectrum of concerns facing people with diseases such as multiple sclerosis (MS) and their families. These concerns include disease management, symptom management, emotional and psychological issues, rehabilitation therapy and exercise, employment issues, education, counseling and instruction on self-help, home care issues and needs, and placement in a long-term care facility.

Neurologists, internists, psychiatrists, physiatrists, urologists, gynecologists, psychologists, speech/language pathologists, social workers, physical therapists, and occupational therapists are also available to address the many problems related to MS.

Consortium of MS Centers An organization of comprehensive multiple sclerosis (MS) centers whose goal is to be the preeminent organization of MS health care providers improving the lives of those affected by this disease.

constipation A condition in which the stool is too hard and difficult to pass. Constipation occurs when the stool moves so slowly through the intestines that too much water is absorbed from the stool by the body. Constipation can prevent any of the stool from being eliminated, or it can result in a partial bowel movement, with part of the waste retained in the bowel or rectum.

Constipation in MS patients may be caused by poor dietary habits or lack of exercise. Common MS symptoms, such as difficulty in walking and chronic fatigue, can lead to slow movement of waste material through the colon. Weakened abdominal muscles can also make the actual process of having a bowel movement more difficult. DEPRESSION can also disrupt the digestive system.

In addition, MS can trigger the loss of myelin in the brain or spinal cord, which may prevent or interfere with the signals from the bowel to the brain indicating the need for a bowel movement. Individuals with MS often have problems with spasticity. If the pelvic floor muscles are spastic and unable to relax, normal bowel functioning will be compromised. Some people with MS do not experience the usual increase in colon activity after eating that propels waste toward the rectum. Finally, some individuals with MS try to solve common bladder problems by drinking less—but restricting fluids only makes constipation worse.

Symptoms and Diagnostic Path

Normal bowel functioning can range from three bowel movements a day to three a week. Despite the widely recommended one movement a day, physicians agree that such frequency is not necessary. The medical definition of infrequent bowel movements is less often than once every three days. Most physicians agree that a movement less often than once a week is not adequate, and one movement every two or three days is a preferable minimum.

Constipation is the most common bowel complaint of individuals who have multiple sclerosis (MS). Many MS symptoms, such as BLADDER DYS-FUNCTION, SPASTICITY, WEAKNESS, immobility, and DEMYELINATION, interfere with communication between the bowel and the brain and can lead to bowel complications.

Patients with bladder problems due to MS should get medical help for these problems first so that adequate fluid intake, which is critical to bowel functions, will be possible and constipation will be less of an issue.

Besides the obvious discomfort of constipation, complications can develop. Stool that builds up in the rectum can put pressure on parts of the urinary system, increasing bladder problems. A stretched rectum can send messages to the spinal cord that further interrupt bladder function. Constipation also aggravates spasticity, making walking more difficult. Constipation can also be the underlying cause of INCONTINENCE, the most distressing bowel symptom.

Severe constipation may lead to impaction, in which a hard mass of stool is lodged in the rectum and cannot be eliminated. This problem requires immediate medical attention. Impaction can usually be diagnosed through a simple rectal examination, but symptoms may be confusing because impaction may cause diarrhea, bowel incontinence, or rectal bleeding. Impaction leads to incontinence when the stool mass presses on the internal sphincter, triggering a relaxation response. The external sphincter, although under voluntary control, is often weakened in patients with MS and may not be able to remain closed. Watery stool behind the impaction thus leaks out uncontrollably.

Treatment Options and Outlook

A number of remedies can improve constipation.

- Stool softeners such as Colace, Surfak, and Chronulac Syrup can be used. Experts do not advise using mineral oil, because it can reduce the absorption of fat-soluble vitamins.

- Bulk supplements, such as natural fiber supplements Metamucil, Perdiem Fiber, FiberCon, Citrucel, or Fiberall, taken daily with one or two glasses of water, are an option. They help fill and moisturize the gastrointestinal tract. They are generally safe to take for long periods.

- Mild oral laxatives such as Milk of Magnesia, Epsom salts, and sorbitol, all of which promote secretion of water into the colon, are reasonably safe. Other mild laxatives include Doxidan and Perdiem. These provide a chemical irritant to the bowel that stimulates the passage of stool. Peri-Colace includes a stool softener. The gentler laxatives usually induce bowel movements within eight to 12 hours. Many over-the-counter laxatives have harsh ingredients, and some are habit forming. Ask your doctor for recommendations even though no prescription is required.

- If oral laxatives fail, a glycerin suppository inserted half an hour before trying a bowel movement may help. This practice may be necessary for several weeks in order to establish a regular bowel routine. For some people, suppositories are needed permanently. Dulcolax suppositories stimulate a strong, wavelike movement of rectal muscles, but they are much more habit forming than glycerin suppositories. Therevac mini enemas are not traditional enemas but rather lubricating stimulants. These agents must be carefully placed against the rectal wall to be effective. If inserted into the stool, no action will occur.

- Enemas should be used sparingly because the body may come to depend on them. They may be recommended as part of a therapy that includes stool softeners, bulk supplements, and mild oral laxatives.

• Manual stimulation may promote elimination by gently massaging the abdomen in a clockwise direction or by inserting a finger into the rectum and rotating it gently. A plastic finger covering or plastic glove should be worn. These techniques may need to be used for several weeks before how well they are working becomes clear. The digestive rhythm is modified only gradually.

See also BOWEL DYSFUNCTION.

contagiousness of MS   Currently no evidence suggests that multiple sclerosis (MS) is infectious or contagious. The role of a virus or VIRUSES, if there is one, affects only people with a genetic predisposition to develop MS.

continuum of care retirement communities Sometimes also called life care communities, this type of facility combines all three levels of care—INDEPENDENT PROVIDERS, ASSISTED LIVING, and nursing home care—in a single setting. These communities provide residents with the independence of retirement home living and the security of long-term care.

Traditionally such communities required a sizeable entry fee, plus monthly maintenance fees, in exchange for a living unit, meals, and eventual health care coverage up to the nursing home level. More recently such communities also have begun to make their services available on a rental basis rather than requiring residents to "buy" a room or cottage using a traditional life care endowment.

contraception and MS   The course of multiple sclerosis (MS) is not affected by birth control pills or intrauterine devices. Women with MS have used the birth control pill, intrauterine devices, and sterilization without complications.

contracture   A permanent shortening of the muscles and tendons next to a joint that can be caused by severe, untreated SPASTICITY in multiple sclerosis and interferes with normal movement around the affected joint. If left untreated, the affected joint can become frozen in a bent position.

cooling strategies   In multiple sclerosis (MS), an increase in body temperature can cause an increase in symptoms such as FATIGUE, spasms, slurred speech, or WEAKNESS. Nerve conductivity slows down when an individual's body temperature rises.

People with MS who are heat sensitive should avoid sunbathing and hot baths or showers and use fans, air conditioners, cool water, icy drinks, and cool showers. They also should keep out of the sun in the middle of the day.

Commercially available cooling garments, including special vests, hats, wristbands, and jackets, can reduce the risk of worsening symptoms on hot days and make outdoor activities more enjoyable. An OCCUPATIONAL THERAPIST, PHYSICAL THERAPIST, or MS nurse can advise on ways to keep cool while exercising.

Copaxone   See DISEASE-MODIFYING AGENTS.

corpus callosum   A bundle of white matter four inches long that contains 300 million myelinated nerve fibers. It is the main bridge between the left and right hemispheres of the brain and carries messages between them. Damage to this area can be the cause of many typical multiple sclerosis symptoms.

corticosteroids   Hormones normally produced in the human body by the adrenal glands that have a number of effects on different organ systems. They are most widely used as an anti-inflammatory medication in the central nervous system and may help suppress the immune system's attack on MYELIN (the protective sheath that insulates nerve fibers) and even improve electrical conduction. Corticosteroids were the first agents successfully used to treat multiple sclerosis (MS) and remain one of the standard treatments for controlling acute attacks. However, their long-term effects on the course of the illness is not known.

Although corticosteroids are very useful for improving acute symptoms in the patient with RELAPSING-REMITTING MS, they do not improve the long-term course of the disease and can lose effectiveness if overused. Physicians generally restrict the use of steroids to severe attacks, when the patient's ability to function is severely limited. There is no consensus, however, on the best form, dose, route, or duration of steroid treatment.

Some corticosteroids (such as prednisone) are usually given by mouth. Others, such as methyl-prednisolone (Solu-Medrol) and dexamethasone (Decadron), are usually given intravenously. A few studies have suggested that short-term treatment with very high doses of intravenous (IV) methyl-prednisolone works more rapidly than adrenocor-ticotropic hormone to reduce symptoms of an acute attack of MS. MS specialists now believe that a three-to-five-day course of high-dose intra-venous steroids is the best treatment for an acute MS attack, providing maximum benefit with the fewest side effects. This treatment may require hospitalization, although it is possible to have IV treatment on an outpatient basis. Depending on the physician's preference, the patient's condition, and the length of the treatment, the IV steroids may be followed by a one- to two-week tapering dose of oral steroids.

No evidence suggests that continuous steroid administration slows progression of MS or improves symptoms over a long period of time. In addition, the long-term use of steroids is associated with sig-nificant potential side effects. However, several stud-ies have found that monthly one-day pulses of intravenous methylprednisolone may help treat patients with SECONDARY PROGRESSIVE MS.

High-dose methylprednisolone given intra-venously is typically administered for major relapses, and oral prednisone is given for mild-to-moderate relapses. A 2001 study on patients with relapsing-remitting MS indicated that methylpred-nisolone might slow brain changes.

Optic Neuritis

Recent studies suggest that a short course of IV methylprednisolone followed by a tapered course of oral steroids may help reverse inflammation and restore vision for patients with OPTIC NEURITIS, an inflammation of the OPTIC NERVE that is often asso-ciated with MS. However, no definitive evidence indicates that IV methylprednisolone produces a more complete recovery than that which would

have occurred without treatment. In fact oral pred-nisone used alone may actually exacerbate optic neuritis, so this drug is now rarely prescribed dur-ing flare-ups.

Side Effects

Side effects of steroids on the central nervous sys-tem can be particularly problematic for patients since they may worsen existing symptoms of MS. These side effects include sleeplessness, MEMORY loss, anxiety, and DEPRESSION. Other possible side effects include stomach irritation, high blood sugar, water retention, restlessness, insomnia, and mood swings. However, most patients tolerate the treat-ment well. Even with short courses of IV steroids, the physician may need to prescribe medications to help the patient sleep and to ease stomach upset.

Oral steroids that have been taken over a period of time should never be stopped abruptly since they can suppress the body's own steroid produc-tion by the adrenal gland. Gradually tapering the dose before discontinuing the medication allows the body time to normalize production. Since a very short course of IV steroids has no effect on the adrenal gland, an oral steroid taper is not usually required.

The side effects of long-term continuous steroid use are serious, including stomach ulcers, weight gain, acne, cataracts, osteoporosis, deterioration of the thigh bone, and chemical diabetes.

cortisol   A steroid hormone naturally occurring in the body that plays a role in fat and water metabolism. Cortisol also affects muscle tone and the excitation of nerve tissue, increases gastric secretion, alters connective tissue response to injury, and impedes cartilage production.

cortisone   A glucocorticoid steroid hormone, produced by the adrenal glands or synthetically, that has anti-inflammatory and immune system-suppressing properties. Prednisone and pred-nisolone also belong to this group. Cortisone is recommended to some patients with multiple scle-rosis to reduce acute inflammations in the central nervous system. However, cortisone treatments carry significant risks and should not be used for long-term treatment.

cranial nerves   There are 12 cranial nerves, any of which may be affected by multiple sclerosis:

1. olfactory nerve (smell)
2. OPTIC NERVE (sight)
3. oculomotor nerve (eyelid/eye muscles)
4. trochlear nerve (eyeball rotation)
5. trigeminal nerve (face and chewing)
6. abducent nerve (eyeball movement)
7. facial nerve (facial expression)
8. vestibulocochlear nerve (hearing and balance)
9. glossopharyngeal nerve (swallowing and taste)
10. vagus nerve (larynx; automatic control of heart, lungs, and gastrointestinal tract; and other autonomic body functions)
11. accessory nerve (shoulders)
12. hypoglossal nerve (tongue)

Credé maneuver   A physical exercise used by many patients with multiple sclerosis to force excess urine out of a distended bladder. While sitting on the toilet, the patient places both hands on the abdomen. As the stomach is relaxed, the patient begins to urinate and simultaneously presses the hands inward and downward. Pressure is continued until fluid is released. Most urologists no longer recommend this procedure.

crutches   Forearm crutches, also called Canadian or Lofstrand crutches, are recommended for people with multiple sclerosis whose balance and strength are severely affected and who have too little strength in their arms to use CANES. This type of crutch provides more stability than canes or standard crutches.

Cruveilhier, Jean (1791–1874)   An eminent mid-19th-century Parisian anatomist who described the pathology of the lesions seen in multiple sclerosis (MS) in much the same way as did Robert CARSWELL. Although the two men worked independently, their illustrations were created at approximately the same time, and there is much debate as to which illustration came first. However, although Carswell's illustrations were published in 1838, Cruveilhier's version was not published until 1842.

Cruveilhier's contribution to the understanding of MS goes beyond his description of its pathology, however, since he was the first to record the clinical history of a patient later found to have neuronal lesions. For example, his notes recall that one patient, "Had been ill six years without cause . . . she noticed that the left leg resisted her will to such a degree that she fell in the street." Cruveilhier described how over several years, the woman developed weakness of both legs and arms, spasms, difficulty in swallowing, and visual disturbances. From this he diagnosed "a lesion of the upper portion of the spinal cord."

CT scan (computerized axial tomography scan)   A diagnostic scan (also called a CAT scan) of the brain made by taking cross-sectional pictures with an X-ray. Although CT pictures of the brain have been useful in determining several types of brain diseases, its usefulness as a diagnostic aid for multiple sclerosis (MS) is limited. The CT scan has largely been replaced by MAGNETIC RESONANCE IMAGING.

The CT scan has limited usefulness because the brain changes typically involved in MS often involve very little tissue—smaller than the smallest volume of tissue that is well visualized by CT scans. Even large areas of DEMYELINATION—destroyed tissue surrounding nerve fibers—may be hard to see with a CT scan because the density of this plaque is virtually the same as surrounding tissue. Moreover, other areas of damage (from tumors, stroke, and infections) look very much like demyelinated plaques.

Cummings, Bruce Fredrick (1889–1919)   An extremely bright zoologist of the early 20th century with a great passion for life who developed multiple sclerosis (MS) and fought a constant battle against his progressive disability. Under the pseudonym W. N. P. Barbellion, Cummings gave a moving personal account of his suffering in his book *The Journal of a Disappointed Man,* published in 1919. The book remains one of the best-known personal testimonies of an MS patient, with entries that detail the gradual incapacitation triggered by the disease.

Cummings eloquently highlights the cruelty of MS and his grief at being relentlessly robbed of his physical abilities, writing on July 5, 1917 in his book, "I am not offering up my life willingly—it is being taken from me piece by piece, while I watch the pilfering with lamentable eyes."

cushingoid features   Long-term use of steroids in the treatment of multiple sclerosis is not recommended because it may cause cushingoid features (round face, obesity around the abdomen) and a rare condition of ASEPTIC NECROSIS OF THE HIP. Steroid overuse also may cause pain, difficulty walking, and heightened risk of osteoporosis.

cyclophosphamide (Cytoxan, Neosar)   A potent immune-modifying medication that can be used to suppress multiple sclerosis (MS), although it is usually given to treat cancer. Cytoxan has been used to treat MS for many years in uncontrolled studies, where it was often (but not always) reported to improve the condition of people with primary or secondary progressive MS.

In spring 2004, doctors at Drexel University reported promising results using huge doses of cyclophosphamide, though researchers believe more patients and time are needed before any victory is declared. The drug was given to MS patients at such high doses that most or all of the person's disease-fighting immune cells were destroyed. The patients' stem cells within their bone marrow survived the drug's onslaught, the doctors say, and were stimulated with drugs to rebuild the immune system from scratch—but without the negative triggers that caused the body to attack its own cells in the first place. Once the immune cells were destroyed, new cells were created that did not recognize the initial stimulus that had triggered them. The immune system was restored but was now able to tolerate whatever trigger caused the autoimmune response in the first place. In this study, several patients with MS-related cognitive problems and coordination troubles experienced an almost-complete disappearance of symptoms in as little as three to six weeks. For example, one patient had the high-dose treatment after other therapies failed and now no longer needs a cane or walker and can walk unassisted.

Just six MS patients completed the chemotherapy, which was administered over three to five days. All had advanced MS and had tried at least three other treatments, including steroids and immune-suppressing drugs, with no benefit. As of yet, scientists do not know how long the benefit will last or whether it leaves patients vulnerable to infections and other problems.

Autoimmune diseases are typically suppressed with interferon, steroids, radiation, and other drugs that stop the production of the cells that treat the body's own cells like they are foreign invaders. The new drug differs by killing the immune cells, not merely suppressing their growth. Patient follow-up and more research is necessary, but the initial results were called "striking and unexpected" by other doctors.

Other studies have shown that, at best, this drug produces only a modest benefit. The drug is currently used only in selected situations. Its use should be discussed with a NEUROLOGIST and decisions should be reached on an individual basis.

Side Effects

Short-term treatment at high doses may cause hair loss, nausea, occasional bladder injury, risk of infection, and temporary MS flares. Long-term side effects include sterility, mutations, and the increased risk of cancer.

cyclosporin A   A drug once used to treat multiple sclerosis (MS) but rarely given today because the risks of this drug outweigh the benefits. Cyclosporin A (also known as cyclosporine) first received attention for significantly reducing rejection rates in organ transplantation.

Unlike most immune-suppressing drugs, it appears to target one type of white blood cell (the helper T cells). Since some evidence suggests that these cells are abnormally active during acute MS attacks and since this drug has been shown to be effective in treating other autoimmune diseases in humans, cyclosporin A was tried in a double-blind, placebo-controlled trial in patients with progressive MS. Unfortunately the side effects were found to be too severe and the benefits too small.

Side Effects

Serious side effects are associated with cyclosporin A, including kidney damage and high blood pressure. Studies suggest that the drug causes twice as many side effects as AZATHIOPRINE.

cytokines   Substances that help to regulate the immune system—a type of signaling chemicals that are messenger molecules of the immune system that can provide both beneficial as well as harmful effects. They may play a role in multiple sclerosis (MS) by mediating MYELIN damage and regulating autoimmune response.

Cytokines are secreted by various white blood cells to regulate all important biological processes, including cell growth, immunity, inflammation, and tissue repair. Interleukins and INTERFERONS are both types of cytokines that are made by immune system cells (such as macrophages and T cells).

MS causes cytokine changes, and experts have found that beta interferon can help some patients. On the other hand, gamma interferon makes some patients with MS worse. This suggests that altering the cytokine level may influence the course of the disease.

Cytoxan   See CYCLOPHOSPHAMIDE.

daclizumab (Zenapax) A genetically engineered human antibody that blocks the interleukin-2 receptor on immune cells. Daclizumab received approval in 1997 for use in kidney transplantation, and it is now being studied as a combination drug for use in patients with multiple sclerosis (MS).

In one study of 11 patients in 2004, when daclizumab was added to INTERFERON (a naturally occurring antiviral protein commonly used to treat MS), the combination therapy produced a 78 percent reduction in new brain lesions and a 70 percent reduction in total lesions, along with other significant clinical improvements. The decrease in new lesions, as well as the total decrease in lesions, occurred gradually over a two-month span. Improvement was also seen as measured by a neurological rating scale and a test-of-hand function. The clinical improvement was unexpected in such a small trial, since a larger number of patients is usually required to show clinical effects.

The study of patients with either RELAPSING-REMITTING MS or SECONDARY PROGRESSIVE MS was led by investigators at the National Institute of Neurological Disorders and Stroke. Findings appeared in the *Proceedings of the National Academy of Sciences*, May 24–28, 2004.

dantrolene (Dantrium) A muscle relaxant used to ease cramping, spasms, and tight muscles caused by certain medical problems such as multiple sclerosis (MS).

Side Effects

Dantrolene has been shown to cause cancer and noncancerous tumors in animals that were given high doses over a long period of time.

Temporary side effects that do not require medical attention, unless they persist or are bothersome, include

- dizziness
- drowsiness or unusual fatigue
- weakness
- nausea, abdominal cramps, diarrhea, or constipation
- blurred or double vision
- chills and fever
- frequent urination
- headache
- loss of appetite
- speech difficulties
- sleep difficulties
- nervousness

Side effects that patients should report as soon as possible include

- seizures
- pain or tenderness
- changes in skin color
- swelling
- shortness of breath
- dark urine or urinary problems
- chest pain
- confusion
- severe constipation
- skin rash or itching
- jaundice (yellow color in the eyes or skin)

Dantrolene will greatly add to the effects of alcohol and other central nervous system depressants. Therefore, patients should not use these when taking dantrolene.

Dawson's fingers   The term used to describe DEMYELINATION occurring along the venous pathways that is commonly seen in patients with multiple sclerosis.

death   The course of multiple sclerosis (MS) varies from person to person; some people have the disease for only the last five years of life, while others may have it for as many as 20 years or more. Most people with MS do not die from the disease. However, very rarely, there is a rapidly progressive course leading to death.

MS itself is almost never the cause of death; death results from complications or infections, or from suicide. Generally speaking the life expectancy of those with MS is at least 95 percent of a healthy person's life.

decubitus ulcer   See BEDSORE.

deep brain stimulation (DBS)   A way to inactivate the thalamus in the brain without destroying this area in order to control tremors typically occurring in patients with multiple sclerosis (MS). DBS is a safer variation of an old surgical treatment method once used to treat these tremors which involved destroying a small area in the thalamus. This surgery was risky, since destruction of the brain could cause severe complications such as paralysis, loss of vision, or loss of speech.

The risks are much lower with DBS. In this method, doctors place an electrode tip in the thalamus, which is connected by a wire to a pacemaker-like device, implanted under the skin of the chest, that generates electrical shocks. The strength of the electrical stimulation is adjusted with four metal contacts that can be used in many different combinations. As the patient's condition changes, the stimulation can be adjusted without requiring a second operation. The stimulator also can be turned off if necessary.

DBS can neither cure MS nor prevent it from getting worse. It is designed to help patients with MS who have significant arm tremors. Although tremor of the head and body may be helped, the decision to have surgery should be based on the goal of decreasing arm tremor. Other MS symptoms, such as VISUAL PROBLEMS, NUMBNESS, or WEAKNESS, are not helped by deep brain stimulation.

DBS has been approved to treat Parkinson's disease and essential tremor. Although it has not been specifically approved to treat MS, this does not mean the treatment is experimental or that it would not be covered by insurance. Many examples of treatments are used every day and are standard and accepted but have not been approved for every application.

Patients should consider surgery only if medication was unable to control the tremor. Ideally, the surgery should be done by experts familiar with this method. Different centers may perform the surgeries in different ways, but the chances of benefit and the risk of complication are directly related to how close the electrode is to the correct target.

deep tendon reflexes   Involuntary jerks normally produced at certain spots on an arm or leg when the tendons are tapped with a doctor's hammer. Reflexes are tested as part of a standard NEUROLOGICAL EXAM in the diagnosis of multiple sclerosis.

dementia   A general term for a group of serious symptoms caused by changes in BRAIN function, that leads to a loss in at least two areas of intellectual function such as language, memory, visual and spatial abilities, reasoning, and judgment. The problems must be severe enough to interfere with a person's daily functioning. Dementia is not a disease itself but describes symptoms that may accompany certain diseases or conditions. Dementia is generally irreversible when caused by disease or injury but may be treatable when caused by drugs, alcohol, hormone or vitamin imbalances, or depression.

Dementia affects many areas of intellectual function and may include changes in personality, mood, and behavior. However, in the beginning a patient may experience problems in only one area, such as:

- repeatedly asking the same questions
- getting lost in familiar places
- being unable to follow directions
- getting disoriented
- neglecting personal safety, hygiene, and nutrition

A person with dementia should be under the care of a neurologist, psychiatrist, family doctor, internist, or geriatrician. The doctor can treat the patient's physical and behavioral problems and can answer the many questions that the person or the person's family may have.

See also COGNITIVE DYSFUNCTION.

demyelinating diseases   A number of conditions involve the damage or destruction of the MYELIN sheath (the fatty insulation covering the nerve fibers) so that nerves cannot conduct electrical impulses.

Multiple sclerosis is the most common demyelinating disease that affects only the myelin of the central nervous system. Some other causes of central nervous system demyelination include viral infections, side effects from overexposure to toxic materials, severe vitamin B_{12} deficiency, autoimmune conditions that lead to inflammation of blood vessels (the collagen-vascular diseases), and some rare hereditary disorders.

Demyelination also can occur in the peripheral nervous system (made up of the nerves outside the brain and spinal cord). Demyelination of the peripheral nervous system can be found in diseases such as GUILLAIN-BARRÉ SYNDROME. However, after some injuries, the myelin sheath in the peripheral nervous system can repair itself.

Some demyelinating conditions are self-limiting, while others may be progressive. Careful examinations may be needed to establish an exact diagnosis among the possible causes of neurologic symptoms.

demyelination   A loss of MYELIN, the fatty sheath surrounding and insulating nerve fibers in the white matter of the central nervous system. Demyelination interferes with nerve function and is the hallmark of multiple sclerosis (MS). It is characterized by the formation of lesions in the brain and spinal cord that cause a variety of intermittent symptoms.

REMYELINATION may not take place or only partially occur. If remyelination does not occur, the nerve will continue to function in an abnormal way, but the axon will remain undamaged. Sometimes after a long period of time, an axon will spontaneously remyelinate and regain function.

The body is capable of remyelination, but the process is slow. Myelin repair is an active area of research at this time. Scars form in areas where myelin has been damaged or lost (which is how multiple sclerosis got its name). Scar tissue can block the formation of new myelin; once axons have gotten scarred, they can never fully regain their former function. Sometimes the underlying axon can wither and entirely lose function; once an axon has withered, it can never repair itself.

Denny-Brown, Derek (1901–1981)   A Harvard University neurology professor who showed that when a damaged nerve was stimulated, it failed to pass the impulse to the connected muscle. He concluded that the DEMYELINATION associated with lesions on the nerve was responsible for the block in conduction. Demyelination was therefore shown to prevent or slow the conduction of impulses through a nerve.

By extrapolating from these observations made in peripheral nerves, experts then understood that the demyelination seen in MS lesions caused the impaired central nerve conduction within the brain and spinal cord, which in turn led to neurological symptoms such as gait problems, limb paralysis, and slurred speech.

dental amalgam and MS   Some have suggested multiple sclerosis (MS) might be caused by heavy metal poisoning from MERCURY leaking from amalgam dental fillings, damaging the immune system and contributing to the demyelinating process. However, no scientific evidence connects the development of MS with dental fillings containing mercury.

Although poisoning with heavy metals such as mercury, lead, or manganese can damage the nervous system and produce symptoms such as tremor and weakness, the damage is inflicted in a different way and the course of the disorder is also different.

depression   A persistent low mood lasting more than two weeks. Depression is a common problem for patients with multiple sclerosis (MS). Depression may occur for several reasons.

First, depression may be the logical result of living with a difficult chronic condition that carries the potential of progression to permanent disability. Depression can also be a side effect of some drugs, such as steroids, that may be prescribed for the treatment of MS. Some evidence also indicates that the interferon medications may trigger or worsen depression in susceptible individuals, although the research on this issue has yielded conflicting results.

Depression may also be caused by the disease process itself since MS damages the MYELIN and nerve fibers deep within the brain. Some evidence suggests that the physiology of MS may predispose people to depression. If MS damages areas of the brain that are involved in emotional expression and control, this could trigger a variety of behavioral changes, including depression.

Finally, depression in patients with MS also may be associated with disease-related changes in the immune or neuroendocrine systems.

Some evidence shows that people with MS are at increased risk for depression when the disease worsens and the person becomes more disabled. Severe depression can be a life-threatening condition because it may lead to suicide. In fact one study found that the risk of suicide was 7.5 times higher among people with MS than in the general population.

Symptoms and Diagnostic Path

It is important to distinguish between clinical depression and grief, a normal emotion that everyone experiences occasionally. Depression requires treatment—grief is normal; clinical depression is not.

Because people with MS often experience losses, such as those of the ability to work, to walk, or to participate in leisure activities, the process of mourning for these losses may resemble depression. The difference between this and a clinical disease, however, is that grief is generally time limited and passes away on its own. In addition, a grieving person may at times be able to enjoy life.

Clinical depression, on the other hand, is persistent and unremitting, with symptoms lasting at least two weeks and sometimes up to several months. It must be diagnosed by a mental health professional, because it is a serious condition that can progress to major depressive episodes and eventual suicide. The symptoms of depression include

- sadness
- loss of interest in everyday activities
- appetite increase or decrease
- sleep disturbances (insomnia or excessive sleeping)
- agitation
- behavior slowing
- fatigue
- feelings of worthlessness or guilt
- concentration problems
- persistent thoughts of death or suicide

Treatment Options and Outlook

Whether a patient becomes depressed in reaction to MS or develops depression as a result of brain changes caused by the disease, effective treatments are available. Studies have found that the best treatment results include both psychotherapy and antidepressant medication.

Modern antidepressants (such as Prozac or Zoloft) can be prescribed by a physician and cause far fewer side effects than standard antidepressant drugs used in the past. Patients should remember, however, that not everyone responds well to the same drug; several drugs may need to be tried before the depression eases. Additionally, any medication typically takes between two to four weeks before beginning to work.

d'Este, Sir Augustus Frederic (1794–1848)   The grandson of King George III of England and the second recorded case of a person suspected to have multiple sclerosis (MS). His personal account of the illness was outlined in his diary, in which he documented the course of his 26-year illness that was retrospectively diagnosed as MS.

Over the course of the diary, beginning with entries in 1822 and ending in January 1848, the obvious decline in handwriting ability is clearly visible as d'Este loses motor control.

d'Este meticulously recorded his symptoms, which began soon after a bout of measles, and included visual impairment, fatigue, and unpleasant sensations. The disease became progressively debilitating with time. An entry made five years before his death noted that he had trouble coordinating his limbs, was numb below the waist, and had spasms at night. An episode at this point triggered the onset of a chronic progressive course with only partial recovery after each relapse.

Eventually, paralyzed in both arms, d'Este died in 1848. His physician was unable to diagnose the illness, since MS would not be recognized until 20 years after his death.

Detrol   See TOLTERODINE TARTRATE.

detrusor–external sphincter dyssynergia (DESD)
A type of BLADDER DYSFUNCTION found in patients with multiple sclerosis (MS) in which there is both a failure to store urine and a failure to empty urine due to a lack of coordination between related muscle groups (the bladder's detrusor muscle and the external sphincter). When working in coordination with one another, the detrusor contracts to expel urine and then the external sphincter relaxes to release it. In DESD, the detrusor and external sphincter contract at the same time, trapping the urine in the bladder.

Also called combined dysfunction, DESD is caused by areas of inflammation, DEMYELINATION, scarring, and/or neuronal damage in the brain or spinal cord that disrupts the normal urinary process by interfering with the transmission of signals between the brain and urinary system.

Symptoms and Diagnostic Path
The problems with urine storage begin when an overactive detrusor muscle begins to contract as soon as a small amount of urine has collected in the bladder. These contractions repeatedly signal the need to urinate even though the bladder has not reached normal capacity. Because of demyelination, the spinal cord is unable to forward the sig-

nals from the bladder all the way to the brain. Without the involvement of the brain, the process of urination becomes less controlled. The urge to urinate becomes a reflex response to the frequent, repeated spinal cord signals.

Problems with emptying the bladder are caused by demyelination in the areas of the spinal cord that usually signal the voiding reflex. Although the bladder fills with urine, the spinal cord is unable to send the appropriate message to the brain to signal the need to urinate or to the external sphincter to signal the need to relax. In the absence of voluntary control, the bladder continues to fill and expand. The eventual result is an enlarged, overly relaxed bladder.

Problems with urine storage can result in urgency, frequency, the urge to urinate during the night, and incontinence. Problems with emptying the bladder may cause uncontrolled urine leaks, a delay in the ability to begin urinating, and incontinence.

Treatment Options and Outlook
A combination of strategies is usually recommended to treat this condition, including intermittent catheterization to remove the residual urine and an anticholinergic or antimuscarinic medication to relax the bladder's detrusor muscle. Occasionally, other medications may also be prescribed, including antispasticity agents to relax the sphincter muscle, including baclofen (Lioresal) or tizannidine hydrochloride (Zanaflex), and alpha-adrenergic blocking agents to promote the flow of urine through the sphincter: prazosin (Minipress); terazosin (Hytrin); tamsulosin (Flowmax). Use of Botox is currently being studied as a treatment.

On the very rare occasions when none of the medications or self-care strategies are enough to manage MS-related bladder symptoms, a surgical procedure called suprapubic cystostomy can be performed. A tube is inserted into the bladder through an opening in the lower abdomen to allow the urine to drain into an external collection bag.

See also BLADDER DYSFUNCTION.

Devic's syndrome   A rare autoimmune central nervous system disorder characterized by a breakdown in the fatty protective covering of the spinal cord (transverse myelitis) and inflammation of the

OPTIC NERVE (OPTIC NEURITIS) causing loss of vision and eye pain. It is considered a special form of multiple sclerosis (MS) with a severe and rapid course.

Symptoms and Diagnostic Path

Individuals may experience VISUAL PROBLEMS and various degrees of paralysis as well as incontinence. The disorder is closely linked with MS and lupus but usually appears before any symptoms of MS are noted. If an isolated disease episode affecting the spinal cord and optic nerve occurs after an infection or common cold, it is considered a postinfectious acute demyelinated encephalomyelitis (ADE) rather than Devic's syndrome.

Devic's syndrome is often fatal. Some patients recover almost completely, while others may have residual deficits. Some severe cases of ADE may be fatal.

Treatment Options and Outlook

No standard treatment for Devic's syndrome currently exists. Generally treatment is symptomatic and supportive. Corticosteroids may be prescribed. Treatment for ADE may include corticosteroids, intravenous immunoglobulin, and intravenous methylprednisolone.

diagnosis　No single lab test or diagnostic method can, by itself, determine if a person has multiple sclerosis (MS). Complicating the diagnosis is the fact that MS produces many symptoms that also can be caused by other diseases. As a result, a diagnosis can be made only by carefully ruling out all other possibilities.

Nevertheless it is important to diagnose MS as quickly as possible to help patients begin to adjust to the condition and to rule out other diseases, such as cancer. Since permanent neurologic damage can occur even in the earliest stages of MS, it is important to confirm the diagnosis so that the appropriate treatments can be started as early in the disease process as possible.

Multiple sclerosis is essentially a diagnosis of exclusion. First, a doctor will conduct a complete physical examination, a discussion of the patient's medical history, and a review of past or current symptoms. Next, the physician performs a variety of tests to evaluate mental, emotional, and language functions, movement and coordination, vision, balance, and the senses. However, there are no tests that are specific for MS, and no single test can be 100 percent conclusive.

A diagnosis of MS requires objective evidence of two attacks (also known as an exacerbations, flares, or relapses)—the sudden appearance or worsening of an MS symptom that lasts at least 24 hours. The two attacks must have occurred at least one month apart in different areas of the central nervous system, and there can be no other explanation for these attacks or symptoms.

Magnetic Resonance Imaging

MAGNETIC RESONANCE IMAGING (MRI) is a painless, noninvasive scan that can reveal detailed pictures of the brain and spinal cord. It is the preferred method of imaging the brain to detect the presence of plaques or scarring caused by MS because it can reveal the central nervous system in great detail. An MRI can detect lesions in different parts of the central nervous system and tell the difference between old and new lesions. The small areas of inflammation in MYELIN-dense areas of the brain and spinal cord show up as dots on an MRI scan that are easily seen by a NEUROLOGIST.

Still, the diagnosis of MS is not made on the basis of an MRI alone, since other diseases create lesions in the brain that look like those caused by MS. Moreover, some lesions are found in healthy individuals—especially older patients—that are not caused by any disease.

On the other hand, a normal MRI cannot rule out a diagnosis of MS, since about 25 percent of patients who have confirmed MS on the basis of other symptoms do not show any lesions with an MRI. Instead these people may have lesions in the spinal cord or lesions that cannot be detected by MRI. Eventually, however, brain or spinal lesions in most people with MS will appear on MRI.

The longer the MRI remains normal, the more questionable the diagnosis of MS becomes. If the MRI findings continue to be normal more than a year or two after the initial diagnosis is made, the neurologist will make every effort to identify another possible cause for the symptoms.

CT Scans

Another type of brain scan is the computed axial tomography (CT) scan. Though CT SCANS are much less effective in diagnosing MS than an MRI, a CT scan can detect other brain problems and so is sometimes used if an MRI is not available.

In this 15-minute test (which may include the use of injected contrast dye), the patient lies on a table with his or her head inside the CT-scan machine. A CT scan should not be done during pregnancy.

Other Tests

Not every patient requires every possible test. However, if a clear-cut diagnosis cannot be made based on the symptoms and the initial tests outlined above, other evaluations may be needed. These may include assessments of visual EVOKED POTENTIALS, cerebrospinal fluid, and blood.

- *Evoked potential tests* These are electrical diagnostic studies that measure the conduction of messages to the brain. They can reveal slowing of nerve transmissions and often provide evidence of scarring along nerve pathways that is not apparent on a neurologic exam. These tests reveal abnormalities in nerve function in about 65 percent of people with MS and are particularly helpful if the MRI scans are normal but symptoms suggest the disease. Evoked potential tests are painless and noninvasive. Small electrodes are placed on the patient's head to monitor brain waves and the response to auditory, visual, and/or sensory stimuli. The time necessary for the brain to receive and interpret messages is a clue to the patient's condition.

- *Cerebrospinal fluid* Obtained by a SPINAL TAP, this fluid is tested for levels of certain immune system proteins (immunoglobulins) produced by B lymphocytes. A large amount of immunoglobulins in the spinal fluid indicates the disease and is found in the spinal fluid of about 90–95 percent of people with MS. However, because B lymphocytes in the cerebrospinal fluid are also associated with other diseases, they cannot be exclusively relied upon as proof of MS.

- *Blood tests* Although no definitive blood test for MS exists, blood tests can rule out other causes for various neurologic symptoms, such as LYME DISEASE, collagen-vascular diseases, certain rare hereditary disorders, and AIDS.

Types of MS

A diagnosis of MS usually specifies one of four different types: relapse-remitting, secondary progressive, primary progressive, and progressive-relapsing.

Relapsing-remitting MS This is the most common form of MS and is characterized by periods of exacerbation in which new symptoms may appear and previous ones may worsen. The attacks are followed by periods of remission when disease activity subsides and may be unnoticeable. A remission may last for months or even years. About 80 percent of MS cases begin as relapsing-remitting.

Secondary progressive MS Within 10 years of the initial diagnosis, more than half of patients with relapsing-remitting MS begin to experience a gradual worsening of symptoms with or without occasional flare-ups, minor remissions, or plateaus. This form of MS is called secondary progressive. Symptoms of 90 percent of patients with relapsing-remitting MS become secondary progressive within 25 years.

Primary progressive MS This type of MS is characterized by a nearly continuous worsening of the disease from the very beginning, with no distinct relapses or remissions. There may be temporary plateaus with minor relief from symptoms but no long-lasting relief. About 10 percent of people with MS have primary progressive MS.

Progressive-relapsing MS This form of the disease is quite rare and takes a progressive course from the onset but is also characterized by obvious acute attacks, with or without recovery. In contrast to relapsing-remitting MS, the periods between relapses are characterized by continuing disease progression. About 10 percent of people with MS have progressive-relapsing MS.

diazepam (Valium) A benzodiazepine that belongs to the group of medicines called central nervous system (CNS) depressants. It is used in multiple sclerosis primarily to ease muscle spasms and SPASTICITY. A physician should check the patient's progress at regular visits to make sure that this medication does not cause unwanted effects.

Diazepam adds to the effects of alcohol and other CNS depressants (such as antihistamines, sedatives, tranquilizers, prescription pain medications, seizure medications, muscle relaxants, and sleeping medications). Therefore a patient taking diazepam should not use these. Stopping this medication suddenly may cause withdrawal side effects.

Side Effects

Temporary side effects that do not require medical attention, unless they continue for several weeks or are bothersome, include

- clumsiness or unsteadiness
- dizziness or lightheadedness
- slurred speech
- abdominal cramps or pain
- blurred vision or other changes in vision
- changes in sexual drive or performance
- constipation or diarrhea
- dry mouth
- fast or pounding heartbeat
- muscle spasm
- trouble with urination
- trembling
- unusual tiredness or weakness

Unusual side effects that patients should discuss with a physician as soon as possible include

- behavior problems, including difficulty concentrating and outbursts of anger
- confusion or mental depression
- convulsions
- hallucinations
- low blood pressure
- muscle weakness
- skin rash or itching
- sore throat, fever, chills
- unusual bleeding or bruising
- unusual excitement or irritability

Symptoms of overdose that require immediate emergency help include

- continuing confusion
- unusually severe drowsiness

- shakiness
- slowed heartbeat
- shortness of breath
- slow reflexes
- continuing slurred speech
- staggering
- unusually severe weakness

Didion, Joan (1934–)   Journalist and novelist who was diagnosed with multiple sclerosis. Didion was born in Sacramento, California, and graduated with a B.A. from the University of California at Berkeley. She has been a journalist, novelist, essayist, and screenwriter since the 1960s and was awarded the 1996 Edward MacDowell Medal and the 1999 Columbia Journalism Award.

After working as a features editor at *Vogue* in the mid-1950s, Didion moved on to become a freelance writer best known for her essays of highly personal commentary on American politics and culture. Collections of her magazine essays include *Slouching Toward Bethlehem* (1968) and *The White Album* (1979). Her critically acclaimed novels include *Play It As It Lays* (1970) and *A Book of Common Prayer* (1977). She contributes journalism and critical essays to magazines like *The New Yorker* and *The New York Review of Books* and collaborated on newspaper columns and screenplays with husband John Gregory Dunne, whom she married in 1964; he died in 2004. Her collection of essays, *Political Fictions,* was published by Alfred A. Knopf in September 2001.

diet   Although eating a healthy diet is important to everyone whether or not they have multiple sclerosis (MS), no specific dietary approach has been found that can affect the frequency or severity of attacks. The recommended diet for people with MS is the same low-fat, high-fiber diet recommended for everyone else.

Maintaining good nutrition takes planning, attention, and some innovation, but a variety of grains, fruits, and vegetables is the foundation to a healthful diet plan. Choices from these groups are rich in vitamins, minerals, carbohydrates, and other substances important for good health—most help create a feeling of fullness and satisfaction to keep the snack urge quiet.

Although good nutrition is essential for everyone, people with MS may have special considerations and needs, since MS symptoms or medications can affect nutritional well-being. Since MS symptoms also can reduce mobility or physical activity, gaining weight might be a problem if eating habits remain the same as activity levels slow down. Added weight can increase FATIGUE, further limit mobility, put a strain on breathing and circulation, and increase the risk for other chronic illnesses.

Being underweight can also compromise health, especially if it is caused by lack of appetite or fatigue that limits food intake. A registered dietitian or doctor can recommend an optimal weight, and reasonable daily calorie intake.

Special foods and preparations may be required if swallowing and chewing are a problem. A speech-language pathologist or nutritionist can provide individual dietary advice and methods for those who are on special feeding regimes.

differential diagnosis Multiple sclerosis (MS) can be mistaken for a number of other neurological conditions, such as spinal cord compression from tumors or spondylosis, Arnold-Chiari malformation, intracranial tumor, central nervous system (CNS) lymphoma, vasculitis of the CNS, acute disseminated encephalomyelitis, transverse myelitis, neurosyphilis, neuro-Lyme disease, vitamin B_{12} deficiency, Friedrich's ataxia, Leber's optic atrophy, neuromyelitis optica, or MOTOR NEURON DISEASE.

diplopia See DOUBLE VISION.

disease management A number of treatment recommendations have been adopted by the executive committee of the medical advisory board of the National Multiple Sclerosis Society regarding use of the current MS DISEASE-MODIFYING AGENTS, including the immunomodulators beta INTERFERON 1b (Betaseron), beta interferon 1a-intramuscular (Avonex), beta interferon 1a-subcutaneous (Rebif), glatiramer acetate (Copaxone), and the immunosuppressant MITOXANTRONE (Novantrone).

The NMSS recommends that therapy be started with an immunomodulator as soon as possible after a definite diagnosis of MS with active disease, and may be considered for selected persons with a first attack who are at high risk for MS. The society also recommends the following:

- A patient's access to medication should not be limited by the frequency of relapses, age, or level of disability.
- Treatment is not to be stopped while insurers evaluate for continuing coverage of treatment.
- Therapy is to be continued indefinitely, unless there is clear lack of benefit, intolerable side effects, new data reveal other reasons for cessation, or better therapy becomes available.
- All of these FDA-approved drugs should be included in formularies and covered by insurers so that physicians and patients can determine the most appropriate agent on an individual basis; failure to do so is unethical and discriminatory.
- Movement from one immunomodulatory drug to another should occur only for medical appropriate reasons.
- Immunosuppressant therapy with mitoxantrone (Novantrone) may be considered for selected relapsing persons with worsening disease.
- Most concurrent medical conditions do not contraindicate use of the immunomodulatory drugs.
- None of the therapies has been approved for use by women who are trying to become pregnant, are pregnant, or are nursing mothers.

disease-modifying agents Five drugs are currently being used in the treatment of multiple sclerosis (MS): INTERFERON beta-1a (Avonex), interferon beta-1b (Betaseron), GLATIRAMER ACETATE (Copaxone), beta interferon 1-a (Rebif), and mitoxantrone (Novantrone). Betaseron was introduced in 1993 as the first disease-altering drug that could be used to treat RELAPSING-REMITTING MS. Avonex and Copaxone followed in 1996, with Rebif in 2002. A sixth drug, natalizumab (formerly known as Antegren; now called Tysabri), had been approved in November 2004 and was voluntarily suspended by the manufacturers on February 28, 2005, after one patient died and another experienced serious side effects after taking a combination of Tysabri and Avonex.

A number of positive outcomes from the use of these treatments have been demonstrated in people with relapsing-remitting disease, including reduction in the frequency of severity of relapses, a drop in the development of brain lesions, and the possibility of a lessened future disability. After several years of experience with the beta interferons and glatiramer acetate, researchers and clinicians with expertise in MS agree that these drugs reduce future disability and improve the quality of life for many individuals with relapsing-remitting multiple sclerosis.

Avonex, Betaseron, and Rebif are biotechnology drugs based on a natural human protein that dampens immune system activity. Copaxone works by a different mechanism; although its action is not fully understood, experts think the medication tricks the immune system by serving as a myelin decoy. All four are injected drugs.

Avonex is administered by deep intramuscular injection once a week into the thigh or upper arm. These injections are usually given in the patient's home by the patient or a family member. Side effects include flu-like symptoms about an hour after the injection and may last 24–36 hours. The flu-like symptoms usually improve with aspirin, Tylenol, or ibuprofen and lessen over time. Rarer side effects include mild anemia and elevated liver enzymes, which may indicate liver inflammation. Blood tests need to be checked on occasion to follow liver function and white blood cell levels.

Betaseron is injected every other day under the skin—usually the thigh, back of the arm, or abdomen. The injection site is changed each injection so that the skin does not become irritated. These injections are usually given in the patient's home by the patient or a family member. Side effects include flu-like symptoms following injection, beginning about an hour after the injection and lasting about eight hours. The flu-like symptoms usually improve with aspirin, Tylenol, or ibuprofen and lessen over time.

A red spot usually develops at the site of the injection. This spot may take several weeks to go away. Very rarely, the red spot may form a scar on the skin. Rarer side effects include elevated liver

enzymes and low white blood cell counts, which make a person susceptible to infection.

Blood tests need to be checked on occasion to follow liver function and white blood cell levels.

Rebif (beta interferon 1a) was approved in March 2002 by the U.S. Food and Drug Administration (FDA) for the treatment of relapsing forms of multiple sclerosis, to decrease the frequency of clinical exacerbations and delay the accumulation of physical disability. Like Avonex, Rebif is the beta-1a form of the human protein interferon, but it can be injected three times a week under the skin, as opposed to Avonex, which must be injected once a week in the muscle. Rotation of injection sites is necessary to avoid injection site complications. As with the other interferon subcutaneous injections, there is possibility of flu-like symptoms following injection, which can be reduced by using aspirin, acetaminophen, or ibuprofen. These symptoms should lessen within the first two to three months. There is usually a red area and possibly some pain at the site of the injection. Very rarely, the red spot may form an ulcer under the skin and leave a scar. Any area of inflammation should be shown to the nurse or doctor. Rarer side effects include elevated liver enzymes and low white blood cell counts, which make a person susceptible to infection. Periodic blood tests are required to follow liver function and white blood cell levels.

Copaxone is different from the interferons, and although the exact mechanism is unknown, it is believed that it blocks the disease process as had previously been shown in animal studies in 1980s. The drug is injected daily, usually in the thigh, back of the arm, or abdomen. The injection site is changed each injection so that the skin does not become irritated. These injections are usually given in the patient's home by the patient or a family member; an autoinjector is available. Copaxone causes few side effects. A red spot often forms on the skin at the site of the injection, which goes away after two or three days. Rarely, patients may have a benign systemic reaction that occurs right after an injection and includes chest pain, flushing, shortness of breath, strong heartbeat, and anxiety. The reaction does not require medical treatment and resolves within 15–20 minutes, although in a few cases it may last up to 45 minutes. This reaction occurs in about 15 percent of patients. Those who get this reaction usually have it only once. Blood tests are not needed for this medication. The medication must be refrigerated but can be at room temperature for up to a week.

Novantrone is recommended for worsening relapsing-remitting MS, PROGRESSIVE-RELAPSING MS, or SECONDARY PROGRESSIVE MS. This drug is administered by IV infusion, usually at three monthly intervals, and it can be given for a limited time only, so to avoid possible side effects to the heart. Novantrone is proven to reduce new lesions, decrease attacks or relapses, and slow the rate of increasing disability. This drug belongs to the general group of medicines called antineoplastics. Prior to its approval for use in MS, it was used only to treat certain forms of cancer. It acts in MS by suppressing the activity of T cells, B cells, and macrophages that are thought to lead the attack on the MYELIN sheath. It is available for careful use in aggressive relapsing disease and for those not responding to immunomodulators. Novantrone was found to delay the time to first treated relapse and time to disability progression, and also reduced the number of treated relapses and number of new lesions detected by magnetic resonance imaging.

Side Effect Treatments

Patients who experience side effects from one of the disease-modifying agents may be able to switch to one of the other two drugs and avoid the side effects. Patients who stop taking the drugs may think they are suffering no consequences, but MS damage can occur steadily and silently for long periods before the next attack.

disease types Multiple sclerosis (MS) tends to take one of four clinical courses, each of which might be mild, moderate, or severe. Researchers are currently trying to identify more precise indicators of the prognosis or predicted disease activity of the four types, as follows:

- RELAPSING-REMITTING MS is characterized by partial or total recovery after attacks (also called exacerbations, relapses, or flares). This is the most common form of MS. Approximately 85 percent of people with MS initially begin with a relapsing-remitting course.

- A relapsing-remitting course that later becomes steadily progressive is called SECONDARY PROGRESSIVE MS (SPMS). Attacks and partial recoveries may continue to occur. Of the 85 percent who start with relapsing-remitting disease, more than half will develop SPMS within 10 years; 90 percent will develop it within 25 years.

- A progressive course from onset without any attacks is called PRIMARY PROGRESSIVE MS (PPMS). The symptoms that occur along the way generally do not remit. Ten percent of people with MS are diagnosed with PPMS, although the diagnosis usually needs to be made after the fact—when the person has been living for a period of time with progressive disability but no acute attacks.

- A progressive course from the outset, with obvious, acute attacks along the way, is called PROGRESSIVE-RELAPSING MS (PRMS). This course is quite rare, occurring in only 5 percent of people with MS.

dizziness A sensation of feeling off balance or lightheaded, a common symptom in flare-ups of multiple sclerosis. This is not the same thing as VERTIGO—an illusion that the patient or the surroundings are spinning. Vertigo more typically develops with ear problems, not with BRAIN or BRAIN STEM problems.

Dizziness is caused by damaged areas in the complex neural pathways that coordinate visual, spatial, and other input to the brain needed to produce and maintain equilibrium.

Patients should consult a physician if dizziness or vertigo becomes annoying. Usually the symptoms respond to an anti–motion sickness drug such as meclizine (Antivert, Bonine, or Dramamine), skin patches that deliver scopolamine, or the antinausea drug ondansetron (Zofran). In severe cases of dizziness or vertigo, a short course of corticosteroids may be needed.

DNA markers Patterns of genetic material that are consistently inherited. Scientists are searching for DNA markers for multiple sclerosis (MS). When one of these markers is identified, scientists focus more intensely on that genetic area; eventually the location of the gene contributing to MS susceptibility can be identified.

As many as 20 markers that may contain genes contributing to MS have been identified, but no single gene has been shown to have a major influence on susceptibility to MS. Research will likely find that other, as yet unidentified genes contribute to MS. After the location of each susceptibility gene is identified, the role that the gene plays in the immune system and neurologic aspects of people with MS will have to be determined. Because the immune system is so intricately involved in MS, many scientists believe that at least some of the susceptibility genes are related to the immune system. Already reports have linked some immune system genes to MS.

Such research could also uncover the basic cause of the disease and help predict its course. This would also lead to earlier diagnoses in families where one or more members already has MS. Many physicians believe that the earlier MS is diagnosed and treatment begun, the better the outcome.

doll's eye sign A condition in which the eyes move up as the head moves down, indicating dissociation between movement of the eyes and of the head; a sign of multiple sclerosis.

donepezil A drug widely used for treating dementia in Alzheimer's disease that has also been shown to help patients with multiple sclerosis (MS) who have mild to moderate cognitive impairment. Most MS patients and their doctors focus primarily on managing the physical symptoms of the disease, yet an estimated 50 percent of patients will face varying degrees of COGNITIVE DYSFUNCTION as well. This may include difficulties with problem solving, attention, learning, and memory, and it can lead to job loss, social withdrawal, and mood changes. Although only 10 percent of all MS patients experience severe cognitive impairment, even mild impairment can significantly interfere with a patient's daily activities.

In spring of 2004, researchers at the State University of New York at Stony Brook demonstrated that donepezil shows promise in treating cognitively impaired patients with MS. This 24-week double-blind clinical trial had 69 participants with MS. All had at least mild impairment on a verbal learning and memory task, and none had severe depressive symptoms. Some were given donepezil 10 mg daily, and some were given a placebo.

The donepezil group displayed greater improvement on the verbal memory function test and experienced a greater reduction in cognitive deficits than did the placebo group. More than 65 percent of the donepezil group reported that their memory had improved with treatment versus 32 percent of those in the placebo group. Cognitive improvement was also seen in almost twice as many donepezil patients, and the drug had no affect on mood or fatigue.

double vision The common term for diplopia—the simultaneous awareness of two images of the same object caused by a failure of both eyes to work together. This is a fairly common symptom in multiple sclerosis. Covering one eye will eliminate one of the images.

Double vision occurs when the pairs of muscles that control a particular eye movement are not perfectly coordinated because of weakness in one or both pairs of muscles. When the visual images are not properly fused, the patient perceives a false image.

Double vision usually goes away without treatment, although in some cases a brief course of corticosteroids may help. Patching one eye can also be useful when driving or performing household tasks, but it is not recommended for long periods of time because it will slow the brain's ability to adjust to the problem. Special lenses are rarely recommended because the symptom tends to be temporary.

dressing Choosing and wearing clothing is a personal, private activity that may become difficult for patients with multiple sclerosis who have significant paralysis in their arms or legs. Patients who need help should be given tactful, sensitive assistance so that they can continue to dress themselves for as long as possible.

Clothing should be loose fitting, comfortable, and easy to put on, with not too many buttons or fasteners. Loose-fitting jerseys, sweats, pullovers, T-shirts, and pants with elastic waistbands are all excellent choices. In order to avoid having to iron (and be near heat sources), clothing should be as wrinkle free as possible.

OCCUPATIONAL THERAPISTS can provide a number of helpful suggestions to make dressing easier. For example, men who have trouble tying a tie can simply loosen the tie, pull it over their head, and store it already tied for next time. Men who have trouble with belts may want to consider suspenders. Women who have trouble fastening a bra may find that front-fastening styles—or one-piece athletic bras that slip over the head—are easier to use. If manual dexterity is a problem, patients could replace tie shoes with slip-ons or sneakers that fasten with Velcro. (However, sneakers provide better traction on slippery floors.) Velcro tabs on all sorts of clothing can make dressing much easier. Patients should be seated while dressing to lessen the chance of falling and make reaching the feet easier. Those who are weaker on one side should dress that side first.

Products to Make Dressing Easier

A number of products can help a person with incoordination, spasticity, sensory problems, or unsteadiness dress themselves. Sock pullers are a device with an extension that can be used to pull up socks without having to bend over. Alternatively, the dressing stick is a device that allows a patient to pull up socks, pants, or underwear. To put on shoes without bending down, an extended shoehorn with a curved handle and extended length can be used. With elastic stretch shoelaces, patients can slip in and out of shoes without having to untie or tie them. Shoe and boot removers can help patients take off shoes without bending down. Zipper pulls are long hooks available in a variety of sizes that can help patients get a firm grip on a zipper. Buttoning aids can be helpful to some patients.

driving Driving is a complex activity that requires quick reactions, memory of traffic laws, good thinking skills, and the ability to make split-second decisions. For these reasons, the ability to drive may be threatened by several of the symptoms that accompany multiple sclerosis (MS): vision problems, fatigue, muscle stiffness, slowed reaction time, and a limited mobility that simply makes getting into and out of the driver's seat difficult.

There are ways the patient can continue driving safely but within limits. These may include not driving at night and avoiding high-density highways or times when he or she is likely to be tired or bothered by extreme heat. A person with MS also may obtain special equipment or vehicle modification to help safely maintain mobility independence for as long as possible.

Choosing a Car

When choosing a car, options can be included such as a minivan with a lowered floor and a ramp or a full-size van with a lift. Specialized modifications allow a person to transfer to the driver's seat or drive from a wheelchair.

Technology may be able to compensate for the loss of strength or range of motion. Examples include reduced-effort steering and/or brake systems to compensate for reduced strength, mechanical hand controls to allow for operating the gas and brake using the upper extremities, and brake/accelerator systems to compensate for reduced strength and/or range of motion of the arms.

Visual Problems

Good eyesight is critical to safe driving, but the vision problems typical in MS patients may be subtle. A person with MS may have 20-20 vision on a black-on-white vision chart but still have episodes of OPTIC NEURITIS when vision is blurry, eye movement is painful, or colors are affected. MS can affect the pathways or circuits in the brain that direct eye movement as well. The MYELIN (the fatty nerve fiber insulation) in the BRAIN or BRAIN STEM is affected by MS, so the pathways for colors, contrast, or shades of gray are affected. MS can also affect the OPTIC NERVE. This can make perceiving contrasts more difficult, which is why night driving is often harder for patients with MS. Patients may need a prescription for eyeglasses that are designed for night driving.

DOUBLE VISION is another MS symptom that may occur; because double vision disappears if one eye is covered, some people use a patch over one eye while driving.

Other patients experience episodes in which objects seem to move, particularly when they are looking to the side or down. Medications for this (GABAPENTIN and BACLOFEN) can ease this bouncing of the eye. Peripheral vision (the far right and left edges of the full field of vision) also can be affected by MS. People are rarely advised by their doctors to stop driving if only their peripheral vision is impaired because drivers can learn to compensate by turning their heads as they turn a corner or move to another traffic lane. Nonetheless, if something is coming in from the side very quickly, a driver with poor peripheral vision may not see it in time to react safely.

Experts advise people with MS to drive only if they are comfortable and their vision is deemed adequate by their doctor.

Physical Changes

WEAKNESS in an arm or leg may affect steering or pushing the foot pedals. Some people with MS find pushing the brake or gas pedals to be hard because they lack sufficient tension in the muscles that extend a part of the body or they have trouble bending their knees enough to move the foot quickly from one pedal to the other. Others have a sensory loss so the foot may slip off the pedal. Fatigue also clearly affects driving.

Heat may also affect a patient's driving ability. Patients who are especially sensitive to the heat should avoid driving soon after getting overheated and should always take a cold drink or ice along on the ride. Air-conditioning also may help.

Cognitive Changes

Driving requires the ability to process many pieces of information simultaneously. However, a person with MS may find that takes longer to absorb, digest, and sort out the important information in order to make quick decisions. Response time has two aspects—the physical part involves how long it physically takes to turn the steering wheel and swerve away from an oncoming car; the cognitive part, how effectively a person can process high-speed incoming information.

MEMORY loss may also affect driving, so that the person forgets familiar routes and fails to recognize landmarks. A person with visuo-spatial problems may have trouble telling left from right.

A neuropsychological evaluation can help determine the degree of cognitive problems in a driver with MS. If the evaluation shows that there

are significant problems, the patient might also want to have a comprehensive driving evaluation. Such a program can be found at most major rehabilitation centers or hospitals.

Drusen disease   A degenerative condition that must be distinguished from OPTIC NEURITIS (inflammation of the OPTIC NERVE) typically seen in multiple sclerosis. Drusen disease mimics optic disc swelling and can cause a visual field loss, but acute visual loss is rare.

dry mouth   A common side effect of some drugs, including some used to treat multiple sclerosis symptoms (especially bladder problems). Dry mouth may make SWALLOWING PROBLEMS worse and contribute to tooth decay and gum disease as well as discomfort. The medication causing the problem may be adjusted, or the patient may need to use mouthwashes, artificial saliva, or other approaches to protect the teeth and increase comfort.

Du Pré, Jacqueline (1945–1987)   World-renowned cellist who burst upon the music scene as a phenomenally talented 16-year-old, whose stellar career was cut short when she was diagnosed with rapidly progressive multiple sclerosis (MS) at the age of 28. Born in Oxford, England, Du Pré grew up in Surrey and became fascinated with the cello after hearing it played on the radio when she was four years old. On her fifth birthday she received a cello, began taking lessons at age six at the London Cello School, and at age seven performed for the first time in public. At age 10 she won the Suggia-Cello Prize at an international competition. At 12 and 13 she performed in BBC concerts in London. By the early 1960s she was a world-famous cellist whose playing was so interpretive that she was often criticized for detracting from the music. However, she also influenced many notable classical musicians with her fervent interpretations of the cello repertoire.

She married Daniel Barenboim in 1967 and just five years later was diagnosed with MS, which halted her brilliant career. She worked only several more years, giving lessons in cello, because her disease was unusually active, progressing rapidly until she died of complications in 1987.

durable power of attorney A legal document that allows an individual (the principal) an opportunity to authorize an agent (usually a trusted family member or friend) to make legal decisions for a time when the patient is no longer able to do so. Durable power of attorney (DPA) forms are available at most office supply stores.

Two types of DPA are available, one for financial affairs and one for health care decisions. The DPA for health care is a legal document that allows a patient to appoint an agent to make all decisions regarding health care, including choices regarding health care providers, medical treatment, and, in the later stages of the disease, end-of-life decisions. It would include the patient's wishes about whether or not to use tube feeding or a ventilator, for example. A DPA for health care does not have to be completed by an attorney, but it requires the signature of the patient and a witness; it does not usually require notarization.

The DPA for property provides for the management of personal property and finances by a designated agent, who would have virtually complete control of the patient's income and assets. The DPA for property does not include precise directives about how the agent should use the income for the patient's behalf. A DPA for property requires the signatures of the patient, a witness, and a notary.

dysarthria A speech disorder, sometimes found in patients with multiple sclerosis (MS), characterized by problems with the clarity or rhythm of speech and caused by muscle dysfunction as a result of damage to the central nervous system or a peripheral motor nerve. A loss of volume control, unnatural emphasis, slurring, poor articulation, or slower rate of speech may occur. Patients with severe dysarthria speak with a lilting quality (also known as scanning). This type of speech sounds labored and is neither lyrical nor spontaneous. Nonetheless, the content and meaning of the spoken words remain normal.

Unlike patients with APHASIA, patients with dysarthria have no problems with the speech centers of the brain. They can select and write out words and sentences; they simply cannot form vocal expression. MS patients with dysarthria

show damage in the CEREBELLUM, which is responsible for coordinating movements. The cerebellum is the area of the brain particularly likely to be damaged in patients with MS.

Some patients with a severe dysarthria problem do not realize their speech is abnormal, although they may realize they have more trouble speaking than other people do. Patients who are aware of their speech problems may benefit from speech therapy, which can improve their speech clarity.

dysdiadochokinesia The medical term for an inability to perform rapidly alternating movements that is usually caused by multiple sclerosis. The condition, which is related to problems in the CEREBELLUM, can be detected by the nose-to-finger NEUROLOGICAL exam.

dysesthesia The impairment of a person's sensitivity to sensation and touch, marked by unusual and occasionally unpleasant sensations, such as tingling.

dyskinesia Abnormal muscular movements caused by a brain disease, such as multiple sclerosis. The disorder may affect the entire body or just one group of muscles. Types of dyskinesia include chorea (jerking movements), athetosis (writhing), tics, tremors, or MYOCLONUS (muscle spasms).

dysmetria A problem with coordination caused by lesions in the CEREBELLUM, characterized by the tendency to over- or underestimate the extent of motion needed to place an arm or leg in a certain position. This tendency, which can also be caused by lesions in sensory nervous pathways leading to the cerebellum or the motor pathways leading from it, is a symptom of multiple sclerosis (MS). Dysmetria that affects the hands can make writing and picking things up difficult or even impossible.

Dysmetria that involves undershooting is called hypometria, and overshooting is called hypermetria.

Dysmetria is a difficult condition to treat, although isoniazid and clonazepam may be effective for some patients.

See also PAIN.

dysmyelination disease The congenital absence of, or defective formation of, the MYELIN sheath protecting the nerves that results in abnormal, delayed, or inadequate MYELINATION of the nerves. This is opposed to DEMYELINATING DISEASES, such as multiple sclerosis, which are characterized by the destruction, loss, or removal of myelin coating the axons and resulting in their inability to transmit impulses. Pelizaeus-Merzbacher disease is one example of dysmyelination disease.

See also DIFFERENTIAL DIAGNOSIS.

dysphasia A term used to describe a problem with the ability to select words (and or to comprehend and read) that is caused by damage to parts of the brain that control speech and comprehension. This symptom may occur in patients with multiple sclerosis.

dysphonia A voice disorder characterized by changes in vocal quality, such as harshness, hoarseness, breathiness, or a hypernasal sound. In patients with multiple sclerosis, dysphonia may be caused by muscle weakness, SPASTICITY, TREMOR, or a lack of muscle coordination (ATAXIA).

dystonia Abnormal muscle rigidity resulting in painful muscle spasms, fixed posture, or strange movements. Generalized dystonia is usually caused by neurological disorders such as multiple sclerosis.

EDSS See EXPANDED DISABILITY STATUS SCALE.

Elavil See AMITRIPTYLINE.

electroencephalography A method of measuring the amount and type of electrical activity in the brain. It is used not so much to diagnose multiple sclerosis (MS) positively (which it does not do well) but to rule out other reasons for the symptoms a patient may be experiencing. Typically an electroencephalogram (EEG) is a reliable indicator of brain wave activity only in superficial brain areas. EEG measurements, which are taken from the scalp, are less reliable in assessing deeper brain structures such as those likely to be abnormal in patients with MS.

Some infectious diseases that can produce symptoms similar to MS also produce striking changes in brain waves as detected by EEG.

electromyography A test that checks the health of muscles and nerves controlling them. In this diagnostic procedure, a needle is placed in a muscle or small plate electrodes are placed on the skin. An electric current is passed through the needle or electrode to stimulate the nerves. The electrical activity detected by the electrodes is displayed on an oscilloscope. The size and shape of the waves reveal how well the muscle responds when stimulated by nerves. The test can also measure the ability of peripheral nerves to conduct impulses and is used to help diagnose or assess nerve injury and reflex responses.

emotional instability See PSEUDOBULBAR AFFECT.

emotional problems Although multiple sclerosis (MS) primarily causes physical symptoms, the disease may have profound emotional consequences as well. At first patients may find it difficult to adjust to the idea of a disorder that is unpredictable, evanescent, and that may ultimately cause significant physical disability. Lack of knowledge about the disease adds to the anxieties commonly experienced by people who are newly diagnosed.

Professional counseling and participating in a support group may help patients and their families cope with the emotional aspects of MS. In many cases the right medication can make the difference between an intolerable and a happy life. An active lifestyle can also help, so the patient should try to continue activities he or she enjoyed before being diagnosed with MS as well as pursue new interests suited to the physical changes the individual is experiencing.

The National Multiple Sclerosis Society can provide a variety of resources to help people deal with the emotional aspects of MS, including support groups, workshops, and other programs geared to maintaining the quality of life of persons with MS. The chapters can also refer patients to community resources.

Depression

Many patients with MS experience DEPRESSION, which may range from feeling a bit blue for a few hours to severe clinical depression that may last for several months. People with MS and all those closely associated with them should be aware that depression in its various forms is common during this disease. In fact studies have suggested that clinical depression occurs more often among people with MS than it does in the general population and that it is even more common in those with MS than among persons with other chronic, disabling conditions. In its most severe forms depression is caused by a chemical imbalance that may occur at any time.

Clinical depression should be suspected if at least five of the following symptoms are present for at least two weeks:

- depressed mood, feelings of hopelessness, and despair
- markedly diminished interest or pleasure in most activities
- changes in appetite and significant weight loss or gain
- insomnia
- restlessness or sluggishness
- fatigue or loss of energy
- feelings of worthlessness or excessive or inappropriate guilt
- diminished ability to think or concentrate, or indecisiveness
- recurrent thoughts of death or suicide

The most effective treatment for depression is generally a combination of psychotherapy and antidepressant medication. Although support groups may be helpful for less severe depressive symptoms and generalized distress, they are no substitute for intensive clinical treatment.

Grief

People with MS often experience losses; for example, they become unable to work, to walk, or to engage in certain leisure activities. The process of mourning for these losses may resemble depression, but grief is usually time limited and gets better on its own. Moreover, a grieving person may at times be able to enjoy some of life's activities. Clinical depression is more persistent and unremitting. Grieving is generally related to changes in self-image triggered by the disease, such as no longer being able to think of oneself as an athlete. However, with time and successful coping strategies, patients with MS can develop an altered self-image. Grief generally gets better over time even without treatment, but supportive counseling, support groups, as well as an understanding and supportive environment can help the process along.

Stress

Life is full of stress, but MS generally adds a great deal more disease-related stress to the mix. MS is unpredictable, and simply anticipating the next exacerbation can be a significant source of stress. MS can also lead to some major life changes such as loss of mobility and interference with work. Thus the person with MS faces significant challenges in coping with a potentially stressful life. Some experts also believe that stress may be a possible trigger to the development of the onset of MS or may trigger exacerbations. However, studies of the effects of stress on MS have had conflicting results.

Stress management programs have become an accepted part of treating many medical disorders. Professional counseling as well as support groups can also help patients in learning how to cope better with stress.

Generalized Anxiety and Distress

MS is a generally disabling, progressive, and unpredictable disease that can cause significant anxiety, distress, anger, and frustration from the very beginning. The tremendous uncertainty associated with MS is one of its most distressing aspects. People with MS never know when and if another exacerbation will occur or how severely they may be affected in the future. The loss of function and altered life circumstances caused by the disease are also significant causes of anxiety and distress. Professional counseling and support groups can be helpful in dealing with the anxiety and distress that may accompany MS.

Moodiness

People with MS may experience rapid and usually unpredictable changes in emotions—especially frequent bouts of anger or irritability. It is unclear if the emotional moodiness observed in MS stems from the distress related to the disease or if it is caused by some changes in the brain. Whatever the cause, moodiness can be one of the most challenging aspects of MS. Family counseling may be very important in dealing with these mood swings since they are likely to affect everyone in the family. Severe mood swings respond well to low doses of the anticonvulsant medication valproic acid (Depakote).

Pseudobulbar Affect

A small percentage of patients with MS experience a more severe form of emotional moodiness in which they experience uncontrollable episodes of laughing or crying that seem to have little or no relationship to actual events or the individual's actual feelings. These changes are thought to result from lesions in emotional pathways in the brain. Family members and caregivers must understand and be prepared for this. They must realize that people with MS may not always be able to control their emotions.

Medications such as AMITRIPTYLINE (Elavil) and valproic acid (Depakote) are used to treat these emotional changes. Studies of other medications are currently under way.

Inappropriate Behavior

A very small proportion of people with MS exhibit inappropriate behavior, such as a lack of sexual inhibition, which is probably caused by MS-related damage to the normal inhibitory functions of the brain. These behaviors may also reflect poor judgment related to COGNITIVE DYSFUNCTION caused by MS. The patient usually cannot control this behavior, and thus it is not a sign of "moral weakness" or sociopathic tendencies.

The treatment of these problems is complex and may require psychiatric medication together with psychotherapy. Family members will probably need supportive counseling since these behaviors are often shocking and disruptive. In some cases the affected individual may require supervision to prevent the behaviors.

employment Multiple sclerosis (MS) can have a significant impact on employment, despite the fact that people with MS may be experienced, well trained, and productive workers who often retain the ability to work long after the illness manifests itself. When working through these issues, an OCCUPATIONAL THERAPIST or a trained employment disability adviser can help the person with MS make planned and purposeful decisions.

An employee (or job applicant) does not have to reveal a diagnosis but may choose to describe problems as "a medical condition." Workplace accommodations and adjustments can be made to compensate for limitations and these cover most employees. The AMERICANS WITH DISABILITIES ACT (ADA) guarantees accommodations as long as they do not present an "undue hardship" for the employer.

The issue in an interview is the match between an individual's abilities, training, and experience and a given job's requirements. Many people will think they should stop working in order to avoid stress. However, people with MS can continue to work and are better off psychologically and physically if employment is maintained. Work situations can be reassessed over time and the job demands, limitations, options, and current performance barriers dealt with as they arise.

Health Insurance

When starting a new job, a person with MS should take advantage of any group health care insurance offered by the employer. It is important that any health care insurance application form be honestly answered and that no attempt be made to hide the MS, but information that is not requested need not be volunteered.

Workplace Accommodations

Accommodations for MS are rarely complex or expensive. The employer will need to do research regarding appropriate accommodations and offer proposals for consideration, such as a telephone headset or a scheduled brief rest period. Accommodations are always negotiated on a case-by-case basis and may not impose a major financial hardship to an employer.

A mutually acceptable accommodation will enable the employer to benefit from the productivity of a valuable employee. Because symptoms typically come and go, people with MS may not always use work accommodations or even need them. Employees should expect the same training and promotion opportunities as would have been given before the diagnosis. The ADA describes several remedies for on-the-job barriers, including

- restructuring of existing facilities
- restructuring of the job
- modification of work schedules

- reassignment to another position
- modification of equipment
- installation of new equipment
- provision of qualified readers or interpreters

The National MS Society recommends an approach in which an employee works with an employer to identify accommodations that support the person's comfort and productivity in the job. This approach is much more likely to produce cooperative solutions to on-the-job needs than is a legal action and is more likely to encourage a positive long-term working relationship with the employer.

Employees with MS are covered by Title I of the ADA if they have a disabling condition (such as MS), they meet the employer's requirements for a job, and they have the capabilities to perform the essential functions of their current job or a job for which they wish to apply.

Employers and the ADA

The ADA prohibits discrimination in employment against otherwise qualified people with disabilities. All employers must comply with Title I of the ADA (except those with fewer than 15 employees, the federal government, Native American tribes, and tax-exempt private membership clubs). Sections 501-504 of the Rehabilitation Act of 1973 prevent the federal government, federal contractors, and any programs receiving federal funds from discriminating against people with disabilities.

The ADA requires that an employer provide a reasonable accommodation, but the employer does not have to provide the most reasonable one requested by the person with MS. Negotiation and needs and agreements are needed to obtain reasonable work accommodation agreements. Because the course of MS is unpredictable, the effectiveness of job accommodations must be monitored on an ongoing basis.

environmental triggers   Experts agree that genes play a role in the development of multiple sclerosis (MS), but environmental factors are believed to trigger the onset of the condition.

Migration patterns and epidemiologic studies have shown that people who are born in a part of the world where people are at low risk for MS and then move to an area with a higher risk before the age of 15 acquire the risk of their new home. Such data suggest that exposure to some environmental agent such as a virus or bacteria that occurs before puberty may predispose a person to develop MS later on.

epidemiology   The study of disease patterns that takes into account variations in geography, demographics, socioeconomic status, genetics, and infectious causes. Epidemiologists contribute to knowledge about multiple sclerosis (MS) by studying the relationships between these factors, as well as patterns of migration, that may be related to areas with high or low rates of MS. Epidemiological studies can help to identify factors that may be related to the risk of developing MS. These factors can then be studied in greater detail as possible clues to the cause of MS.

There appear to be many factors that combine to increase the risk of developing MS, possibly including infectious agents and environmental, genetic, and immune-system factors. First, MS occurs around the world with much greater frequency in higher latitudes (above 40° latitude) than in lower latitudes, which lie closer to the equator. In the United States, MS occurs more often in the northern states than in the south. Nationwide, there are an estimated 400,000 people with MS. An individual who is born in an area with a higher risk of developing MS and moves to an area of lower risk acquires a risk similar to that of the lower-risk area if the move occurs prior to adolescence. MS is more common among Caucasians (particularly those of northern European ancestry) than other ethnic groups and is almost unheard of in some populations, such as the Inuit. MS is also two to three times as common in women than in men. Although certain outbreaks or clusters of MS have been identified, the cause and significance of these outbreaks is not known. In certain populations, a genetic marker, or trait, has been found to occur more often in people with MS than in those who do not have the disease. Thus far, however, no specific gene has been identified that definitely confers susceptibility to MS. Large-scale research is continuing to try to identify the multiple genes that appear to make people susceptible to MS.

These and other studies have contributed to the opinion that early exposure to an environmental agent might be a triggering factor in people who are predisposed by genetic factors to develop MS.

epilepsy A brain disorder in which clusters of nerve cells in the brain sometimes signal abnormally. The normal pattern of neuronal activity becomes disturbed, causing strange sensations, emotions, and behavior or sometimes convulsions, muscle spasms, and loss of consciousness. This is brought about by brief abnormal electrical discharges in an injured or scarred area of the brain. Epilepsy can be caused by anything that affects the brain, including lesions, tumors, or strokes.

The risk in the general population of developing epilepsy is about 3 percent; the risk of experiencing any type of seizure at some point (including a fever-related seizure) is 10 percent, according to the Epilepsy Foundation. Although some published studies have suggested that seizures occur more commonly in people with multiple sclerosis (MS), experts still do not agree about this. A recent population-based study conducted of Olmstead County, Minnesota, did not find seizures to be more common in people with MS than in the general population.

Symptoms and Diagnostic Path

Seizures may take several forms:

- Generalized tonic-clonic seizures are brief episodes of unconsciousness with uncontrollable jerking movements of the extremities.
- Generalized absence seizures are momentary lapses of consciousness without abnormal movements.
- Partial complex seizures are periods of stereotyped repetitive activity. The person appears to be awake but does not respond to external stimuli.

All of these forms result from sudden changes in the transmission of electrical signals from one cell to another.

Paroxysmal symptoms in MS are brief, sudden attacks of abnormal posturing of the extremities, loss of tone in the legs ("drop attacks") or other manifestations that may appear similar to an epileptic seizure but are of different origin. Examples of paroxysmal symptoms include paroxysmal pain (such as TRIGEMINAL NEURALGIA), tonic spasms of an arm or leg, LHERMITTE'S SIGN (electric shock–like sensation down the spine when the neck is flexed), and UHTHOFF'S SIGN (transient blurring of vision associated with exertion and elevated body temperature).

Treatment Options and Outlook

Anticonvulsants are medications that are designed to prevent convulsions and other types of seizures. Seizures occur in 3 to 5 percent of people with MS, which is somewhat higher than the incidence of epilepsy in the general population. Seizures may occur as part of the disease but may also be related to infection, fever, or abrupt cessation of certain medications.

Epstein-Barr virus (EBV) A very common virus that causes infectious mononucleosis and other disorders and that some experts suspect may be linked to multiple sclerosis (MS). In one study researchers found that 83 percent of a group of children with MS had been exposed to the Epstein-Barr virus, compared to 42 percent of a control group of children without MS. The study included 30 pediatric MS patients and 53 healthy control children. Blood samples from the children in the study were examined to determine exposure to EBV.

Although the findings, which were published in the *Journal of the American Medical Association,* did not indicate that the Epstein-Barr virus is the cause of multiple sclerosis, it does suggest an association between the two.

Once Epstein-Barr virus has infected the body, it remains semidormant in both the immune system and in the throat. It then retains the ability to infect new people via the saliva—hence its nickname "the kissing disease." It does not appear to be transmissable via blood or through the air. In more than half the U.S. population, EBV infections do not cause symptoms. In others, though, the virus often causes infectious mononucleosis with fever, sore throat, and swollen lymph glands. It is rarely fatal in temperate regions, but in the tropics it is associated with two forms of cancer (Burkitt's lymphoma and nasopharyngeal carcinoma).

Experts began to suspect a link between Epstein-Barr virus and MS because several studies have shown that people with MS have higher-than-normal levels of antibodies to the Epstein-Barr virus. As early as 1981, experts suggested that EBV might be linked to MS; several subsequent studies noted that the onset of MS often follows infectious mononucleosis. What makes a link difficult to determine is the fact that people do not usually develop MS during or immediately after their first EBV infection, although the vast majority of people with MS have been previously infected by the virus. Most people have EB antibodies, but most do not develop MS.

Other studies have found higher-than-expected antibodies to EBV proteins, EBV serum DNA, or anti-EBV killer T cells in people with MS. These studies have found significantly higher levels of antibodies to viral proteins such as Epstein-Barr nuclear antigens (EBNA-1 and EBNA-2), viral capsid antigen (VCA), and diffuse early antigen (EA-D). One study found that people with the highest levels of antibodies to EBNA were 33 times more likely to develop MS than people with the lowest levels. Further evidence comes from another study showing that people with MS have elevated counts of anti-EBV killer T cells, suggesting that these cells cross-react with both a section of protein on the EBV and with the same section of protein in myelin. Two studies have found that very few people with MS have no evidence of previous EBV infections. One study also demonstrated that active EBV replication is rarely seen in people with stable MS but is correlated with MS relapses.

Direct action by Epstein-Barr virus in the central nervous system is thought to be an unlikely cause of MS because studies have failed to find any evidence of active virus in MS lesions. Instead, some experts have suggested that a small section of one of the viral proteins resembles a small section of one of the proteins in myelin. Such small sections are known as epitopes and are the means by which the immune system identifies foreign invaders for destruction. Experts suggest that when the immune system detects the identical epitopes in myelin, it is unable to recognize that they belong to self-proteins and attacks them. This results in the damage seen in MS lesions. Such recognition is known as acquired immunity and involves cells known as lymphocytes.

There are two main types of lymphocytes: T cells, which orchestrate the immune response, and B cells, which release antibodies. Both of these cell types are believed to be involved in MS. Usually the immune system does not allow autoreactive lymphocytes (ones that attack their own body) to develop. However, it seems that one myelin protein, myelin oligodendrocyte glycoprotein, is not protected by this process. Further support for the theory comes from the discovery of T cells that are reactive to both EBV and myelin. Additionally, it has been demonstrated in mice that a virus can precipitate EXPERIMENTAL AUTOIMMUNE ENCEPHALOMYELITIS, an animal model of MS.

Increased antibodies to many different viruses have been found in the blood and cerebrospinal fluid of people with MS. This may not necessarily represent disease-causing infection by these viruses. It is more is likely to be the result of non-specific immune activation. The role of a virus as triggering agent of MS is unproven.

erectile dysfunction (ED)   The repeated inability to get or keep an erection firm enough for sexual intercourse. ED can be the total inability to achieve erection, an inconsistent ability to do so, or a tendency to sustain only brief-duration erections. Any disorder—such as multiple sclerosis (MS)—that causes injury to the nerves in the brain, spinal column, and area around the penis has the potential to cause ED.

Within the penis are two chambers filled with spongy tissue that contain smooth muscles, fibrous tissues, veins, and arteries. The urethra, which is the channel for urine and ejaculate, runs along the underside of the chambers. Erection begins as impulses from the brain and local nerves relax the muscles of the penis so that bloods flows in, filling the open spaces in the spongy tissue and making the penis expand. Erection is reversed when muscles in the penis contract, stopping the inflow of blood and opening outflow channels. Since an erection requires a sequence of events, ED can occur when there is a problem with any one or more of these events.

Treatment Options and Outlook

Erectile dysfunction is treatable, and more men have been seeking help and returning to normal sexual activity because of improved, successful treatments.

Drugs for treating impotence can be taken orally, injected directly into the penis, or inserted into the urethra at the tip of the penis. SILDENAFIL (Viagra) was the first oral pill to treat ED. Approved in 1998, Viagra is taken an hour before sex and works by enhancing the effects of nitric oxide, a chemical that relaxes smooth muscles in the penis during sexual stimulation, boosting blood flow.

Levitra, a new pill for erectile dysfunction, has recently been approved—the first new medication for ED since Viagra was approved in 2000. Levitra works by targeting an enzyme important for maintaining an erection. The approval was based on clinical trials that did not include men with MS, but two of the trials did have volunteers with diabetes. Levitra improved sexual function in all the trials. Another recently approved drug to treat erectile dysfunction is Tadalafil, which helps to maintain an erection that has been created by stimulation.

Although these three drugs improve the response to sexual stimulation, they do not trigger an automatic erection as injected drugs do. Patients have also claimed that other oral drugs are effective, including yohimbine hydrochloride, dopamine and serotonin agonists, and trazodone, but no scientific studies have proved the effectiveness of these drugs in relieving ED.

Many men gain potency by injecting drugs into the penis, causing it to become engorged with blood. Drugs such as papaverine hydrochloride, phentolamine, and alprostadil (Caverject) widen blood vessels. However, these drugs may create unwanted side effects, including persistent erection (known as priapism) and scarring. Nitroglycerin, a muscle relaxant, can sometimes enhance erection when rubbed onto the surface of the penis.

A system for inserting a pellet of alprostadil into the urethra is marketed as MUSE. The system uses a prefilled applicator to deliver the pellet about an inch deep into the urethra at the tip of the penis. An erection will begin within eight to 10 minutes and may last 30–60 minutes. The most common side effects of the preparation are aching in the penis, testicles, and area between the penis and rectum; warmth or burning sensation in the urethra; redness of the penis due to increased blood flow; and minor urethral bleeding or spotting.

Mechanical vacuum devices cause erection by creating a partial vacuum around the penis, which draws blood into the penis, engorging and expanding it. The penis is placed into a plastic cylinder, and a pump draws air out of the cylinder. An elastic band is placed around the base of the penis, preventing blood from flowing back into the body, to maintain the erection after the cylinder is removed and during intercourse. A variation of the vacuum device is a semirigid rubber sheath placed on the penis that remains there during sex.

If the above treatments are not successful, surgery may be used to implant a device to cause the penis to become erect, to reconstruct arteries to boost blood flow to the penis, or to block off veins that allow blood to leak from the penile tissues. Implanted devices can restore erections in many men with ED. However, they carry risks of breaking down and causing infection, although mechanical problems have diminished in recent years because of technological advances. Malleable implants usually consist of paired rods, which are inserted surgically into the twin chambers running the length of the penis. The user manually adjusts the position of the penis and, therefore, the rods. Adjustment does not affect the width or length of the penis.

Inflatable implants consist of paired cylinders surgically inserted inside the penis that can be expanded using pressurized fluid. Tubes connect the cylinders to a fluid reservoir and pump, which are also surgically implanted. The patient inflates the cylinders by pressing on the small pump, located under the skin in the scrotum. Inflatable implants can expand the length and width of the penis somewhat. They also leave the penis in a more natural state when not inflated.

See also SEXUAL PROBLEMS.

esophageal reflux   See GASTROESOPHAGEAL REFLUX.

essential fatty acids   Substances that cannot be made by the body and that therefore must be included in the diet to avoid malnutrition. Some people believe that a low-fat diet rich in fatty acids (such as primrose oil [LINOLEIC ACID], sunflower seeds, safflower seeds, corn, or various fish oils) may help patients with multiple sclerosis (MS) because the acids are important in nerve and MYELIN repair.

Although a lack of fatty acids can cause nervous system problems, experts have not been able to prove that eating a lot of essential fatty acids can affect the MS condition.

So far special diets have not suppressed MS exacerbations or improved REMYELINATION of damaged nerve pathways.

estriol   A form of the hormone estrogen that rises to high levels during PREGNANCY. The role of estriol in multiple sclerosis is uncertain.

Pregnant women with MS are known to experience lower exacerbation rates during pregnancy, particularly during the second and third trimesters when the estriol level is highest. Some MS researchers, wondering what causes the protective effect of pregnancy, have focused on estriol, which is also known to affect the immune system.

During pregnancy, the mother's immune system naturally changes so it will not reject the "foreign" baby, also lessening the likelihood that the immune system will attack the mother's central nervous system.

In a pilot study funded by the National MS Society, 12 nonpregnant women, half with relapsing-remitting and half with SECONDARY PROGRESSIVE MS, were given six months of estriol. (The trial had a crossover design, so all 12 eventually received the treatment.) Brain scans documented an 80 percent drop in inflammatory lesions in the six women with RELAPSING-REMITTING MS while they were on the active treatment. Inflammatory protein levels also dropped. The six women with secondary progressive MS did not improve significantly.

Future longer studies will assess the use of estriol with more women. If the results confirm estriol's benefit, researchers will conduct still longer studies for three to five years. Only longer studies can establish whether estriol can also reduce relapse rates and whether or not it is safe for long-term use.

If it proves both effective and safe, it would be the first oral drug treatment for MS.

Research published in the April 2004 issue of the *Journal of Neuroimmunology* suggests that there is a potential role for estriol treatment in men as well as in women. The study found that experimental autoimmune encephalomyelitis (EAE) severity in both women and men was eased with estriol treatment as compared to placebo. Also, pro-inflammatory cytokine production slowed down with estriol treatment in both women and men. These data, say the study authors, support a potential role for estriol treatment for men in addition to women with MS.

ethnicity and MS   Multiple sclerosis is found throughout the world, but it is most common in Caucasian people of northern European origin, especially those of Scottish and Scandinavian descent. It is extremely rare among Asians and Africans.

evening primrose oil   See LINEOLIC ACID.

evoked potentials   A group of tests that measures electrical activity in certain parts of the brain in response to stimulation of specific sensory nerve pathways. These tests are often used to help make a diagnosis of multiple sclerosis (MS), because they can pinpoint dysfunction along these pathways that is too subtle to be noticed or to show up on a NEUROLOGIC EXAMINATION.

People with MS have damaged MYELIN, the fatty sheath protecting nerve fibers in the central nervous system. This damage slows, garbles, or halts nerve impulses altogether, producing the symptoms of MS.

In order to measure evoked potentials, wires are placed onto the scalp over the areas of the brain being tested. The examiner then provides specific types of stimulation and records the person's responses. Evoked potential testing is harmless, painless, and very sensitive in detecting damaged areas.

It usually takes about two hours to do all three types of evoked potentials. The results are interpreted by a neurologist or neurophysiologist with specialized training in the use of these tests. A fourth type of test (motor evoked potentials) can detect lesions along motor pathways of the central nervous system, but they are not widely used to diagnose MS.

Although evoked potentials are used to help diagnose MS, other conditions also produce abnormal results, so the tests are not specific for this condition. The information the tests provide needs to be considered along with other laboratory and clinical information before a diagnosis of MS can be made.

Types of Evoked Potential Tests

Visual evoked response (VER)   Also known as the visually evoked potential (VEP) test, this test measures the speed of the brain's electrical activity in response to visual stimuli. It is a test to determine the presence of OPTIC NEURITIS or other evidence of DEMYELINATION along the optic nerve or the optic pathways.

VERs are very sensitive at measuring slowed responses to visual events and can often detect dysfunction not possible to find through clinical evaluation. Typically the patient is unaware of any visual problems. Because this test can identify silent lesions and demyelination, it is a very useful diagnostic tool.

A definite diagnosis of MS requires at least two distinct demyelinating episodes in two different central nervous system sites separated by at least one month. This test can often provide evidence of such episodes when other tests—including MAGNETIC RESONANCE IMAGING—cannot.

In this test, the patient must focus on a black-and-white checked pattern in the center of a TV screen. Each square in the pattern alternates between black and white at measured intervals. The patient wears a patch on one eye for a while and then on the other so that the speed of both optic nerves can be measured. Each pattern reversal stimulates a nerve transmission along the optic nerve, the optic chiasm, and the optic tract, which eventually stimulates the brain to generate a large electrical potential that is detectable on the electroencephalogram (EEG) sensors. White matter lesions anywhere along this pathway will slow or even stop the signal. Between 85 and 90 percent of people with a definite diagnosis of MS, and 58 percent of people with probable MS, will have abnormal VEP test results.

Other conditions causing a similar abnormal test result would include Friedreich's ataxia, vitamin B_{12} deficiency, and neurosyphilis.

Brain stem auditory evoked potentials (BAEP)   This test measures the speed of impulses along the auditory portion of the eighth cranial nerve—the nerve that transmits auditory information from the ear to the brain stem. Lesions in the pons area of the brain stem can slow down nerve impulses from the ear, which can be detected in changes in EEG brain activity.

In the test, the patient is fitted with electrodes to the earlobe and skull and then lies down in a darkened room to prevent visual signals from interfering with measurements. A series of clicks and beeps are played back to the patient, which can be detected as a series of clicks in each ear. About 67 percent of people with definite MS and 41 percent of people with probable MS will have abnormal BAEP test results.

This test has many similar names, including brain stem auditory evoked response (BAER), auditory brain response (ABR), and auditory evoked potential (AEP).

Sensory evoked potentials (SEP)   Short electrical impulses are administered to an arm or leg. The SEP (also called the somatosensory evoked potential test) involves strapping an electrical stimulus around an arm or leg. A low-voltage current is switched on briefly, and electrodes on the back and skull painlessly measure the response at particular junctions. The speed of various nerves can be measured in this way; points where the signal slows down suggest lesions where the myelin has been destroyed. An estimated 77 percent of people with definite MS and 67 percent of people with probable MS will have abnormal SEP test results. Abnormalities with SEPS are not specific for MS and can be abnormal due to other disease processes.

exacerbation   A sudden worsening of a multiple sclerosis (MS) symptom or the appearance of new symptoms. To be considered an exacerbation, the condition must last at least 24 hours and be separated from a previous exacerbation by at least one month. The most common disease course in MS, called RELAPSING-REMITTING MS, is characterized by clearly defined acute exacerbations followed by complete or partial recovery with no progression of the disease between attacks.

A true exacerbation of MS is caused by an area of inflammation in the central nervous system followed by DEMYELINATION—the destruction of MYELIN, the fatty sheath that surrounds and protects the nerve fibers. Demyelination causes an abnormal area called a plaque, which slows, distorts, or halts nerve impulses, producing MS symptoms.

An exacerbation may be mild or may significantly interfere with the individual's daily life. Exacerbations usually last from several days to several weeks, although they may extend into months. Most experts believe that a short course of corticosteroids will shorten an exacerbation or make it less severe. Of course, not every exacerbation means that MS is getting worse. Sometimes an increase in symptom activity has nothing to do with the underlying MS but is caused by other things, such as stress, fever, infection, or hot weather that can temporarily aggravate MS problems. This is referred to as a PSEUDOEXACERBATION.

exercise   Exercise is a good way to help manage many symptoms of multiple sclerosis (MS). Although exercise will not affect the disease process, a good exercise program can help develop the maximum potential of muscle, bone, and breathing. Exercise can also help patients avoid complications, such as bladder and bowel dysfunction, osteoporosis, permanent muscle contractions, ulcerations of the skin, or abnormal blood clotting.

In fact studies have shown that patients who participated in an aerobic exercise program had better cardiovascular fitness, improved strength, better bladder and bowel function, less fatigue and depression, and a more positive attitude. People with MS who do not get enough exercise can experience weakened muscles, decreased bone density with an increased risk of fracture, and shallow, inefficient breathing.

However, MS symptoms can temporarily worsen during physical activity, if the person becomes overheated, so any program must be planned carefully. People with MS also should be careful not to overexercise since overheating can trigger symptoms and worsen fatigue. Cooling strategies are an important part of an exercise plan. A doctor or physical therapist should be consulted to determine the best form of physical activity for a particular patient.

Which Exercise to Choose

There is not one specific exercise that is best for people with MS. The most important factor when patients choose an exercise program is to find something they enjoy, because maintaining an exercise program is difficult if the person does not like the activity. Other factors to consider are access to equipment, safety with transfers to and from equipment, and group versus individual exercise. An exercise program also needs to be appropriate to a patient's ability and limitations and may need to be adjusted as MS worsens.

A physical therapist experienced with the unique and varied symptoms of MS can help design, supervise, and revise an exercise program.

Stretching and range-of-motion exercises are important because they can alleviate some muscle SPASTICITY. Specific exercises that strengthen and increase the endurance of muscles that control breathing functions may be helpful. (It is not yet known if such exercises reduce lung complications over the long term.) Pool exercises with water temperature less than 82°F are particularly helpful since water can support the body while the cool water dissipates heat.

Exercise Tips

Exercise programs must be designed to stimulate working muscles while avoiding overload and overheating, which can block nerve conduction. Periods of exercise should be timed to avoid the hotter times of the day and prevent excessive fatigue. Patients should also avoid exercising first thing in the morning, when they are tired or sleepy, or after eating a large meal. Patients should not exercise for at least seven hours after drinking alcohol, especially those with GAIT PROBLEMS or balance problems.

Patients should drink lots of water before and after every exercise session, and they should urinate before beginning. Warm-up and cool-down exercises are vital, and patients who wear ORTHOTIC devices should keep them on while exercising. Patients should work out on a soft surface (a rubber mat or rug), wearing light, padded shoes. The exercise area should be large and well ventilated, free from objects that the patient could bump into. Frequent rests during exercise are important for patients with MS.

Wheelchair Exercises

Even patients who use wheelchairs can—and should—exercise as often as possible. Before beginning an exercise program, wheelchair-bound patients should discuss a program with their doctor and PHYSICAL THERAPIST and find out which exercises would be the most useful. Just as with other MS patients, those in a wheelchair should not exercise to the point of exhaustion. Patients who have lost the use of their legs can instead concentrate on their arms and upper torso. Exercise is particularly recommended for these patients because sitting in a wheelchair for long periods of time can trigger problems such as stiffness, poor circulation, BEDSORES, sluggish bowels, and depression. Exercises involving range of motion, stretching, strengthening, balance, and aerobics are all important for someone who is not ambulatory.

See also WATER EXERCISE.

expanded disability status scale (EDSS) One of the oldest and most widely used rating systems for judging the condition of people with multiple sclerosis (MS). The EDSS is an expansion and refinement of the KURTZKE DISABILITY STATUS SCALE (DSS), both of which were developed by neurologist John Kurtzke, M.D.

The EDSS is measured in one-half-step increments, from 0.0 (normal) to 10.0 (death). In order to rate a person on the EDSS, a neurologist first performs a standard neurological examination to test strength, coordination, vision, walking, and so on. The neurologist next summarizes the results of the neurological examination in several functional system scores such as strength and SPASTICITY, vision, bowel and bladder, and so on. Finally, the neurologist uses the functional system scores, along with the patient's ability to walk, to rate the individual on the EDSS.

Although it is widely used in research, the EDSS is limited to some extent because it appears to be measuring different functions at different levels. Scores on the less severe end of the scale are more dependent upon nuances in a number of MS symptoms; those in the middle range are more dependent upon walking; those in the more impaired range depend upon self-care ability. Most important, evidence indicates that the EDSS may not be sensitive enough to symptom changes that occur over time.

Although a few neurologists use the EDSS to track the course of individual patients, it is mostly used as a benchmark in clinical trials. In spite of its limitations, the EDSS represents a familiar and widely used standard.

Expanded Disability Status Scale

- 0.0: normal neurological exam
- 1.0–1.5: no disability but with some abnormal signs on the neurological exam
- 2.0–5.5: disability is present but able to walk without mechanical or human assistance
- 6.0: needs a single cane, crutch, or brace in order to walk
- 6.5: needs two canes, two crutches, or two braces in order to walk
- 7.0–7.5: may be able to take a few steps but needs a wheelchair for mobility
- 8.0: not able to walk; restricted to a wheelchair
- 8.5–9.5: restricted to bed
- 10.0: death due to MS

experimental autoimmune encephalomyelitis (EAE) An autoimmune disease induced in laboratory rodents that produces symptoms similar to human multiple sclerosis (MS). Before testing on humans, a potential treatment for MS may first be tested on laboratory animals with EAE in order to determine the treatment's efficacy and safety.

extensor spasm A symptom of SPASTICITY in which the legs straighten suddenly into a stiff, extended position. These spasms, which typically last for several minutes, occur most commonly in bed at night or on rising from bed.

extrapyramidal system   A network of nerve pathways that link nerve nuclei in the surface of the cerebrum, the basal ganglia deep within the brain, and some of the brain stem. It is a collective term for those structures involved in the central nervous control of motor function other than the pyramidal tracts and their connections.

Damage to any part of this system, as can happen with the lesions of multiple sclerosis, may interfere with voluntary movements or muscle tone.

eye movements   See NYSTAGMUS.

eye problems   Many signs of multiple sclerosis (MS) involve the eyes, including changes in the ability to see clearly (visual acuity), abnormal pupil responses, changes in the appearance of the optic nerve, unusual eye movements, pale optic disks, DOUBLE VISION, limits in the field of vision, and visual field disturbances.

If the optic nerve is damaged, the pupils will not respond normally to light. Normally pupils con-strict in bright light to reduce the amount of light entering the eye. In patients with a damaged optic nerve, the affected eye does not respond as quickly to bright light, producing a reaction called MARCUS GUNN PUPIL. In this case, the pupil constricts in the abnormal eye when a bright light is shined into the normal eye. The pupil then dilates when the light is shined into the abnormal eye, because this eye is stimulated more by light perceived by the good eye. The Marcus Gunn response may be the only abnormal symptom in patients with mild MS.

Unusual eye movements are another type of problem often seen in MS patients. These may appear as severe or slight up-and-down or side-to-side eye movements when the patient looks up and down or side to side, respectively. There are different patterns of these unusual eye movements (called NYSTAGMUS). One particularly typical pattern of nystagmus is called internuclear ophthalmoplegia, in which looking-to-the-side nystagmus appears only in the eye looking inward but does not appear when the eye turns inward to focus on an incoming object.

facial pain   See TRIGEMINAL NEURALGIA.

Faeroe Islands outbreak   Although multiple sclerosis (MS) is not believed to be contagious, one of the most widely quoted epidemiological studies of MS uncovered a much higher prevalence of MS in the Faeroe Islands (between Iceland and Scandinavia) after the wartime occupation by 1,500–2,000 British troops between 1941 and 1944.

Four separate CLUSTERS OF MS outbreaks occurred between 1943 and 1989 in the Faeroe Islands. The incidence of MS increased each year for 20 years after the war, leading some researchers to think that the troops might have brought with them some disease-causing agent.

Some scientists have classified the Faeroe Islands cluster as an epidemic, although other researchers have challenged this view. In any case, the MS prevalence clearly and substantially increased in the Faeroes following the British occupation. Furthermore, the relationship between MS in the Faeroe islanders and the presence of British soldiers is strongly supported by the fact that the cases of MS all occurred in islanders who lived close to British bases. This demonstrates that the environmental factor can be transported from one area to another. Similar outbreaks were reported in the Shetland and Orkney Islands, in Iceland, and in Sardinia.

Falana, Lola (1942–)   An entertainer diagnosed with multiple sclerosis (MS) in 1987, which effectively ended her show-business career. During the 1970s, Falana made millions as a Las Vegas singing star. After her diagnosis, she left that career to work for the poor and concentrate on being a poet, motivational speaker, civic activist, and Catholic evangelist.

She was born Loletha Elaine Falana on September 11, 1942, in Camden, New Jersey, after her Cuban father came to the United States to work as a welder. At age five, Falana was singing in the church choir. Music was so much a part of Falana's life that she left Germantown High School a few months before graduation to begin her career in show business.

She was working at dancing jobs in Harlem when one day Sammy Davis, Jr., spotted her and cast her as the lead dancer in his Broadway musical *Golden Boy.* Falana sang on her first record, *My Baby,* for Mercury Records in 1965 and starred in the Broadway musical *Dr. Jazz* in 1975, for which she was nominated for a Tony Award. She also made regular appearances on *The New Bill Cosby Show, Laugh-In,* Bob Hope specials, and other variety shows. When she was tapped as the commercial pitchwoman for Faberge's product Tigress, she became the first African-American spokesperson for a major perfume.

By the late 1970s Falana was a Las Vegas star. In 1984 she joined the cast of the CBS soap opera, *Capitol,* but three years later she was diagnosed with MS. At first crippled and partially blinded, Falana recovered somewhat over the next two years and returned briefly to Las Vegas until 1989, when she permanently retired from show business.

famous people with MS   A number of well-known people from all walks of life have been diagnosed with multiple sclerosis (MS), including

• Sir AUGUSTUS FREDERIC d'ESTE: a grandson of King George III of Great Britain who provides the second documented case of a person with MS

- JOAN DIDION: journalist and novelist
- JACQUELINE DU PRÉ: cellist
- LOLA FALANA: singer
- DONNA FARGO: country and western singer
- ANNETTE FUNICELLO: singer, dancer, child star, and former Mouseketeer
- ROMAN GABRIEL: football player, Los Angeles Rams, 1962–72
- TERI GARR: actress
- LENA HORNE: singer and actress
- DAVID HUMM: NFL quarterback, Oakland Raiders
- BARBARA JORDAN: Congresswoman, professor, civil rights activist
- LIDWINA of SCHIEDAM: Dutch patron saint of ice skaters and the earliest written record (c. 1400) of someone with MS
- ALAN OSMOND: Osmond Brothers singer
- RICHARD PRYOR: comedian and actor
- JAMES SCOFIELD: poet
- PAUL WELLSTONE: U.S. senator, Minnesota
- MONTEL WILLIAMS: talk show host

In addition, a number of well-known celebrities have or had close relatives with the disease. They include

- baseball player Wade Boggs (sister)
- singer Gloria Estefan (father)
- designer Tommy Hilfiger (sister)
- TV news anchor Larry Kane (mother)
- journalist Stone Phillips (wife)
- author J.K. Rowling (mother)
- actor Adam Sandler (cousin)

fampridine-SR   See AMINOPYRIDINE.

Fargo, Donna (1949–)   Country and western singer who was diagnosed with multiple sclerosis (MS) in 1979.

Born November 10, 1949 in Mt. Airy, North Carolina, Donna Fargo was the daughter of a tobacco farmer. She began singing in church as a child and

grew up to become a school teacher. She was discovered by her future husband, record producer Stan Silver, when she was singing in a Los Angeles club.

Fargo wrote and recorded the 1972 country/pop hit "Happiest Girl in The Whole USA." The song became a pop-and-country best seller and won Fargo a Grammy; she followed up with a string of hits, including "Funny Face." In 1979 she discovered she had MS, but she continued performing and recording.

fatigue   Feeling of pervasive tiredness. Fatigue is typical among people with multiple sclerosis (MS), affecting up to 80 percent of patients. It can significantly interfere with a patient's ability to function at home and at work and is the most common reason why they have to quit their jobs. The cause of MS-related fatigue is not known.

The fatigue common with MS is not like the tiredness that healthy people experience. MS-related fatigue usually occurs every day and may appear early in the morning even after a restful night's sleep. It tends to get worse as the day progresses and may be aggravated by heat and humidity. MS-related fatigue appears easily and suddenly, is generally more severe than normal fatigue, and is more likely to interfere with daily responsibilities. However, MS-related fatigue does not appear to be directly linked with either depression or the degree of physical impairment.

In addition to the primary fatigue or lassitude caused by MS, there are many other factors that can contribute to feelings of tiredness. Patients who feel very tired during the day may actually not be getting enough sleep at night because of pain, depression, or medication reactions.

Treatment Options and Outlook
Primary MS fatigue can be improved with a variety of medications; the most commonly prescribed are AMANTADINE (Symmetrel) and MODAFINIL (Provigil). Although neither is approved specifically by the U.S Food and Drug Administration for the treatment of MS-related fatigue, each has been shown in clinical trials to relieve the symptoms of fatigue for many people with MS.

Symmetrel was originally prescribed to treat Parkinson's disease and Asian flu. Although researchers know that Symmetrel helps release the neurotransmitter dopamine from the basal ganglia in the brain, they are not sure why this would dramatically improve exhaustion in MS patients, as it clearly does. Physicians have found that patients who take this drug experience a definite improvement in energy and their general outlook on life. In addition, this drug can improve tremor; it is therefore sometimes prescribed just for this reason.

The side effects of this drug are typically minor, including dry mouth and jitteriness. Blurred vision can occur, which may cause problems for patients who are already experiencing the visual inflammation (OPTIC NEURITIS) common in MS. Other side effects include CONSTIPATION, DIZZINESS, and a skin condition called livedo reticularis, which produce purple blotches on the skin.

Other drugs that may be prescribed include the central nervous system stimulants PEMOLINE (Cylert) or methylphenidate (Ritalin) or certain antidepressants. However, pemoline has various side effects that require careful monitoring, and clinical trials with this drug have shown conflicting results.

Occupational therapy can help patients simplify tasks at work and home. Physical therapy can help people learn energy-saving ways of walking (with or without assistive devices) and performing other daily tasks. Sleep regulation, which might involve treating other MS symptoms and using sleep medications on a short-term basis, can help ease fatigue in some patients. Alternatively, psychological interventions such as stress management, relaxation training, support groups, or psychotherapy may help. Managing how hot the patient becomes is also important since overheating can worsen fatigue.

Caffeinated drinks may improve fatigue as well, although the initial energy boost they provide is usually followed some hours later by a concomitant letdown.

fatigue impact scale A test that provides an assessment of the effects of FATIGUE in terms of physical, cognitive, and psychosocial functioning.

fecal incontinence The lack of ability to control bowel movements. This condition does not usually occur in patients with multiple sclerosis (MS). However, some individuals who lose strength and sensation below the waist can no longer control their bowel movements. Some people with MS report that a sensation of abdominal gas warns them of impending fecal incontinence. Even in those who maintain good bowel control, taking drugs to manage other problems (such as antibiotics to treat bladder infections) may irritate the intestines and cause fecal incontinence.

Treatment Options and Outlook

Incontinence can usually be managed over time, especially if a regular schedule of elimination can be established. When the bowel becomes used to emptying at specific intervals, accidents at other times are less likely. Eating a regular diet can help develop a rhythm that makes the situation easier to manage. Right after eating, the intestinal activity will increase, and a bowel movement is likely to occur. Sitting on the toilet at that time may avoid accidental soiling.

Dietary irritants such as caffeine and alcohol can contribute to the problem and should be eliminated. In addition, medications that reduce SPASTICITY in striated muscle (especially baclofen [Lioresal] and tizanidine [Zanaflex]) may also contribute to the problem.

Anticholinergic drugs can ease symptoms if a hyperactive bowel is the underlying cause of incontinence. In addition to drugs, biofeedback may help train an individual to be sensitive to subtle signals that the rectum is filling. Meanwhile, protective underwear can be used to prevent embarrassing accidents.

In a few rare instances, fecal incontinence becomes such a significant problem that the patient may elect to have a colostomy, in which the intestines are surgically altered so they can void into a bag on the front of the abdomen. Patients who face years of bowel problems may prefer this method rather than having to live in diapers. However, because bowel control may improve over time, a colostomy should not be performed unless the patient has tried other methods for at least a year.

fertility and MS   Multiple sclerosis (MS) does not affect the basic fertility of either men or women, nor does it lead to an increased number of spontaneous abortions, stillbirths, or congenital malformations. Several studies of large numbers of women have repeatedly demonstrated that pregnancy, labor, delivery, and the incidence of fetal complications are no different in women who have MS than in control groups of women without the disease.

However, sexual problems may interfere with the ability of a man with MS to father a baby. Dry orgasms—a condition that may impair fertility—have been reported by men with MS in several studies. These problems have been successfully treated with medication or through techniques to harvest sperm for insemination. Men who are concerned about fertility issues should consult a urologist experienced in this area.

finger-to-nose test   A test of coordination problems (DYSMETRIA) and INTENTION TREMOR, two common symptoms in multiple sclerosis, that is part of the standard NEUROLOGICAL EXAMINATION. In this test, the person is asked to close the eyes and touch the tip of the nose with the tip of the index finger.

flaccid big bladder   A serious type of BLADDER DYSFUNCTION that can occur among patients with multiple sclerosis. This happens due to damage of the MYELIN covering of nerves near the voiding reflex center (a group of nerves found along the lower spinal cord). When myelin in this area is damaged or removed, it can eliminate signals that order the bladder to contract when urination is necessary. As a result, the bladder becomes flaccid and unable to empty on cue. Eventually the bladder becomes so stretched that it overflows, leading to dribbling and incontinence. Sometimes, if the urine remains for too long in the bladder, infections can result.

Treatment Options and Outlook

In this type of condition, treatment is aimed at helping the bladder empty more efficiently or at lowering the number of times a patient must urinate a day. Several drugs can help, although these medications are usually more helpful for a SPASTIC SMALL BLADDER than a flaccid large one. In some cases, taking the antispasticity drug Lioresal

(BACLOFEN)—used by patients with SPASTICITY problems—can be effective. More commonly the drug oxybutynin (Ditropan) may be prescribed once or twice a day. It can be taken as needed, such as before leaving the house. However, this drug has a narrow therapeutic range before it becomes toxic, so dosage levels must be carefully monitored.

Another commonly used drug is Pro-Banthine, an anticholinergic antispasmodic muscle relaxant that is less effective—but less toxic—than oxybutynin. Pro-Banthine works by blocking nerve impulses in the parasympathetic nerve endings, blocking muscle contractions and bladder spasms. Although it has fewer side effects than oxybutynin, it may cause drowsiness, rapid heartbeat, and CONSTIPATION. This drug should not be taken with megadoses of vitamin C or antacids, which may make Pro-Banthine less effective.

The antidepressant imipramine (Tofranil) is occasionally prescribed to relax the mechanism that opens the bladder. This drug also can boost mood and combat depression.

All of these medications also reduce the frequency of bathroom trips by increasing the volume of urine passed each time.

Alternatively, the nasal spray DDAVP (desmopressin acetate) is a different kind of medication that reduces the amount of urine in the kidneys.

If medication does not control the flaccid big bladder, the next step is catheterization. INTERMITTENT SELF-CATHETERIZATION, in which a catheter is placed by the patient, is safe and effective. For those who cannot manage this, however, an INDWELLING CATHETER may be used. This type of catheter is placed by a doctor and left in place.

flexor spasm   Involuntary, sometimes painful contractions of the flexor muscles, which pull the legs upward into a clenched position. These spasms, which last two to three seconds, are symptoms of SPASTICITY. They often occur during sleep but can also occur when the person is awake and in a seated position.

flu vaccine   The vaccine to protect against influenza is given every year. The injectable vaccine can be given safely to patients with multiple sclerosis (MS) without increased risk of triggering a flare-up of symptoms. However, the nasal spray flu vaccine—a live vaccine—should not be given to patients with MS.

See also IMMUNIZATIONS AND MS.

focal deficits Impaired strength or sensation over parts of the body.

foot drop A weakness in the muscles of the foot and ankle that interferes with a person's ability to flex the ankle and walk with a normal heel-toe pattern. Instead the toes touch the ground before the heel, causing the person to trip or lose balance. Foot drop is a neurological disturbance caused by a malfunction either in the central nervous system or in a peripheral nerve.

See also ORTHOTICS; PHYSICAL THERAPIST.

forearm crutch A crutch designed to fit around the forearm just below the elbow with a flexible cuff, instead of under the arms, allowing the patient to use the hands without dropping the crutches. Unlike normal underarm crutches, forearm crutches do not put constant pressure on the underarm, which can cause nerve damage. Forearm crutches can be used by patients with multiple sclerosis (MS) whose balance and strength are severely affected and who have too little strength in their arms to use CANES. Crutches also provide more stability than canes.

Forearm crutches are more appropriate for people with long-term needs, such as MS patients. Cuffs that adjust in length above the handgrip afford the most comfort. Some forearm crutch models have telescoping mechanisms that retract the shaft for easy transport.

See also ASSISTIVE DEVICES; WALKERS; WHEEL-CHAIRS.

forgetfulness Minor MEMORY lapses are usually completely normal and are probably not a symptom of multiple sclerosis (MS). Many perfectly healthy individuals experience moments of forgetfulness; forgetting the whereabouts of everyday items such as glasses or car keys is normal. Patients with MS who begin to have more serious instances of forgetfulness may want to consult a physician.

forms of multiple sclerosis The clinical course of multiple sclerosis (MS) usually falls within one of four categories, although a patient may progress from one pattern to another. The categories include RELAPSE-REMITTING MS, PRIMARY PROGRESSIVE MS, PROGRESSIVE-RELAPSING MS, and SECONDARY PROGRESSIVE MS.

The primary progressive (PP) form of MS is characterized by disease progression with occasional plateaus and temporary minor improvements.

The progressive-relapsing (PR) form of MS is characterized by progressive disease at the onset with acute relapses, with or without full recovery. Periods between relapses are characterized by continuing symptom progression. This is considered to be a rare form of the disease.

The relapsing-remitting form of MS is characterized by clearly defined disease relapses (flare-ups) with full recovery or with residual deficits after recovery. During the periods between relapses, the disease does not get gradually worse.

The secondary progressive (SP) form of MS is characterized by initial relapsing-remitting disease followed by progression with or without occasional relapses, minor remissions, and plateaus.

France All of France falls within the high-frequency zone for multiple sclerosis (MS). The nationwide prevalence rate is at least 50 per 100,000 population, and there is evidence of geographic clustering of the disease. The geographic distribution of MS within the 95 departments and the 21 regions of France was defined from a 1986 nationwide prevalence series derived from questionnaires. This indicated a significant clustering of high-frequency regions in the northeastern part of the country, with most significantly low areas in the south and west. Distributions were similar to those for MS death rates by department and region for 1968 through 1977, indicating geographic stability over time. However, evidence also indicated diffusion over time. The 1986 prevalence distribution was also compared with all published prevalence rates for communities in France.

free radicals   Highly reactive forms of oxygen created in cells during normal metabolic processes that are capable of causing damage in brain and other tissues. When free radicals interact with the lipids that compose cell membranes and vessel walls, they convert the lipids to inactive solids that cause slow but steady cellular death. Because free-radical oxidants are so destructive, the brain and blood must have an ample supply of antioxidants in order to survive. Antioxidants are chemicals that oxygen finds more attractive than the structural components of cells. In a sense, antioxidants sacrifice themselves to preserve the body.

Since free radicals are the natural result of the body's metabolic reactions, the body is able to neutralize them with various antioxidant enzymes that it produces. For example, superoxide radicals are created in brain cells as a by-product of energy production in the mitochondria. These free radicals are immediately broken down by the superoxide dismutase, which is one of the body's own antioxidant enzymes. Humans also depend on essential antioxidants from the daily diet.

The environment has become a perpetual source of free radical contamination, primarily from radiation and the chemical pollution in the air, water, and food. Americans today are overwhelmed with more free radicals than their bodies can neutralize.

Some patients use antioxidant vitamins or supplements (vitamins A, E, or C; coenzyme Q10; pycnogenol; or grape seed extract) to try to treat symptoms of multiple sclerosis (MS) since the destruction of myelin in the disease process may be partly due to chemical damage from free radicals. Some experts warn, however, that antioxidants can trigger production of inflammatory components of the immune system (such as T cells and macrophages) and therefore may pose some danger to MS patients.

The safety of taking antioxidants for people with MS has not been established. One small, five-week study indicates that antioxidants are safe for people with MS, but the study is too small and short to be conclusive. In addition, antioxidant vitamins stimulate the immune system in laboratory experiments and in some groups of people. In MS, where an overactive immune system appears to be part of the disease process, stimulation may be dangerous.

The most reasonable course may be for people to obtain antioxidants by eating two to four servings of fruits and three to four servings of vegetables every day. If antioxidant supplements are used, it may be best to use them in moderation. There is limited evidence suggesting that antioxidants may be beneficial, and there is also some evidence suggesting potential harm.

The details of the immune system are complex, but in general it may be best to assume that in MS, immune stimulation may be dangerous and immune down-regulation may be beneficial. Accordingly, supplements that are supposed to "boost" or "improve" immune function may be the worst choice for people with MS.

Frerichs, Friedrich Theodor von (1819–1885)   German pathologist who brought medical recognition of multiple sclerosis (MS) a step closer by elaborating in 1849 on the clinical description of MS provided by Jean CRUVEILHIER and identifying specific symptoms and key features of the illness.

Ten years after the first illustrations of neuronal lesions had been published, experts still did not know much about the clinical symptoms of MS. Frerichs's clinical account for the first time recognized that remissions were a characteristic feature of MS. In addition, he described unusual eye movements (NYSTAGMUS) as a symptom of the disease. This visual sign was later incorporated into the famous triple description of symptoms called Charcot's triad.

Frerichs also provided the first medical description of mental disorders in MS, recognizing the possible impact of the disease on cognitive behavior and other higher functions of the brain.

frontal lobe   The front part of the brain and an important center of voluntary and planned motor behaviors, such as voluntary movement of the eyes, the trunk, and the many muscles used for speech. The motor speech area is usually in the frontal lobe of the left hemisphere no matter which hemisphere is dominant.

Functional Independence Measure (FIM)   A test of function in multiple areas, including feeding, grooming, bathing, dressing, toileting, transferring, walking, comprehension, expression, social interaction, and problem solving.

Funicello, Annette (1942–) Singer, dancer, child star, and former Mouseketeer who was diagnosed with multiple sclerosis (MS) in 1987. Because of the disease, she retired from her stage and screen career.

Annette Joanne Funicello was born October 22, 1942, in Utica, New York, and moved to California when she was four. Eight years later, Walt Disney was in the audience as she performed at age 12 as the lead dancer in a school production of *Swan Lake*. One last slot remained to be filled to complete the 24 original Mousekeeters planned as part of the *Mickey Mouse Club* TV program of the 1950s, and she was asked to audition for the remaining Mousekeeter opening. Funicello was introduced to America with the rest of the Mouseketeers in a national TV special in 1955 that coincided with the opening of Disneyland.

She went on to star in several Walt Disney movies, including *Babes in Toyland* and *The Monkey's Uncle*. She became a successful pop music recording artist in the late 1950s and early 1960s. During the 1960s she and actor Frankie Avalon starred in a series of beach party movies.

She first noticed signs of what would be diagnosed as MS while working on the 1987 film *Back to the Beach;* five years later she made her diagnosis public. She established the Annette Funicello Fund for Neurological Disorders at the California Community Foundation in 1993 and a year later published her autobiography, *A Dream Is a Wish Your Heart Makes.*

gabapentin (Neurontin) An antiepileptic drug used to control some types of seizures in epilepsy. Although not approved for this purpose, it is also used in patients with multiple sclerosis (MS) to control neuropathic pain caused by MS lesions and to reduce abnormal sensory sensations that occur in the absence of stimulation (DYSESTHESIA). Gabapentin may also be effective in easing SPASTICITY.

Side Effects

Side effects that typically go away as the body adjusts to the medication and do not require medical attention unless they continue include:

- blurred or double vision
- dizziness
- drowsiness
- muscle aches
- swelling of hands or legs
- tremor
- unusual fatigue or weakness
- diarrhea
- frequent urination
- indigestion
- low blood pressure
- slurred speech
- sleep difficulty

Patients should consult a doctor as soon as possible if any of the following side effects occur:

- clumsiness or unsteadiness
- continuous uncontrolled eye movements
- depression or mood changes

- memory problems
- hoarseness
- lower back pain
- painful or difficult urination

Symptoms of overdose requiring immediate attention include:

- double vision
- severe diarrhea
- dizziness or drowsiness
- slurred speech

Patients taking gabapentin should not use alcohol and other central nervous system depressants that may cause drowsiness (such as antihistamines, sedatives, tranquilizers, prescription pain medications, seizure medications, and muscle relaxants), because the combination will intensify their effects. Stopping this drug abruptly may cause seizures.

Gabriel, Roman (1940–) Football player for the Los Angeles Rams from 1962 to 1972, who retired after the 1977 season and has been diagnosed with multiple sclerosis. Born August 5, 1940, in Wilmington, North Carolina, he was a starting quarterback at North Carolina State University.

gadolinium The common name given to a range of compounds of the chemical element gadolinium that are used to enhance MAGNETIC RESONANCE IMAGING (MRI) and distinguish between old and new lesions. In multiple sclerosis (MS), gadolinium-enhanced lesions that appear on MRI tend to be associated with an inflammatory response, which is typical of the relapsing-remitting form of the disease. This inflammatory response is seen less often in the secondary progressive and the primary progressive forms.

Compounds of gadolinium are used in MRI scans and work by altering the local magnetic field in MS lesions, thus enhancing the MRI image. Gadolinium is harmless except to the very small number of people who have an allergic reaction to it (about one per 20,000).

gadolinium-enhancing lesion A lesion appearing on MAGNETIC RESONANCE IMAGING after injection of the chemical compound GADOLINIUM, which reveals a breakdown in the BLOOD-BRAIN BARRIER. This breakdown of the blood-brain barrier indicates either a newly active lesion or the reactivation of an old one.

gait problems Difficulty in walking is among the most common movement limitations in people with multiple sclerosis (MS). It is usually related to weakness, SPASTICITY, loss of balance, sensory deficits, and FATIGUE.

Muscle WEAKNESS is one of the most common causes of gait problems, leading to toe drag, FOOT DROP, and other gait abnormalities. Weakness in both legs is known as paraparesis; weakness in only one leg is monoparesis. Patients who feel weak may compensate by using appropriate exercises and assistive devices, including braces, canes, or walkers.

Muscle tightness or spasticity can also interfere with gait. Antispasticity medications such as baclofen or tizanidine are usually helpful in treating this symptom. Stretching exercises are also helpful.

BALANCE PROBLEMS typically cause a swaying gait known as ATAXIA (or gait ataxia). People with severe ataxia may be helped by using an assistive device.

Some people with MS have such severe NUMBNESS in their feet that they cannot feel the floor or know where their feet are. This is referred to as a sensory ataxia.

Treatment Options and Outlook

Most gait problems can be improved with physical therapy, by using appropriate assistive devices,

and in some cases, with medications. Each person's gait disorder needs to be evaluated by a health care professional to determine an appropriate therapy program.

gamma globulin A family of antibodies that is increased in the spinal fluid of many, but not all, people with multiple sclerosis (MS). Gamma globulin is a protein found in the blood that helps fight infection. Its presence in spinal fluid indicates the body is mounting an attack on what it believes is an infection. In the case of patients with MS, the attack is typically against the body's own MYELIN.

Garr, Teri (1944–) Offbeat actress, best known for her comedic roles, who was diagnosed with multiple sclerosis in 1999. Born December 11, 1944, Garr began her career as a dancer and danced professionally with the San Francisco Ballet when she was 13. She began in films doing background work, including several Elvis Presley films. Since then Garr has been seen in more than 50 films and numerous television shows, including *Star Trek* and *Friends.*

She is now a spokeswoman for a pharmaceutical firm involved in producing MS drugs. She rarely appears on film or TV.

gastroesophageal reflux Also called acid reflux, this painful condition occurs when the sphincter muscles at the top of the stomach (the gastroesophageal sphincter) do not close properly, allowing stomach acid to flow backward into the esophagus.

Symptoms and Diagnostic Path

Gastroesophageal reflux causes sensations of heartburn, a sour taste in the mouth, pains in the middle of the chest, coughing and choking when lying down, and asthma symptoms during sleep. Gastroesophageal acid can also reach the larynx, causing laryngitis. This can occur in patients with multiple sclerosis if lesions are in the medulla oblongata region of the brain stem where the 10th cranial nerve begins.

Normally the gastroesophageal sphincter opens to let each bit of food into the stomach and closes behind it, preventing the acid from flowing back;

any small amounts that leak back are neutralized by saliva. However, in gastroesophageal reflux, so much acid flows back that the saliva cannot neutralize it, and the acid burns the esophageal lining. The esophageal epithelium is often damaged by this process.

Increased stomach pressure makes gastroesophageal reflux worse by squeezing even more acid out of the stomach. This increased pressure can be caused by a full stomach, obesity, bending forward, lifting heavy objects, pregnancy, or lying down.

Gastroesophageal reflux is usually diagnosed from a history of symptoms. A barium meal or pH probe can help confirm a diagnosis.

Treatment Options and Outlook

Reflux can be managed by avoiding fatty foods, acidic foods such as citrus and tomato products, strong spices, caffeinated or carbonated drinks, chocolate, mint, alcohol, or nicotine. Eating smaller, more frequent meals rather than three large ones can help reduce stomach pressure, and bedtime snacks should be avoided. Raising the head of the bed by six to eight inches with blocks under the legs of the bed helps gravity to prevent acid from leaving the stomach. Patients also should avoid lifting heavy objects and bending forward.

If these methods do not work, several medications may be prescribed to help this condition. These include antacids after meals and at bedtime: Tagamet (cimetadine), Zantac (ranitidine), Pepcid (famotidine), Axid (nizatidine), Prilosec (omeprazole), or Reglan (metoclopramide).

See also PREGNANCY AND MS.

gender Multiple sclerosis (MS) affects about twice as many women as men for reasons that scientists do not yet fully understand.

About 8.5 million people in the United States have some form of autoimmune disease. Of these, 6.7 million (almost 80 percent) are women. The reasons for a sex bias in MS and other autoimmune diseases may relate to several factors that include sex-related differences in immune responsiveness, response to infection, the effects of sex hormones, and sex-linked genetic factors.

Most experts believe that MS involves a misdirected immune system attack against the MYELIN coating that insulates nerve fibers in the brain and spinal cord. Scientists believe that the immune response in MS is regulated by immune cells known as T cells, which produce messenger cytokines (proteins that affect the immune system). In MS, the cytokines produced are inflammatory and are known as T helper 1 (Th1) cytokines. Th2 cytokines, which can suppress inflammation, are overwhelmed by the Th1 response.

Recent studies suggest that certain sex hormones may affect the production of cytokines. Some scientists suspect that the increased incidence of MS in women is in part due to a gender-related increase in Th1 cytokines in women. In fact in some studies, women with MS showed significantly stronger immune system attack to a myelin protein that may be a target of the immune response in MS.

genes in MS Genetic factors appear to make certain individuals more susceptible than others to getting multiple sclerosis (MS), although no evidence indicates that MS is directly inherited. If scientists understood how genes contribute to determining who gets MS, they could provide major clues to the cause and even point to ways of preventing and treating the disease.

Two types of evidence support the connection between genes and MS susceptibility. First, population studies suggest that people from different ethnic groups have different tendencies to develop MS. Typically the disease affects people of northern European heritage. Other ethnic groups, including Eskimos, African blacks, and southeast Asians, are less likely to have MS.

The second type of evidence comes from studies of families in whom MS occurs more often than chance would dictate. The average person in the United States has about one chance in 750 of developing MS. However, relatives of people with MS—children, siblings or nonidentical twins—have a higher chance, ranging from one in 100 to one in 40. The identical twin of someone with MS, who shares all the same genes, has a one in three chance of developing the disease. In other words, the risk to the general population, if no one else in the family has MS, is 0.1 percent. The risk to a child of a mother with MS is 3–4 percent. The risk to an identical twin of someone with MS is 31 percent. Although family evidence strongly suggests that genes are important for determining who may get MS, there must still be other factors. Otherwise, the identical twin of a person with MS would always get MS if genes were the only factor involved.

These other factors determining susceptibility to MS may well be exposure to germs or viruses. Genetic factors may determine who is susceptible to the unknown outside trigger.

Genes contain the instructions for making the proteins of which all living things are made and that all organisms use to carry out their functions. Most of the trillions of cells in a person's body have two complete sets of genes, one inherited from the mother and one from the father. Each set, including 30,000–40,000 genes, contains all the instructions needed to build all human proteins. The complete set is known as the human genome. Genes are passed from one generation to another by being copied from the parents' genes. The cells that copy genes are able to correct most copying errors, but sometimes these cells make mistakes. Because the genome is copied many times for each generation, there are many slightly different versions of all the human genes. Much of this variation is harmless and is partly what gives each person his or her unique characteristics. Except for identical twins, no two people have exactly the same sequence of DNA bases in their genes. Sometimes, however, a difference in a single gene can be responsible for a disease that is inherited.Since the 1970s, scientists have been developing ways to isolate and determine the chemical structure of genes.

See also GENETIC TESTS AND MS.

genetic tests and MS   Genetic information from a simple blood test may help doctors detect changes in people with multiple sclerosis (MS) and improve diagnosis and treatment for these patients, according to a 2004 American and Israeli study. Preliminary results indicate that gene microarrays, which can measure the expression of thousands of genes at once, can help identify different states of MS without using more invasive procedures such as spinal taps. These microarrays could then perhaps be used to predict the course of disease and, potentially, the response to treatment.

In the study, scientists found significant differences, in more than 1,000 genes, between control subjects and people with MS. The scientists identified a different subset of more than 200 genes that become more or less active in people with MS flare-ups.

More research is needed to determine whether gene microarray results can help predict what type of disease course will be experienced by a person newly diagnosed with MS or whether a person with MS in remission is likely to experience a relapse.

See also GENES IN MS.

geographical factors   The risk of developing multiple sclerosis (MS) is quite different in different parts of the world. In fact, there is a specific geographical area in which cases of MS occur at much higher rates than in other places. Worldwide, MS has more prevalence in higher latitudes, between 40 and 60 degrees north and south latitude. It is five times more prevalent in temperate climates than in tropical climates. The high-frequency zones for MS (affecting 50–120 people out of every 100,000) include central Europe, Italy, Canada, Russia, Israel, northern United States, New Zealand and southeastern Australia. Lowest frequency zones for MS (affecting only five out of every 100,000 people) are found in the countries of Asia, Africa, and South America.

Middle-risk areas are southern Europe (except Italy), southern United States, northern Australia, northern Scandinavia, the Caucasian sections of South Africa, and maybe Central America. Low-risk areas include parts of Africa and Asia, the Caribbean, Mexico, and possibly northern South America. Whether this pattern is related to environmental factors, genetics, or both is unclear.

MS also shows large differences in prevalence within some individual countries in the high-risk area. In Norway, for example, MS is up to five times more common in the inland farming areas than in the relatively nearby coastal fishing areas. In Canada, MS is at least twice as prevalent in the Prairie provinces (100–225 per 100,000) as it is on the island of Newfoundland (50 per 100,000). It is also much higher in Pincher Creek, Alberta, for unknown reasons. Saskatchewan has the highest rate on the prairies.

In the United States, MS occurs more frequently in states that are above the 37th parallel than in states below it. From east to west, the 37th parallel extends from Newport News, Virginia, to Santa Cruz, California, running along the northern border of North Carolina to the northern border of Arizona and including most of California. The MS prevalence rate for the region below the 37th parallel is 57–78 cases per 100,000 people. The prevalence rate for those above the 37th parallel is 110–140 cases per 100,000 people. Nationwide, an estimated 400,000 people have MS.

girdle sensations The sensation of feeling a tight band around one's trunk that is sometimes experienced by people with multiple sclerosis. It is usually caused by a lesion on the spinal cord. Sensations that feel so tight the patient cannot take a complete breath can be treated with intravenous methylprednisolone.

glatiramer acetate See DISEASE-MODIFYING AGENTS.

glial cells One of the types of cells that make up the supportive tissue of the brain and central nervous system (CNS). The glial cells protect, support, and feed neurons, outnumbering them 10 to one; the brain contains more than 100 trillion glial cells. Some of these glial cells act as a sort of bed for neurons. Unlike neurons, glial cells do not generate electrical impulses, but they do play an important supportive role in maintaining efficiency along the brain's nerve network. They help to form a covering to protect the large neurons in the spinal cord. MYELIN is placed around the axons of some neurons by a particular type of glial cell, and axons covered by this myelin sheath conduct impulses up to 12 times faster than those without it.

The areas of the brain that contain myelin-covered axons are called the WHITE MATTER, because the myelinated axons look white.

Two main types of glial cells are in the CNS. OLIGODENDROCYTES produce, maintain, and repair the myelin sheath of the axons. ASTROCYTES, named for their characteristic starlike shape, provide both mechanical and metabolic support to neurons. Other types of glial cells are outside the CNS.

glucocorticoids Steroid hormones that are produced by the adrenal glands in response to stimulation by adrenocorticotropic hormone from the pituitary. These hormones, which can also be manufactured synthetically (prednisone, prednisolone, methylprednisolone, betamethasone, dexamethasone), play both an immunosuppressive and an anti-inflammatory role in the treatment of multiple sclerosis flares. The hormones damage or destroy certain types of T lymphocytes that are involved in the overactive immune response and interfere with the release of certain inflammation-producing enzymes.

gout A disease characterized by an increased level of uric acid in the blood and the sudden onset of acute arthritis. Some experts believe that multiple sclerosis (MS), which is associated with low uric acid, and gout, which is associated with high uric acid, are mutually exclusive. A study of 20 million Medicare and Medicaid records found no overlap between MS and gout.

grief and MS Patients diagnosed with multiple sclerosis (MS) may experience a grief reaction typical for any type of loss. The five stages in the grieving process, as described by Elisabeth Kübler-Ross in writing about bereavement, include denial, anger, bargaining, DEPRESSION, and acceptance.

However, not every patient with MS will grieve, and not all who do will go through the process in an orderly fashion. Some patients skip steps or go back and forth from one step to another. These feelings are part of a normal, healthy adjustment to the diagnosis.

See also EMOTIONAL PROBLEMS.

grooming aids See ASSISTIVE DEVICES; BATHROOM AIDS.

Guillain-Barré syndrome (GBS) A DEMYELINATING DISEASE that destroys the covering (MYELIN) of the peripheral nerves that lead from the brain stem and spinal cord to the rest of the body. Multiple sclerosis (MS) is a demyelinating disorder that destroys the myelin of the brain and the spinal cord (central nervous system [CNS]).

Myelin is the fatty sheath that surrounds and insulates nerve fibers. However, myelin in the peripheral nervous system is different from that in the central nervous system. Peripheral system myelin has a different biochemical makeup and different antigens (molecules on the cell's surface that provoke an immune response) than that in the CNS. In GBS, the damage is caused primarily by antibodies to a component of peripheral myelin.

GBS usually develops after a viral infection such as the flu. Although most cases of GBS are acute and occur just one time, a chronic relapsing form is characterized by repeated episodes. GBS is usually diagnosed by clinical examination, analysis of the cerebrospinal fluid, and sometimes electrodiagnostic studies. The diagnostic criteria are different than those for MS.

Although GBS may lead to paralysis and can be life threatening because it can interfere with breathing, treatment can be effective and patients usually recover. Treatment involves a process called plasmapheresis—separating the blood components to remove the attacking antibodies—and administering immune globulin. Treatment may take many months, but most patients with GBS make a good recovery with little or no residual effects.

headache Although headache is not a common symptom of multiple sclerosis (MS), some reports suggest that people with MS have an increased incidence of certain types of headache. One report noted that migraine headaches were more than twice as common in a group of MS patients than in a matched group of people without MS. Other investigators found a prior diagnosis of migraine in one-third of the MS group being studied. A third study found that 20 percent of a sample group of people with MS had a family history of migraine, compared with 10 percent of controls, which suggested that there may be a common trigger for both MS and migraines. Sometimes vascular or migraine headaches have been reported as the first symptom of MS.

health care MS team An interdisciplinary team involved in the care and management of people with multiple sclerosis (MS). They include a neurologist, family physician, MS nurse, PHYSICAL THERAPIST, OCCUPATIONAL THERAPIST, speech-language pathologist, social worker, counselor, neuropsychologist, and spiritual adviser.

In addition to establishing the initial diagnosis, a neurologist prescribes treatments for MS and symptom management. Regular annual visits to the neurologist are recommended for assessment and monitoring of MS. The neurologist will refer the patient to other specialists such as a urologist, gastroenterologist, gynecologist, psychiatrist, or pain specialist.

The family physician provides primary health care, including general health checkups, immunizations, and preventive care. People with more severe progressive MS tend to rely on their neurologists for primary health care.

The MS nurse coordinates health care services and oversees initial and long-term management issues, teaches self-care, including administration of medications, and advocates for needs with insurance companies and other agencies.

The physical therapist (PT) focuses on exercise programs to reduce and prevent serious complications, such as contractures (frozen joints) and osteoporosis, and to ease SPASTICITY and tremor. PTs provide information on equipment such as WHEELCHAIRS, scooters, hoists, CANES, braces, and WALKERS. They teach safe, effective ways to use these devices, including the best ways to transfer in and out of bed, a car, a shower, and more. PTs will help their clients create personal exercise programs for increasing stamina and preventing losses. Occupational therapists (OTs) focus mainly on skills that require upper body function. OTs are specialists in tools, techniques, or equipment to conserve energy and compensate for disabilities that interfere with dressing, grooming, personal hygiene, eating, driving, using computers, and other ordinary activities. They may consult with architects or builders about renovations and home adaptations to support independence. OTs may also contribute to coping with cognitive problems.

A speech-language pathologist evaluates and treats speech and SWALLOWING PROBLEMS by training the person with MS and caregivers how to eat safely, prepare easy to swallow food, and manage feeding tubes if necessary. They teach the use of speech amplifiers or telephone aids, and, like OTs, may contribute to coping with cognitive problems.

The social worker assesses social needs and links clients to appropriate resources in areas of income maintenance, insurance, entitlement programs, housing, long-term care options, living wills, and estate planning. Mental health professionals help individuals and family members develop problem-solving skills, grieve for losses, recreate self-esteem, handle changing relationships, learn to live with uncertainty, and find ways to be productive. The neuropsychologist specializes in cognition problems and can set up programs to compensate for weaknesses identified in comprehensive neuropsychological testing.

Finally, spiritual advisers may support efforts to make sense of MS within a set of personal beliefs. The choice of advisors and the sources of support are intensely personal matters but the need to pay attention to this aspect of life with MS cannot be overemphasized.

health care proxy   A legal document (also called a health care power of attorney or a medical power of attorney) that allows individuals to convey their wishes regarding medical treatment. The designated agent will then be allowed to make health care decisions in accordance with the person's wishes. The person writing the health care proxy has the right to place specific limitations on the agent's authority. Specific desires to limit the agent's authority should be explained in the proxy.

Without a formally appointed person, many health care providers and institutions will make critical decisions for the incapacitated person, not necessarily based on what the person would want. In some situations, a court-appointed guardian may become necessary unless the person has a proxy, especially when the health care decision requires that money be spent for care.

Health Status Questionnaire (SF-36)   One of the most widely used assessments of health-related quality of life that can discriminate between subjects with different chronic conditions and between subjects with different severity levels of the same disease. The so-called Short Form-36 also has demonstrated sensitivity to significant treatment effects. There is no single overall score for the SF-36; instead, it asks questions in eight areas—physical functioning, role limitations due to physical problems, pain, general health perceptions, vitality, social functioning, role limitations due to emotional problems, and mental health. The test produces two summary scores—one assessing physical health and the other mental health.

The SF-36 is one of the components of the MULTIPLE SCLEROSIS QUALITY OF LIFE INVENTORY to serve as a generic health-related quality of life measure that could provide a basis for comparison between the people with MS and those without the disease.

The SF-36 is a structured, self-report questionnaire that the person can generally complete with little or no intervention from an interviewer. However, people with visual problems or upper extremity impairments may need to have the SF-36 administered as an interview.

hearing loss   An uncommon symptom of multiple sclerosis (MS) that occurs in about 6 percent of patients. In very rare cases, hearing loss has been reported as the first symptom of the disease. Deafness due to MS is exceedingly rare, and most sudden episodes of hearing problems caused by MS tend to improve.

Hearing loss may take place during an acute worsening of MS symptoms. Hearing loss is usually associated with other symptoms that suggest damage to the BRAIN STEM (the part of the nervous system that contains the nerves that help to control vision, hearing, BALANCE, and equilibrium).

Hearing deficits caused by MS are thought to be due to inflammation or scarring around the eighth cranial nerve (the AUDITORY NERVE) as it enters the brain stem. However, plaques at other sites along the auditory pathways could also contribute to hearing problems. Plaques are abnormal areas that develop on nerves whose myelin (the fatty sheath that surrounds and protects nerve fibers) has been destroyed. Plaques cause the nerve impulses to be slowed or halted, producing the symptoms of MS. Because hearing deficits are so uncommon in MS, people with MS who do develop hearing loss should have their hearing thoroughly evaluated to rule out other causes.

heat   In many cases, high temperatures tend to worsen multiple sclerosis (MS) symptoms temporarily, significantly weakening the patient, because body overheating causes damaged nerves to function less efficiently than usual. Overheating may occur when the weather is very hot or humid or if the person has a fever, sunbathes, gets overheated from exercise, or takes very hot showers or baths.

Some people with MS notice that their vision becomes blurred when they get overheated (a phenomenon known as UHTHOFF'S SIGN). These temporary changes can result from even a very slight elevation in core body temperature (no more than a half of a degree) since a higher temperature further impairs the ability of a demyelinated nerve to conduct electrical impulses. (MYELIN is the protective sheath that surrounds and protects nerve fibers.)

Because patients with MS are so susceptible to heat, for many years the hot bath test was used to diagnose the condition. In this test, a patient with suspected MS was submerged in a hot tub of water. The appearance or worsening of neurologic symptoms was taken as evidence that the person had MS.

Handling Heat Problems

Heat typically causes only temporary worsening of symptoms and does not cause actual damage to the tissue. The symptoms can be quickly reversed when exposure to the high temperature is eliminated. Active cooling can help reduce fatigue and improve stability. The adverse effects of heat may be eased if the person with MS remains in air-conditioned surroundings as much as possible during periods of extreme heat. If an air conditioner is needed to help minimize the symptoms of MS, the cost of this equipment may be tax deductible if there is a prescription from a physician. In addition, the home of a patient with MS should also be kept slightly cool in winter. Patients may want to avoid hot baths or swimming in heated pools.

Patients may also try a variety of products that use special cooling bandanas, scarves, baseball caps, and neck wraps. A selection is available at the Web site of the National MS Society at http://www.nationalmssociety.org/IMSApril04-SummersComing.asp. These products cool the head and neck, lowering core body temperature and reducing MS symptoms during daily activities. The effects may vary depending on the season.

Doctors recommend that people with MS who are sensitive to temperature try to avoid extremes of either hot or cold and that people who are considering moving to a different climate try to visit first to see if the climate change really helps. Plans may have to be changed if the weather seriously worsens MS symptoms.

In order to remain cool, people with MS should

- avoid outdoor activities in warm weather between 10 A.M. and 4 P.M.
- carry cold drinks in insulated containers that attach comfortably to a belt, waist-pack, backpack, or shoulder strap
- wear lightweight shoes (when the feet are cool, the rest of the body tends to be cool too)
- wear vests, hats, or kerchiefs that hold "blue ice" gel packs or materials that can be chilled for long-lasting coolness
- dress in layers, in order to add or remove clothing as body temperature changes
- use air conditioners, electric fans, or a battery-powered, handheld mini-fan
- refresh with a mist of water from a plastic spray bottle
- lower body temperature immediately before and after exercise with a cool soak or shower, run cool water over wrists, or apply cold paper towels to neck and forehead
- relax in a swimming pool if the water temperature is 80 to 84 degrees

See also CLIMATE.

heat exhaustion A condition that occurs when the body loses too much fluid and overheats, which often happens in people with multiple sclerosis. Less commonly heat exhaustion may result when the body loses too much salt. Symptoms include thirst, dizziness, nausea, and vomiting.

See also CLIMATE.

heavy metals See DENTAL AMALGAM AND MS.

heel-knee-shin test A diagnostic for multiple sclerosis (MS). In this test, the patient places the ball of the heel onto the knee of the other leg and then moves it down the shin. If the patient displays uncoordinated, clumsy movements (ATAXIA), this may indicate a problem in the CEREBELLUM, common in patients with MS.

hemianopia   Blindness for half the field of vision in one or both eyes. Hemianopia, which occurs rarely in patients with multiple sclerosis, causes visual loss on the right or left visual fields of both eyes. When looking straight ahead, a person with hemianopia may see everything on the right clearly and see nothing to the left (or vice versa). Spectacle-mounted prism devices may improve vision for both types of field loss.

hemiparesis   Sensory loss or WEAKNESS of the face, arm, and leg on one side of the body, which is common in multiple sclerosis.

hemiplegia   Paralysis of one side of the body.

hemopoietic stem cell transplantation   See BONE MARROW TRANSPLANTATION.

herpesvirus 6 (HHV-6)   A form of herpesvirus that causes roseola, a benign disease in children, and also causes encephalitis (brain inflammation) in persons with weakened immune systems. Some experts suspect that this type of herpesvirus might be related to multiple sclerosis (MS). Although many different VIRUSES have been implicated in causing MS, no definitive proof has yet linked any one virus to the autoimmune reaction that is believed to be the process responsible for the MS symptom of DEMYELINATION (the destruction of MYELIN, the fatty sheath that surrounds and insulates nerve fibers in the central nervous system).

A number of studies have reported higher-than-normal rates of HHV-6 infection in MS patients. However, some experts argue that nearly everyone harbors this virus and that there is still no evidence of a link between the virus and MS. Other herpes viruses also can infect brain cells: herpes simplex 1 and 2 (the causes of oral and genital herpes), varicella-zoster virus (the cause of chicken pox and shingles), and cytomegalovirus.

Viruses are known to cause DEMYELINATING DISEASES in animals and humans. Demyelination slows or halts nerve impulses and produces the symptoms of MS. Data from epidemiological studies suggest that exposure to an infectious agent may be involved in causing MS. Some viruses are

known to have a long latency period between time of infection and appearance of clinical symptoms, as is thought to be the case in multiple sclerosis.

Heuga, Jimmie (1944–)   Former Olympic ski racer who was diagnosed with multiple sclerosis (MS) in 1970 at the height of his racing career. Jimmie Heuga founded the HEUGA CENTER in 1984 to teach people with MS how to use EXERCISE to help manage this disease. Heuga wanted to share the principles that transformed his life into one of health and well-being.

When Heuga was first diagnosed, people with MS were advised to avoid physical activity. By defying conventional wisdom, Heuga began a program of exercise, nutrition, and psychological motivation that improved not only his physical condition but also his outlook on life. Heuga's success revolutionized the management of MS.

HHV-6   See HERPESVIRUS 6.

high-fat diet and MS   No study has ever proven that a high-fat diet causes multiple sclerosis (MS). In fact, studies of the diet of people diagnosed with MS reveal that their nutritional intake is the same as people who do not develop the condition. Most North Americans who are diagnosed with the disease eat a diet typical of this culture, including meat, dairy foods, fruits, and vegetables.

Hispanics and MS   Cases of multiple sclerosis occur infrequently in South America, but relatively more often in Hispanic Americans. Multiple sclerosis remains far more common in Caucasian Americans than among Hispanic Americans. This supports the idea that environmental factors play a role in development of the disease.

history of multiple sclerosis   The first documented case of multiple sclerosis (MS) was described in a 1421 text, when St. LIDWINA OF SCHIEDAM presented with symptoms at the age of 16 after she fell while skating. Historical texts reveal that she was afflicted with a debilitating disease that sounds a great deal like MS. Another four centuries passed, however, before scientists truly began to study the disease.

Early Studies—19th Century

The effects of MS were first described in the 1830s, and MS was first identified as a distinct disease in the 1860s. The 19th-century doctors did not understand what they saw and recorded, but drawings from autopsies done as early as 1838 clearly show what we today recognize as MS. The first studies of myelin and glial cells in brain tissue were begun in 1860. Eight years later, Jean-Marie CHARCOT—the founder of neurology and a professor at the University of Paris—was the first to correlate MS clinical symptoms with a central nervous system pathology. After carefully examining a young woman with an unusual tremor, he noticed other neurological problems such as slurred speech and abnormal eye movements. He compared these symptoms to those of other patients he had seen. When the patient died, he examined her brain and found the characteristic scars or plaques of MS. Charcot named the disease *sclerose en plaques* and wrote a complete description of the brain changes typical of the condition. He was baffled by its cause, however, and frustrated by his inability to treat the symptoms using electrical stimulation and the nerve stimulant strychnine. He also tried injections of gold and silver, which worked for syphilis but proved useless in treating MS. He also tried zinc and sulfate to no avail.

Once the scientific method took hold in medicine, MS was among the first diseases to be described scientifically. As the 19th century drew to a close, other physicians around the world came to understand that MS was a specific disease. Five years after Charcot first identified it, MS was recognized in England by Dr. William Moxon; this recognition was followed five years later in the United States by Dr. Edward Seguin. By the end of the 19th century, scientists knew that the disease was more common in women than men, that it is not directly inherited, and that it can produce many different neurological symptoms.

Unfortunately, observation of the disease was limited by the lack of a deeper understanding of biology and better research tools. In the 19th century, the existence of the immune system was still unknown. Doctors thought that a person would not get the same disease twice because the disease had depleted the materials in the body it needed to live. During the 19th century scientists first learned that bacteria cause many diseases. However, the understanding of viruses did not occur until the early 20th century when scientists began to develop techniques for growing and studying bacteria and viruses in the laboratory.

Improvements in Research—1900–1980

In 1906, the Nobel Prize for medicine was awarded to Dr. Camillo Golgi and Dr. Santiago Ramon y Cajal, who perfected new chemicals to enhance the visibility of nerve cells under the microscope. Equipped with this new technology, Dr. James Dawson at the University of Edinburgh in 1916 performed detailed microscopic examinations of the brains of patients who had died with MS, noting the inflammation around blood vessels and the damage to the myelin. Unfortunately, scientists knew so little about the brain's function that the meaning of these changes could not be understood.

In the decade after World War I, MS researchers became more sophisticated in their methods, noting abnormalities in spinal fluid.

The first electrical recording of nerve transmission, by Lord Edgar Douglas Adrian in 1925, established techniques needed to study the activity of nerves and launched a series of experiments to determine just how the nervous system works. His efforts earned him six Nobel Prizes. Researchers were realizing how important myelin was in nerve conduction and that nerves without the protective myelin sheath cannot transmit electrical impulses. Scientists still did not understand the cause of MS, wondering if it could be some form of toxin or poison that triggered the myelin breakdown. Because most MS damage occurs around blood vessels, it seemed reasonable that a toxin circulating in the bloodstream leaked out into the brain, even though no researcher could locate such a toxin.

In 1928, scientists discovered that myelin is produced by oligodendrocyte glial cells. Five years later, scientists developed the first animal model of MS (acute EXPERIMENTAL AUTOIMMUNE ENCEPHALOMYELITIS [EAE]). Now that they had an animal model of the disease, they could spend more time studying the possible immunology and treatment of MS. Because EAE demonstrated how the body can generate an immunologic attack against itself, research about EAE paved the way for modern theories of autoimmunity.

Unfortunately, most doctors ignored the importance of EAE and continued to try to find the toxin that caused MS. Years would pass before the link between the immune system and MS was understood.

As World War II galvanized scientific research, scientists in 1943 made the first detailed description of the composition of myelin. The first research grant from the Society for the Advancement of Multiple Sclerosis Research (now the National MS Society) was awarded in 1947 to Dr. Elvin Kabat at Columbia University to study the relationship between the body's immune defense system and the impact of MS on the central nervous system.

Dr. Kabat identified abnormal immunologic proteins in the spinal fluid of people with MS, which appeared as patterns known as OLIGOCLONAL BANDS. These bands would become a diagnostic test for MS as well as evidence that MS and the immune system were connected.

In 1950, the society persuaded Congress to establish the National Institute for Neurologic Disorders and Stroke (NINDS). From then on, NINDS, the National MS Society, and members of the International Federation of MS Societies supported virtually every major MS study. By this time, the first prevalence studies of MS in the United States had begun. Soon afterward came the first well-defined MS diagnostic criteria—guidelines that are still used by some today. At the same time, a rating scale for determining the level of disability and the parts of the nervous system affected by MS was refined by Dr. John Kurtzke.

The first studies of treatments for MS were completed in 1969, when researchers discovered that people having an acute attack of MS could recover more quickly if they were given adrenocorticotropic hormone. This early type of intramuscular steroid therapy paved the way to the modern steroid therapy still used today for acute exacerbations.

As treatment research was progressing, scientists were still trying to uncover the cause of MS. During the 1960s, scientists began to focus on two primary ideas about the cause of MS that are still being studied today. The first focused on the fact that white blood cells that react against a component of myelin, called MYELIN BASIC PROTEIN, were discovered in MS. This suggested that the disease might involve a direct immune system attack on myelin. The second idea came from studies that showed that people with MS have altered antibodies against viruses. This led scientists to wonder if the viruses involved in MS were somehow altering the immune system and inducing it to damage myelin.

Scientists still grapple with these two ideas, since MS may combine features of both an infectious and an autoimmune disease. In the 1970s, though, studies were unable to locate specific viruses in the brain, cerebrospinal fluid, and blood of those with MS.

Research was still making headway in the attempt to develop treatments. Steroids to suppress immune activity were now widely used to treat MS attacks, and the first small studies were performed using interferons (substances that modulate the immune system). The first studies of beta interferon for MS began at the end of the 1970s. At the same time, scientists mixed protein fragments and used this mixture to treat first animals and then humans with MS. The product was named copolymer 1 and is today called Copaxone, an approved disease-modifying treatment.

Major Advances in Treatment—
1980 Through Today

In the 1980s, scientists began to use MAGNETIC RESONANCE IMAGING (MRI) to reveal MS lesions in living patients—an important step forward in diagnosing this baffling neurological disease. By 1984, it became apparent that MRI could actually show MS attacks within the brain, including many that did not cause any symptoms. By 1988, sequential MRI scans showed that MS is a constant, ongoing disease that continues to destroy myelin in the brain even though symptoms may appear only sporadically.

Scientists began to understand in more detail how white blood cells are activated by foreign substances to mount attacks. One activating trigger can be a virus. Scientists also learned that parts of some viruses look so much like normal human tissue that white blood cells will inadvertently attack the self-tissue when they attack the virus. This is yet another mechanism by which viral infections could indirectly lead to the destruction of myelin.

At about the same time, the white blood cell type that causes the actual damage to myelin in MS was finally identified. It is the macrophage ("big eater" in Greek).

The first studies of identical and fraternal twins were begun in the 1980s and extended knowledge about the genetics of MS. Psychosocial and mental health issues, as well as the cognitive changes occasionally caused by MS, began receiving long overdue research attention.

The 1980s may legitimately be called the treatment decade in MS. The number of clinical trials exploded. Guided by the National MS Society, scientists reached a consensus on the design of and how to conduct research for new treatments. For the first time, the emphasis could shift away from palliation, where the aim is to help people with MS feel as good as possible for as long as possible, and go instead toward attempts to control or cure the underlying MS.

Major clinical trials conducted during this decade led to approvals of the first drugs in history shown to affect the course of this disease. In 1983, researchers reported a treatment breakthrough: a temporary control of CHRONIC-PROGRESSIVE MULTIPLE SCLEROSIS using the immunosuppressive drug Cytoxan, although this treatment remained quite controversial through the 1980s.

In the 1990s after years of research, the first effective drugs were finally introduced. INTERFERON beta-lb (Betaseron) was introduced in 1993, followed by interferon beta-1a (Avonex) in mid-1996, and glatiramer acetate for injection (Copaxone) in late 1996. By 2002, a variation of interferon beta-1a (Rebif) was introduced, giving U.S. patients four options for reducing disease activity and preventing many attacks. Since then another therapy has been added: MITOXANTRONE (Novantrone), an intravenous infusion given at three monthly intervals for a limited time due to possible side effects to the heart.

In addition, scientists were able to transplant myelin-making oligodendrocytes into myelin-deficient mice, resulting in the production of new myelin.

Even though almost 140 years have passed since the "discovery" of MS, the cause of MS is still not known, nor can it be conclusively diagnosed. Some experts believe that MS may actually be several different diseases. Whether or not this is true may be revealed by research yet to come.

See also CARSWELL, ROBERT.

Hoffmann's sign   A symptom of multiple sclerosis that indicates lesions in the corticospinal tract. In this test, a nail is tapped on the third or forth finger. A positive response would be flexion of the last part of the thumb. This sign is similar to BABINSKI REFLEX but involves the hands rather than the feet.

home adaptations   Many changes can be made to the home of a person with multiple sclerosis (MS) to help make it easier to maintain independence and conserve energy. An OCCUPATIONAL THERAPIST or rehabilitation specialist can recommend a variety of devices that are designed to make home care and daily activities more comfortable.

Maneuvering Space

The person with MS and an occupational therapist should identify any potential access problems, especially looking at levels of living space both inside and outside the home. Mobility aids require a certain amount of open space to maneuver, and CANES, CRUTCHES, and WALKERS also require ample turning space. WHEELCHAIRS and scooters have a considerably wider turning radius, which varies with the design. Improving access reduces FATIGUE, even if an aid is not used.

The "easy-reach zone" for most wheelchair users begins about 15 or 16 inches from the floor and ends about 51 or 52 inches from the floor. Standing, the zone begins at knee level and ends a few inches higher than the individual's height (not outstretched arms). Therefore, each work or storage area needs to have devices and items with easy reach.

Storage/Tools

Storage adaptations may include hanging baskets, rolling storage carts, peg boards, hooks, and so on. People with limited balance or vision tend to avoid open spaces, preferring to keep in contact with walls and furniture. Furniture and wall hangings should be stable and not obstruct the person's ability to move about the house.

Adding weight to tools, containers, and hand appliances may make things usable for the person with weakness or tremor. Lightweight tools and containers help with weakness and fatigue, but heavier objects give more sensory input (both touch and pressure). Weight may help some tremor and coordination problems. Some objects can be weighted, perhaps with sand or lead pellets.

Doors and Handrails

Doors and handrails are important features for each home environment. All outside doors should be 36 inches wide, and all inside doors should be at least 32 inches, including bathroom and closet doors. Most doors can be widened a couple of inches by replacing standard hinges with offset hinges. Some doors can simply be removed. The door frame also can be removed to provide more width. Some doors can be replaced with curtains if privacy is an issue. A sliding door or a pocket door that slides into the wall may be an option. Folding doors are another alternative if there is no room for a door to swing open, but they narrow the doorway by several inches. If the door cannot be modified, a crank device can be added to a folding manual wheelchair which can briefly narrow the width of the chair.

If a door is difficult to open or close, the hardware can be changed. Lever-style handles are usually easier to use than round doorknobs. Temporary metal or rubber handles, found in adaptive equipment catalogs, are useful if traveling or living in a rental property. The more expensive options are electric or hydraulic door openers.

Bathroom Safety

The installation of grab bars in the bathroom and in the bedroom are priorities for an individual's safety and ease of activities. There are several ways to elevate a toilet seat. The three-in-one commode can be used as a bedside commode, a shower chair, or placed over the toilet as an elevated toilet seat. Other options include a variety of permanent or portable elevated seats, with or without arms or backs and of different heights.

If constructing or remodeling a bathroom with a tub, the faucets should be centered in the middle of the long wall of the tub rather than at one end. An 18-inch tile-covered seat at one or both ends of the tub, and level with the tub, facilitates transfers and storage. The ideal bathroom would have a tub and a roll-in shower.

Beds, Chairs

Beds and chairs are easier to rise from if they are high. Low chairs are best avoided, especially if the seats slant back and down. Transferring to and from a wheelchair is best when seats are at the same level, so the person can slide easily from one to the other using a sliding board. This is easier than standing up, turning, and sitting again.

Adjustable hospital beds are a big investment, but they have important advantages. Some are available that do not look like institutional furniture, and these beds can be raised to change the bedclothes or to permit a person to "stand down" from the bed when rising. The bed also can be lowered to reduce the risk of injury from falls during occupancy, allow access to nightstands, or facilitate smooth transfers. The maximum and minimum heights and ease of operation should be checked before purchasing a bed.

Kitchen Safety

Removal of doors and cabinets under the sink in the kitchen allows wheelchair access, and, if the cabinet base is left in place, this can become a footrest if a scooter is used. Exposed pipes should be covered with insulating material to prevent bumps and burns.

Kitchen countertops usually need to be lowered for wheelchair users. This major carpentry job should be carefully planned. Even if a wheelchair is not used, one low section is useful so that the person with MS can sit while doing kitchen work.

A stove with controls at the front or center of the cooktop are better as this avoids reaching around hot pans to access controls. Smooth cooktops are easiest to clean.

Desks and Tables

By raising a desk or table sitting posture can be improved and at the same time the surface can be used to stabilize arms, improve coordination, and reduce tremor. It is often necessary to raise tables and desks to allow access to a wheelchair or scooter.

Flooring and Stairs

High doorsills, the edges of carpets or rugs, and other changes in the floor covering can impede access and it is often best to remove doorsills. Special little ramps are available in catalogs for unavoidably high doorsills.

The thicker the carpet, the more difficult it is to pick up heavy feet or propel a wheeled mobility device. Smooth non-skid floors are always best for people with mobility problems, and it is a good idea to remove all slippery rugs and mats. If rugs are left in place, they should be firmly secured to the floor with double-sided carpet tape, non-slip backing or matting, and/or metal or other edging. Any worn rugs, mats, or carpet should be removed.

Stairs can be avoided by using ramps, electric stair chairs, or elevators. Ramps and outdoor grades should not rise more than one inch per foot, and ramps should be 30 to 40 inches wide. Stairs and long ramps need sturdy handrails on both sides.

Transfer Lifts

Permanent or portable transfer lifts can pick up, move, and put down a person almost anywhere. Mounted on ceilings, walls, or wheels, they provide access to a pool or tub, to vehicles, or from bed to chair. Some can be operated independently.

Wall Switches/Outlets

The location of wall switches and electric outlets is important. When designing rooms, outlets can be placed in whatever location is best. Extensions can be placed on existing switches and electric outlets to bring them into easy reach. Planning enough electric outlets so that an appliance does not have to be unplugged to plug in another appliance will aid the person to access outlets easily and reduce fatigue and frustration.

Curtains/Drapes

Short strings or control rods on blinds or curtains can be replaced with longer ones. They can also be operated by remote control.

Communication

Access to the telephone is essential for safety, as well as for social and business reasons. Portable telephones are good investment for people with mobility difficulties because they provide easy access to communication and avoid unnecessary movement. Some models clip on to the belt and have small headphones in place of a receiver, and while cellular phones are more expensive, they operate even if phone or power lines are down.

Phone directories can be visually and physically difficult; so can dialing. Disability exemptions are provided by most local and some long-distance carriers. This eliminates charges for directory assistance and operator-assisted calls. Preprogrammed numbers are accessible with the press of one button. These may be obtained through the local telephone company.

Environmental Control

Environmental control units (ECUs) can provide bedside or chairside control of many electrical functions. With an ECU, lights can be operated, as well as fans and other small appliances, heat, air-conditioning, the telephone, the hospital bed, and audiovisual equipment. It is possible to open and close curtains and answer the door and admit visitors. ECUs can be operated by voice, computer, push buttons, breath—even by eye movement. The simplest systems, providing push button or computer control, are "X-10 Powerhouse" compatible. These are inexpensive, expandable, and available at major retailers.

Lighting

For people with visual problems, assessing and adapting the lighting throughout the home helps avoid abrupt changes, such as going from a dark hallway to a bright bathroom full of shiny surfaces. The use of nightlights can make changes less drastic inexpensively. It is important to maximize contrast in work spaces through the use of light-colored containers and cutting boards when preparing dark food. A dark non-skid mat or towel under a container often helps identifying objects.

Safety Issues

While everyone should consider the safety of the home, it is especially important to plan for emergencies if MS causes cognitive, mobility, or vision problems. Crime, fire, and accident prevention should be the first goal, so emergency measures will never actually be needed.

Access and ability to operate the phone, essential doors and locks, window latches, and mobility aids in times of emergency are integral to safety. Local police and fire departments can help the person with MS or the caregiver conduct a safety inspection and give advice on emergency exit routes.

Installing wide-angle peep holes in solid doors at eye level allows a door to be answered from a chair or scooter. The residence from the outside should not easily show that someone with a disability lives there.

Electric door locks and intercom systems may be well worth the investment. This enables communication with a visitor without opening the door and ensures that the door will lock automatically behind guests as they leave. Some designs also function as an intercom throughout the house.

Comfort

Temperature, humidity, and ventilation affect comfort and influence how a person feels. Temperature extremes should be avoided; 68 degrees Fahrenheit is considered the ideal temperature for working indoors. Different textures have inherent temperatures; metals, ceramics, and smooth surfaces feel cool; fabrics, carpets, and textured surfaces are perceived as warm.

Resources

There are several sources to explore for technical and financial help. Every state has a department of vocational rehabilitation. Some have independent-living programs that provide evaluation and advice on structural modification or equipment to allow people with disabilities to live successfully at home. Many cities have independent-living centers—nonprofit consumer organizations with extensive information and referral services offering advice on living at home with a disability. MS organizations have information on equipment discounts, entitlement programs, local resources, and emergency equipment loans. Any adaptation or renovation to help cope with MS may be tax deductible.

If a person with MS meets low-income requirements, state and local departments of human resources may have programs that provide housekeeping and/or attendant care and financial assistance for adapted equipment and structural modifications.

Lions Clubs specialize in helping people with visual problems. Scout troops earn badges for service to people with disabilities. High school vocational departments may give credit for building projects. Most states have a service agency for the blind. Anyone with a visual impairment is generally eligible for their services.

home health care The delivery of clinical, social, and supportive services at home or in the community to help certain patients, such as those with multiple sclerosis, maintain or regain the highest possible level of health, function, and comfort. An essential element of home health care's success has been the emphasis on patient and family education.

Home health care services can help prevent hospitalizations or institutionalization. Home health care professionals offer comprehensive care in the community along with solid clinical, educational, and supportive services. Services are usually provided by home care organizations or from registries and independent providers. Home care organizations include home health agencies; homemaker and home care aide agencies; staffing and private-duty agencies; and companies specializing in medical equipment and supplies, pharmaceuticals, and drug infusion therapy. Several types of home care organizations may merge to provide a wide variety of services through an integrated system.

Home care services are usually available 24 hours a day, seven days a week. Depending on the patient's needs, services may be provided by one person or a team of specialists.

home health care agency A home care provider that can provide Medicare and Medicaid home health services; such an agency is usually certified by Medicare as meeting federal minimum requirements for patient care and management. Patients who need skilled home care services usually get their care from a home health care agency. Because of legal requirements, services provided by these agencies are highly supervised and well controlled.

Some agencies deliver a variety of home care services through physicians, nurses, therapists, social workers, homemakers, home care aides, and volunteers. Other agencies focus on delivering nursing and one or two other specialties. If a patient needs care from more than one specialist, home health care agencies can put together a caregiving team to administer comprehensive services.

hormone replacement therapy A type of therapy sometimes administered to women who are postmenopausal. Some scientists suspect that hormonal changes may affect neurologic symptoms in multiple sclerosis (MS).

In one study based on questionnaires completed by 30 women with MS attending an MS meeting in London, researchers found evidence to support the idea that hormone replacement therapy (HRT) may have a beneficial effect on MS symptoms in women who have already gone through menopause. Among 19 postmenopausal women, 54 percent reported that their symptoms became worse with menopause. Of those who had tried HRT, 75 percent said it had helped reduce their symptoms. The researchers suggest that the results of the small study support the possibility that the drop in estrogen levels that accompanies menopause may have an adverse effect on the MS disease process. Thus HRT may have a beneficial effect on MS symptoms.

Further research is warranted in this area, particularly given the findings from the Women's Health Study in 2002 and 2004 that the overall risks of HRT may outweigh the benefits for all women. These studies revealed that estrogen replacement alone and that combination estrogen-progestin therapy may cause problems ranging from a higher risk of heart disease and stroke to breast cancer.

See also HORMONES.

hormones Chemical substances produced by the body that circulate in the bloodstream and control numerous body functions. Hormones may affect— and may be affected by—the immune system and therefore may have some effect on multiple sclerosis (MS). For example, both estrogen and progesterone, two important female sex hormones, may suppress some immune activity. The male hormone testosterone may also suppress the immune response.

MS is a disease that is more common in premenopausal women than in other groups. Although what effects hormonal changes have on neurologic symptoms in MS is not entirely clear, it has long been observed that certain other disorders, such as epilepsy or migraine headaches, are worse just before and during menstruation. To see if a correlation exists between neurologic symptoms in women with MS and the menstrual cycle, researchers at an MS clinic distributed a questionnaire to female patients. Of the 149 women with MS who answered the questionnaire, 70 percent reported that their MS symptoms seemed to change at a regular time in their cycle. Most of those who reported a change indicated that the change, usually involving a worsening of their symptoms, occurred within one week of the onset of menstruation—usually involving WEAKNESS, imbalance, FATIGUE, and DEPRESSION. Other self-report studies have replicated these data.

More recently, MAGNETIC RESONANCE IMAGING (MRI) studies done in women with MS at different points in the menstrual cycle indicate that disease activity as measured on MRI may vary according to differing hormonal environments. These findings have all come from small, uncontrolled studies. Much more research is needed to characterize the relationship between MS and the menstrual cycle.

During PREGNANCY, estrogen and progesterone levels are very high, which may help explain why pregnant women with MS usually have fewer exacerbations. In addition, the higher testosterone levels in men may partially account for the fact that women with MS outnumber men with MS by two to one. Manipulation of sex hormones in animal models of MS as well as in models of some other autoimmune diseases has been shown to prevent or ameliorate these diseases.

Both testosterone and ESTRIOL, an estrogen hormone that is produced during late pregnancy, have been shown to have a beneficial effect on experimental allergic encephalomyelitis, the animal model of MS. Based on these findings, scientists conducted a small trial of estriol in women with MS. Estriol appeared to reduce MRI activity in women with RELAPSING-REMITTING MS but not in those with SECONDARY PROGRESSIVE MS.

No large-scale studies have been conducted on the effects of birth control pills or hormone replacement therapy in postmenopausal women with MS. The effects of such hormonal therapies on MS are unknown. One study has suggested that the use of birth control pills by women has no effect on the rate of development of MS.

Horne, Lena (1917–) Singer and actress who was diagnosed with multiple sclerosis. Horne was born June 30, 1917, in Brooklyn, New York, the daughter of an actress and a hotel operator. She was raised primarily by her paternal grandmother, Cora Calhoun Horne. Lena Horne made her professional debut at the age of 16 as a singer in the chorus at Harlem's Cotton Club, learning from the composers Duke Ellington, Cab Calloway, and Harold Arlen. Arlen was later to compose "Stormy Weather," a big hit for him as well as for Horne.

Horne's fame, however, could not prevent the anticommunist extremists from hounding her for her civil rights activism, which marked her in their minds as a communist sympathizer. Like many politically active artists of the time, Horne was blacklisted and unable to perform on television or in the movies. For seven years the attacks continued, but Horne worked as a singer, appearing in nightclubs and making some of her best recordings. *Lena Horne at the Waldorf Astoria*, recorded in 1957, is still considered to be one of her best. Though the conservative atmosphere of the 1950s took their toll on Horne, by the 1960s she had returned to the public eye and was again a major cultural figure.

In 1963, she participated in the March on Washington and performed at rallies throughout the country for the National Council for Negro Women. Horne then spent 10 years touring, recording, and acting in TV and the movies.

Sadly, in the early 1970s her father, son, and husband all died within a period of 12 months, and Horne retreated almost completely from public life. Not until 1981 did she fully return, making a triumphant comeback with a one-person show on Broadway. *Lena Horne: The Lady and Her Music* chronicled Horne's early life and her almost 50 years in show business. It ran for 14 months and became the standard by which one-woman shows are judged. Throughout the past 20 years, Horne's performances have been rare yet welcome occurrences.

hot bath test A once-common test for multiple sclerosis (MS) in which a person suspected of having the disease was immersed in a hot tub of water. If neurologic symptoms appeared or got worse, these symptoms were taken as evidence that the person had MS. The test is no longer widely performed, as more sophisticated diagnostics have been developed.

See also CLIMATE; DIAGNOSIS; HEAT.

housekeeping aids A variety of helpful aids for housecleaning are available from hardware stores and medical supply stores. Long-handled carpet sweepers, dust brooms, and dusters may make cleaning easier. For moving furniture, castors for furniture legs or special pads to help slide furniture are both available. Automatic extension arms with a grip on one end (some with magnets) can be used to grab onto small items out of reach on shelves. People with weak grips may find using a push button pusher that can be fitted onto spray cans to be helpful.

See also ASSISTIVE DEVICES; HOME ADAPTATIONS; OCCUPATIONAL THERAPIST.

Humm, David (1952–) Former Oakland Raiders quarterback who was diagnosed with multiple sclerosis in 1988 and lost the use of his legs in 1997. Humm played 10 seasons in the NFL with the Raiders, the Buffalo Bills, and the Baltimore Colts, and he played on two Super Bowl teams with the Raiders.

hydroxyzine (Atarax) An antihistamine used to relieve allergy symptoms that can also relieve the symptoms of itching seen in some patients with multiple sclerosis (MS). Itching is one of the sensory symptoms (DYSESTHESIA) that can be associated with MS.

Side Effects

Temporary side effects that occur as the body adjusts to the medication include drowsiness, thickened mucus, blurred vision, difficult urination, dizziness, dry mouth, fast heartbeat, sensitivity to sunlight, appetite changes, nightmares, ringing or buzzing in the ears, skin rash, stomach upset, and nervousness or restlessness.

Side effects that should be discussed with a doctor as soon as possible include fast or irregular heartbeat, sore throat and fever, unusual bleeding or bruising, and unusual tiredness or weakness.

Symptoms of overdose include clumsiness or unsteadiness, seizures, severe drowsiness, feeling faint, flushing, hallucinations, shortness of breath, and sleeping problems. Since distinguishing between certain common symptoms of MS and some side effects of hydroxyzine may be difficult, patients should be sure to consult a doctor if an abrupt change of this type occurs.

hyperbaric oxygen treatment A type of treatment for multiple sclerosis (MS) in which the patient is placed into a chamber filled with highly concentrated, high-pressure oxygen in an effort to force oxygen into body tissues. Within the chamber, the oxygen exceeds the usual oxygen pressure at sea level.

Although this type of treatment is useful in treating infections caused by germs that flourish without oxygen, it has been ineffective in suppressing DEMYELINATION. Early reports of amazing responses to hyperbaric oxygen treatments in MS patients have not been supported with subsequent in-depth studies. MS experts do not believe that it is effective in MS. In the past, some thought the treatment decreased the severity and frequency of flare-ups in a few patients but worried that many years later adverse effects from the treatment may appear. This method is very expensive and is not usually covered by health insurance. It has been evaluated in several controlled double-blind studies and found to be ineffective in MS.

hypermetria See DYSMETRIA.

hypometria See DYSMETRIA.

imipramine (Tofranil) A tricyclic antidepressant drug used to treat bladder control problems and nerve pain in patients with multiple sclerosis. One of the safest anticholinergic drugs, it can relieve bladder symptoms by blocking reflexes in the bladder wall or spinal cord. (Imipramine is also often used to help stop bed-wetting in children). A 100 mg dose of imipramine at night may help control bladder activity the next day.

Side Effects

Side effects that typically go away as the body adjusts to the medication and do not require medical attention unless they continue for several weeks include

- blurred or double vision
- dizziness
- drowsiness or unusual fatigue
- muscle aches, weakness, or tremor
- swelling of the hands or legs
- diarrhea or frequent urination
- indigestion
- low blood pressure
- slurred speech
- sleep difficulty

Patients should check with a doctor as soon as possible if any of the following side effects occur:

- clumsiness or unsteadiness
- continuous, uncontrolled eye movements
- depression or mood changes
- memory problems
- hoarseness

- lower back pain
- painful or difficult urination.

Symptoms of overdose requiring immediate attention include

- double vision
- severe diarrhea
- dizziness
- drowsiness
- slurred speech

Because this medicine will add to the effects of alcohol and other central nervous system depressants that may cause drowsiness (such as antihistamines, sedatives, tranquilizers, prescription pain medications, seizure medications, and muscle relaxants), patients should not combine them.

immune system and MS The immune system is what the body depends upon to defend itself against germs. Scientists believe that when a person develops multiple sclerosis (MS), the immune system somehow goes awry, mistakenly attacking the patient's own MYELIN-covered nerves. Exactly how this occurs is not well understood.

The immune system is an elaborate network of white blood cells (leukocytes). When an antigen (such as a virus) first enters the body, the immune system produces a protective chemical called an "antibody" to fight the invading antigen. Antibodies are made by white blood cells (lymphocytes), which are produced in bone marrow and circulate in the blood, seeking to identify and protect against invading germs. The next time that person's body encounters the same virus, the immune system recognizes the antigen and releases the specific antibodies that react to that virus and destroy it more quickly than the first time the antigen was encountered. The immune system is capable of producing antibodies in the exact shape of the antigen, which enables the antibody to destroy the invader.

Scientists have identified two basic types of lymphocytes—B cells and T cells. B cells produce antibodies that neutralize components of invading germs (such as mumps); the T cells act more directly against the germs. Some T cells are cytotoxic T cells, which create holes in the antigen. Other T cells are helper T cells, which boost the role of other immune system cells and activate macrophages—chemicals that ingest every invading antigen they find. Secretions from the helper T cells also trigger the release of natural killer (NK) cells, which also fight viral infections in an unknown way. The suppressor T cells halt the attack the immune system once the invading antigens are completely destroyed.

Scientists are only beginning to decode the complex interactions of the many subsets of the immune system. In addition to the delicate interaction between B cells, T cells, macrophages, and antibodies, the immune system also differentiates between self and nonself components. This is why transplanted organs are rejected by the body: The immune system instantly recognizes that this organ is nonself—not a genetic original—and therefore tries to destroy it.

Some experts believe that MS is caused by an immune system problem in which the person's own MYELIN is somehow perceived as nonself. Scientists know that B cells, T cells, and macrophages accumulate around MS lesions—but whether these cells are actually causing the damage is unclear.

Other experts suspect that a person's immune system may be involved in MS as the result of an attempt to fight off some type of MS virus. No direct evidence indicates that there is such a thing as an MS virus that theoretically hides in myelin, thus triggering the person's immune system to destroy the myelin in an attempt to kill the virus. Some evidence does suggest, however, that myelin and a virus may be chemically similar. If the person's immune system could not tell the difference between the virus and the myelin, the immune system might start to fight off the virus and then turn on the myelin—the virus's identical twin. Once sensitized to myelin, the immune system could continue to attack the myelin, even long after the initiating virus has left the body. If a biochemical similarity triggers such a cross-reaction, this would explain why scientists have never found a specific MS virus.

immunizations and MS Immunizations (also known as vaccinations) are commonly given to people to protect against serious illness. When a person is vaccinated, the body's immune system makes certain protective proteins called antibodies that circulate in the bloodstream to protect against the disease for which the person was vaccinated. For example, a flu shot triggers the body to produce antibodies to protect against the flu.

Immunizations that are safe for people with multiple sclerosis (MS) include

- flu shot
- diphtheria/tetanus
- hepatitis B
- varicella (chicken pox)
- measles and rubella (German measles)

MS patients should delay getting vaccinated if they are having a serious flare-up and have trouble attending to daily activities. Patients should wait at least four weeks after the relapse before getting vaccinated.

Patients who are taking drugs that suppress the immune system should not be vaccinated. If a patient is given a live vaccine when the immune system is suppressed, the patient may get the disease that the vaccination is designed to protect against. Note, however, that interferon and Copaxone are not immune system suppressors. A patient taking these drugs for MS can be safely vaccinated.

immunocompetent cells White blood cells (B and T lymphocytes and others) that defend against invading substances in the body.

See also IMMUNE SYSTEM AND MS.

immunosuppressants Drugs that work by blocking certain factors in the immune system that contribute to the inflammatory process; these drugs are being investigated for use in patients with progressive multiple sclerosis (MS). Each of these drugs can produce serious side effects, including susceptibility to infection, and evidence of their benefits is uncertain. Still, they may help some patients with severe MS.

Mitoxantrone

MITOXANTRONE (Novantron) has been approved for the treatment of secondary progressive MS since two studies suggested that it may be of some help in reducing progression and relapse rates. Cumulative doses can have toxic effects on the heart, however, and so the drug should be used for only a limited period.

Methotrexate

In some patients, low doses of the immunosuppressant METHOTREXATE may slow the course of chronic-progressive MS, particularly in those with secondary progressive MS. So far, however, studies have found beneficial effects on only the upper body. Although this drug, like all immunosuppressants, can have toxic side effects, it may be taken in low doses for MS and so the side effects are generally minimal.

Azathioprine

AZATHIOPRINE (Imuran) is designed to suppress the immune system and reduce the number of cells attacking the myelin sheath covering the nerves. It is administered with or without steroids and is sometimes used as an alternative to patients with relapsing-remitting MS who do not respond to either beta interferon or glatiramer acetate. One study reported that 40 percent of patients had experienced no relapse after taking the drug for three years, a significant decrease. However, others report only modest benefits. The drug has no effect on the progression of disability.

Cyclophosphamide

CYCLOPHOSPHAMIDE (Cytoxan) blocks cell growth and also suppresses the immune system. Some studies have reported benefits for patients with chronic-progressive MS. In particular, two small 2001 studies suggested that monthly intravenous administration of cyclophosphamide or combining it with beta interferon may help some patients with rapidly deteriorating MS. However, cyclophosphamide has many side effects, including hair loss, nausea, vomiting, infertility, lung scarring, and blood abnormalities. Thus it should be considered only for patients who do not respond to other treatment.

Cladribine

CLADRIBINE (Leustatin) may be effective in delaying progression in patients with chronic-progressive MS. It has no significant effect on relapsing-remitting MS.

Drugs Without Benefit

Other immunosuppressant drugs that have shown little or no obvious benefits, or unacceptably high side effects, include sulfasalazine, CYCLOSPORIN A, acyclovir, and oral BOVINE MYELIN.

immunosuppression A form of treatment that can be administered to patients with multiple sclerosis to slow or inhibit the body's natural immune responses, including those directed against the body's own MYELIN.

impotence See ERECTILE DYSFUNCTION.

Imuran See AZATHIOPRINE.

incontinence Loss of bladder or bowel control that may occur in more severe cases of multiple sclerosis (MS). When an MS patient first shows signs of incontinence, a doctor should make sure the problem is not caused by an infection, which is a treatable cause of incontinence.

Urinary incontinence may be controlled by monitoring the frequency of both liquid intake and urinating. Once a schedule has been established, the patient may be able to anticipate incontinence episodes and get to the toilet before they occur. Going to the bathroom at regular intervals, especially after meals, before bedtime, and upon arising—and every two hours during the day—may help.

See also BLADDER DYSFUNCTION; BOWEL DYSFUNCTION.

independent providers   Nurses, therapists, aides, homemakers, and companions who are privately hired by individuals. Aides, homemakers, chore workers, and companions are not required to be licensed or to meet government standards except in cases in which they receive state funding.

The responsibility for recruiting, hiring, and supervising the independent provider rests with the client and his or her family. This also means that finding backup care, in the event that the provider fails to report to work or to fulfill job requirements, is the client's responsibility. Clients also pay the provider directly and must comply with all applicable state and federal labor, health, and safety requirements.

Inderal   See PROPANOLOL.

indwelling catheter   A type of catheter that remains in the bladder on a temporary or permanent basis, used when INTERMITTENT SELF-CATHETERIZATION is impossible or ineffective. The most common type of indwelling catheter is a Foley catheter, a flexible rubber tube inserted into the bladder to allow the urine to flow into an external drainage bag. A small balloon is inflated after insertion to hold the Foley catheter in place. Indwelling catheters require monitoring and care to avoid complications such as infections and bladder stones. Silicone catheters are changed every three to four weeks or at regular intervals to avoid infections. Six to eight glasses of fluid is essential in order to irrigate the bladder and reduce the risk of infection and stone formation. Carbonated drinks should be avoided, as they make the urine alkaline, which encourages stones. Low-grade infections are common with indwelling catheters, and long-term antiseptic treatment or short-term antibiotics may be required.

See also BLADDER DYSFUNCTION.

infections and MS   Since everyone is exposed to numerous VIRUSES and bacteria during childhood, and since viruses are known to cause DEMYELINATION and inflammation, some experts believe that a virus or other infectious agent may trigger multiple sclerosis (MS). Although many infectious microorganisms have been investigated, no one agent has emerged as a proven trigger. However, there are several reasons to suspect a link between viruses and MS.

First, the disease has a distinct geographical distribution, which suggests there could be a contagious aspect to the condition. The number of MS cases increases the farther the distance from the equator in either direction. Second, MS "clusters" also occur in certain areas, such as the clusters that occurred between 1943 and 1989 in the Faeroe Islands. During World War II, this region was occupied by British troops. The incidence of MS in the islands rose each year for 20 years after the war, leading some researchers to think that the troops might have brought with them some disease-causing agent.

The third reason to suspect a viral basis to MS is that some viruses are strikingly similar to the myelin protein, confusing the immune system and causing the T cells to continue to attack their own protein rather than the viral antigen. In addition, more than one antigen may be involved; and some may trigger the disease while others may keep the process going.

It is also possible that different MS patients may be affected by different organisms and that infections cause some, but not all, cases of MS. Organisms at the top of the suspect list are those that can affect the central nervous system. Scientists are studying more than a dozen viruses and bacteria, including measles, hepatitis B, and canine distemper, to determine if they are involved in the development of MS. The top three suspects are HERPESVIRUS 6, *CHLAMYDIA PNEUMONIAE*, and EPSTEIN-BARR VIRUS. So far, however, no germ has been definitively linked to MS.

inflammatory response   The immune system's response to invading organisms or substances is inflammation. Invaders may include viruses, bacteria, fungi, allergens, or, in the case of autoimmune diseases, the body's own tissue.

In multiple sclerosis (MS) and other autoimmune diseases, the inflammatory response appears to be triggered without any kind of germ or invading substance. In the case of MS, certain immune system cells seem to be mistakenly identifying the insulating sheath around nerves (myelin) as a foreign invader.

When an invading organism is first recognized, the immune system launches a response, mobilizing a number of different white blood cells at the site of the infection. A number of physiological changes help to destroy invaders, including:

- increased blow flow to the area to mobilize white blood cells at the site of infection
- thinning of the blood capillary walls to allow the white blood cells to squeeze through
- an increase in local temperature (fever) to kill germs

As the attack continues, a large number of immune system-signaling molecules (chemokines) are released by white blood cells to coordinate the immune response and to call more white blood cells to the site. Once the invader has been vanquished, the body halts the immune response by depriving the white blood cells of nutrients, and making them "commit suicide" (a process called apoptosis). Apoptosis is triggered when special cellular messenger molecules (cytokines) arrive to tell the white blood cells to die and by not sending other cytokines that tell the white blood cells to keep living.

insurance Most people with multiple sclerosis (MS) (60 to 65 percent) are covered by employer-sponsored or other private insurance plans; 20–25 percent are covered by Medicare; 5–10 percent are covered by Medicaid; and 5–10 percent are uninsured.

intention tremor A condition in which goal-directed movements produce shaking in the moving body parts, especially the hands, a condition that is quite common in multiple sclerosis (MS). In order for a person to move a finger to perform a fine task, such as holding a pencil, the nerve transmissions are sent down the motor nerve pathways, informing the arm muscles to move. The brain gets feedback about the movement from sensors in the joints and muscles that it uses to control the movement and gently guide the pencil. People with intention tremor get the feedback more slowly, send corrective transmissions to the muscles more slowly, process the whole thing more slowly in the CEREBELLUM (the part of the brain responsible for coordination), or experience any combination of the three. This makes the hand constantly overshoot the target, resulting in tremor.

Intention tremor is more obvious when performing delicate, fine movements than when carrying out larger ones. Although intention tremor is quite common in MS, it is associated with a number of other conditions, including Parkinson's disease, trapped peripheral nerves, and some drug treatments. Intention tremor is related to ATAXIA and in MS is often caused by lesions in a part of the brain called the CEREBELLUM.

Symptoms and Diagnostic Path
Intention tremor is often detected by neurologists using FINGER-TO-NOSE TESTS. The NEUROLOGIST holds up a finger, and the patient moves his or her finger from his or her nose to the doctor's finger and back to the nose. A tremor may easily be detected using this simple test.

Treatment Options and Outlook
Intention tremor is difficult to treat. Isoniazid, ondansetron (Zofran), propranolol, and primodone are drugs that have been tried with moderate results. Some people with MS find that CANNABIS (marijuana) is effective for tremors. Physical therapy is often useful, and wearing wrist weights can often mask the tremor. DEEP BRAIN STIMULATION with a "gamma knife" (focused radiation) to stimulate or destroy parts of the brain (particularly the thalamus) has been tried, but such options are used only as a last resort for very severe tremors that do not respond to other treatments.

interferon A group of proteins that are normally produced by cells in response to viral infection. Two types of interferon are used to treat multiple sclerosis (MS): interferon beta-1a and interferon beta-1b (Avonex, Rebif, and Betaseron). They were first described in 1957 and were named for their ability to interfere with viruses that are replicating.

Interferons alpha and beta are produced mainly by white blood cells and certain connective tissue cells called fibroblasts. Another type of interferon, interferon gamma, is produced primarily by activated T cells (a naturally occurring substance in the body that promotes inflammation and that some experts believe may be involved in MS flares). Once tried as a treatment for MS, interferon gamma was found to make the disease worse. Interferon beta can counteract the effects of interferon gamma.

Interferon Beta-1a (Avonex)

This medication is approved by the U.S. Food and Drug Administration (FDA) for the treatment of patients with relapsing forms of MS to slow the accumulation of lesions in the brain and lessen the frequency and severity of flare-ups. Avonex is produced from a type of naturally occurring interferon beta (a type of protein). The human-made variety of this interferon is made up of exactly the same amino acids as the natural interferon beta found in the human body.

In studies of patients with relapsing MS, those taking the medication experienced fewer flares and had fewer and smaller active lesions in the brain when compared with the group taking a placebo. In a subsequent study of patients who had experienced a single demyelinating event and who had MS-like lesions in the brain, Avonex significantly delayed the time to a second flare and thus delayed time to a clinically definite diagnosis of MS.

Avonex is injected once a week, usually in the large muscles of the thigh, upper arm, or hip.

Side effects Common side effects include flu-like symptoms (fatigue, chills, fever, muscle aches, and sweating) that disappear after the first few weeks of treatment. If these symptoms continue, become more severe, or cause significant discomfort, patients should discuss their symptoms with a doctor.

Symptoms of depression, including ongoing sadness, anxiety, loss of interest in daily activities, irritability, low self-esteem, guilt, poor concentration, indecisiveness, confusion, and eating and sleep disturbances, should be reported promptly.

Since flu-like symptoms are a fairly common side effect during the initial treatment, experts recommend that the Avonex injection be given at bedtime. Taking acetaminophen (Tylenol) or ibuprofen (Advil) right before each injection and for 24 hours afterward can help ease the flu-like symptoms.

Precautions Avonex should not be used during PREGNANCY or by any woman who is trying to become pregnant. Women taking Avonex should use birth control measures at all times.

No increase in depression reports occurred during studies of the drug. However, since depression and suicidal thoughts are known to occur with some frequency in MS and have been reported with high doses of various interferon products, experts recommend that patients with a history of severe depression be closely monitored while taking Avonex. There also have been postmarketing reports of depression, suicidal thoughts, or new or worsening psychiatric disorders.

Rebif: Another Interferon Beta-1a

In March 2002 the FDA approved a third form of interferon, called Rebif, indicated for the treatment of patients with relapsing forms of MS to decrease the frequency of flares. Like Avonex, Rebif is the beta-1a form of the human protein interferon. However, unlike Avonex's once-a-week, intramuscular injection regimen, Rebif is injected three times a week subcutaneously.

Interferon Beta-1b (Betaseron)

This drug also lessens the frequency and severity of MS attacks and reduces the accumulation of lesions in the brain. It was approved by the FDA in 1993 to reduce the frequency of flares in relapsing-remitting MS. In 2003, the FDA extended the approval of Betaseron to "relapsing-forms of MS," including people with secondary progressive MS who continue to have relapses.

Betaseron works by reducing the body's immune response that is misdirected against its own myelin, the fatty sheath that surrounds and protects nerve fibers. This destruction, known as demyelination, slows or halts nerve impulses and produces the symptoms of MS. Damage to the myelin sheath is also associated with destruction of the nerve fibers themselves.

Betaseron is produced from one of the naturally occurring interferons (a type of protein). In a clinical trial of 372 ambulatory patients with relapsing-remitting MS, those taking the currently recommended dose of the medication experienced fewer exacerbations, a longer time between exacerbations, and exacerbations that were generally less severe than those of patients taking a lower dose of the medication or a placebo. Additionally, patients on interferon beta-lb had no increase in total lesion area, as shown on magnetic resonance imaging, in contrast to the placebo group, who had a significant increase.

Betaseron is injected between the fat layer just under the skin and the muscles beneath every other day.

Side effects Common side effects include flu-like symptoms (fatigue, chills, fever, muscle aches, and sweating) and injection site reactions (swelling, redness, discoloration, and pain). Most of these symptoms tend to disappear over time. If they continue, become more severe, or cause significant discomfort, though, the patient should discuss these problems with a physician.

The patient should contact a physician if the injection sites become inflamed, hardened, or lumpy. Patients should not inject into any area that has become hardened or lumpy.

Depression has been reported by patients taking Betaseron, including symptoms of sadness, anxiety, loss of interest in daily activities, irritability, low self-esteem, guilt, poor concentration, indecisiveness, confusion, and eating and sleep disturbances. Some patients have attempted suicide. Patients who feel suicidal or who experience any of these symptoms for longer than a day or two should contact a physician promptly.

Managing symptoms Since flu-like symptoms are a common side effect associated with the initial weeks of taking Betaseron, experts recommend that patients take the medication at bedtime. Taking acetaminophen (Tylenol) or ibuprofen (Advil) 30 minutes before each injection will also help ease flu-like symptoms.

Because swelling, redness, discoloration, or pain at the injection site are fairly common, experts recommend that patients rotate the sites according to a schedule provided by a physician. Skin damage at the injection site occurs in about 5 percent of patients during the first four months of therapy.

In order to avoid infection and other complications, patients should report any break in the skin, which may be associated with blue-black discoloration, swelling, or drainage of fluid from the injection site. A physician must decide whether to continue treatment while the skin lesions are being treated.

Precautions Betaseron should not be used during pregnancy or by any woman who is trying to become pregnant. Women taking Betaseron should use birth control measures at all times. Because of the potential of Betaseron to affect the functioning of the liver and thyroid gland and to alter the levels of white blood cells, red blood cells, and platelets in a person's system, blood tests are recommended at regular intervals. During a clinical trial, four suicide attempts and one completed suicide occurred among those taking interferon beta-1b. Although no evidence indicates that the suicide attempts were related to the medication itself, it is recommended that individuals with a history of severe depressive disorder be closely monitored while taking Betaseron.

interferon beta-1a See INTERFERON.

intermittent self-catheterization (ISC) A procedure in which a patient periodically inserts a catheter into the urinary opening to drain urine from the bladder. ISC is used in the management of BLADDER DYSFUNCTION to drain urine that remains after voiding, prevent bladder distention, prevent kidney damage, and restore bladder function.

See also INDWELLING CATHETER.

internuclear ophthalmoplegia A disorder of eye movements caused by a lesion in an area of the brain called the medial longitudinal fasciculus. This condition is associated with jerky eye movements (NYSTAGMUS) in one eye when the other one moves outward. It can also, but not always, cause DOUBLE VISION (diplopia). Multiple sclerosis (MS) is the most common cause of internuclear ophthalmoplegia, and in MS it usually affects only one eye.

See also VISUAL PROBLEMS.

intramuscular injection Injection characterized by a long needle that is injected deep into the muscle.

intravenous immunoglobulin G (IVIG) A sterile solution of concentrated antibodies taken from healthy people and injected into a vein of a person with low antibody levels to prevent bacterial infections. Although it is not currently approved for use in multiple sclerosis (MS), there is some evidence that IVIG reduces annualized exacerbation rates. Immunoglobulins are antibody proteins secreted by white blood cells (called B lymphocytes) and by plasma cells in response to the presence of antigens (foreign substances in the body).

Early clinical trials of treating MS with IVIG produced variable results. However, a subsequent two-year Austrian study of patients with RELAPSING-REMITTING MS showed a small but significant improvement on the EXPANDED DISABILITY STATUS SCALE. In a second study in Israel, fewer patients had flare-ups, but there was no effect on lesions shown on magnetic resonance imaging. Another study in 1998 showed fewer brain lesions in treated patients with relapsing-remitting MS than in nontreated patients.

A recent meta-analysis of the various IVIG studies conclude the drug may be a valuable alternative for the treatment of relapsing-remitting MS for those patients who cannot or will not take one of the approved injectable medications. More research is needed to establish the role of IVIG in the management of MS and to determine the ideal dosage level.

Ishihara Test for Color Blindness (ITCB)   A test of color vision.

isoniazid (Laniazid)   An antituberculosis drug that is used for patients with multiple sclerosis who have certain types of tremors.

Side Effects
Temporary side effects that do not require medical attention unless they persist include

- nervousness and restlessness
- sleep difficulties

- dizziness
- rapid heartbeat
- flushing and sweating
- headache
- nausea
- trembling
- weakness
- pink or red saliva

Side effects that patients should report to a physician as soon as possible include chest pain and irregular heartbeat.

itching   Itching may occur as a symptom of multiple sclerosis. It may present as one of many different abnormal sensations, including PINS AND NEEDLES, burning, stabbing, or tearing pains. These sensations are known as DYSESTHESIAS. Dysesthetic itching may occur in sudden, brief, but intense periods over any part of the body or face. It is different from the generalized itching that can accompany an allergic reaction since there is no external skin rash or irritation at the site.

Treatment Options and Outlook
Corticosteroid ointments will not help ease this type of itch, but several medications can help dysesthetic itching. These include anticonvulsants, such as carbamazepine (Tegretol), diphenylhydantoin (Dilantin), and GABAPENTIN (Neurontin). Antidepressants such as amitriptyline (Elavil) and monoamine oxidase inhibitors or the antihistamine hydroxyzine (Atarax) also may help.

joint position sense function test A sensory exam often included in a NEUROLOGICAL EXAMINATION in which people are assessed for multiple sclerosis. People are told to stand up, shut their eyes, and position their feet together. Healthy individuals will receive enough information from their joints to keep their balance and remain standing; patients with sensory loss in the joints will tend to lose their balance during this test. In a variation of this test, the doctor moves a patient's big toe while the person's eyes are closed, asking the patient whether the toe is extended up or down. Patients with sensory problems involving the joints will have trouble with this test.

Jordan, Barbara (1936–1996) Congresswoman, professor, and civil rights activist who was diagnosed with multiple sclerosis (MS) and who died of pneumonia at the age of 59.

Barbara Charline Jordan was born February 21, 1936, in Houston, Texas, to impoverished parents, Ben and Arlyne Jordan. Early in life she distinguished herself in school. Jordan graduated magna cum laude from Texas Southern University in 1956 and earned her law degree from Boston University in 1959. She then returned home to Houston to practice law. She was elected to the Texas senate in 1966, becoming the first female African American to do so. In 1972, she was elected president pro tempore of the Texas senate—the first African American elected to preside over a legislative body anywhere in the country. When Jordan was elected to the U.S. House of Representatives in 1972, she became the first African-American woman to represent a previously Confederate state in Congress. In 1976, Barbara Jordan became the first African-American woman to deliver a keynote

address at a political convention. As a member of the House Judiciary Committee, Jordan was in the national spotlight during the Watergate hearings that would eventually lead to the resignation of President Nixon.

Jordan retired from politics in 1979 after three terms in Congress and accepted a position on the faculty at the University of Texas at Austin. Her battle with MS was taking its toll on her health.

Barbara Jordan lived with Nancy Earl in their home in Texas. The two had met on a camping trip in the 1960s and lived together for two decades. In 1976, they built a house in Austin.

Jordan addressed the Democratic National Convention again in 1992 in New York. Two years later she was awarded the Presidential Medal of Freedom, the nation's highest civilian honor. Despite her declining health, she continued to teach and serve in public office, including a post on the presidential task force on immigration reform.

Jordan died of pneumonia on January 17, 1996, at the Austin Diagnostic Medical Center. She was eulogized by President Clinton and former Texas Governor Anne Richards. Jordan was buried at the Texas State Cemetery—an honor reserved for Texas heroes. She was the first African-American woman to be buried there.

journaling The practice of keeping a journal is used by some people with multiple sclerosis as a nonmedical coping strategy. A written or tape-recorded account of symptoms can help individuals keep track of when problems occur, the management tools that work best for specific symptoms, medication schedules, and many other issues. Some patients find that recording thoughts and feelings may also be helpful.

Kabat, Elvin A. (1914–2000) American immunochemist best known for his immunological studies of multiple sclerosis (MS).

Throughout the 20th century, research has continued to map the precise cause and effects of MS as investigative methods became more sophisticated with advancing technology. During the 1940s, Dr. Kabat used electrophoresis to study samples from MS patients at Columbia University. Dr. Kabat compared the electrophoretic pattern of proteins in the cerebrospinal fluid (CSF) with controls, finding that the CSF from MS patients contained a higher proportion of gamma globulins. His key finding confirmed that there was an immunological component to MS, a concept first postulated in the late 19th century. Subsequent research has tried to explain why the immune system generates this inappropriate response, and potential treatments have focused on trying to suppress the immunological activity that leads to DEMYELINATION (the destruction of the protective sheath that covers nerve fibers).

Klonopin See CLONAZEPAM.

Kurtzke disability status scale One of the most common scoring systems used to estimate the progression of multiple sclerosis. Few if any patients, however, will experience every single step on the scale, especially in the advanced stages. It is also possible that not every patient will follow each step chronologically; a patient may reach the sixth step and then improve, moving back to step two or three.

0 Normal neurological exam results without any symptoms of disease

1 No symptoms but slightly abnormal signs

2 Slight disability in one body function

3 Moderate disability in one body function, but patient can walk independently

4 Severe disability in one body function, but patient can still walk independently

5 Severe disability with severely impaired ability to walk; patient cannot work a full day

6 Aids such as a cane are required for walking

7 Patient is confined to a wheelchair and can walk only a few minutes a day

8 Patient is fully confined to a wheelchair or bed and cannot walk at all; arm movements remain intact

9 Patient is fully confined to bed and has little or no use of limbs

10 Death

See also EXPANDED DISABILITY STATUS SCALE.

laboratory testing for multiple sclerosis   There is no single test that results in a diagnosis of multiple sclerosis (MS); therefore, tests performed in the diagnosis process are interpreted for each individual case. The following tests are used in the diagnosis process in addition to a clinical history and a clinical neurological examination. These tests also help exclude other possible diseases.

- *Magnetic resonance imaging (MRI)*   This highly specific brain scan is sensitive in detecting the destruction of MYELIN (the protective covering of nerves). MRI also helps track the progression of MS over time.

- *Cerebrospinal fluid*   Checking this fluid can reveal a substance called oligoclonal bands, which indicate that a chronic inflammatory process in occurring in the central nervous system. More than 90 percent of people with clinically definite MS will have oligoclonal bands. A spinal tap also can exclude other diseases similar to MS.

- *Evoked potentials*   These tests may demonstrate reduced transmission of impulses across nerve fibers caused by demyelination. Visual evoked potentials are the most sensitive to MS-related damage and can help confirm a diagnosis.

- *Blood studies*   Blood tests are usually normal in people with MS; abnormal results may indicate a diagnosis of another disease.

language areas of the brain   The areas of the brain associated with language reception, comprehension, processing, and production are still not fully understood. However, functional BRAIN SCANS have helped explain how the brain interacts with language. Some of these areas may be affected by multiple sclerosis.

Broca's Area

Most studies agree that this area of the frontal lobe in the dominant hemisphere is primarily related to speech production. Broca's area is usually associated with maintaining of a list of words and parts of words used in producing speech and their associated meanings. It has been linked to articulation of speech and to semantic processing, or assigning meanings to the words people use.

The original area described in 1861 by Pierre Paul Broca to be the "seat of articulate language" has now been further studied and subdivided by functional imaging studies (functional magnetic resonance imaging [fMRI] and positron emission tomography [PET] scans) into smaller subsections that each participate differently in language tasks. Semantic processing has been linked to the upper portion of the area, while articulation falls within the center of Broca's original region of importance. Broca's area is not simply a speech area but is associated with the process of articulating language in general. It controls not only spoken but also written and signed language production.

M1-Mouth Area

This area of the brain is responsible for controlling the physical movements of the mouth and articulators used to produce speech. It is part of the motor cortex and controls the muscles of the face and mouth just as the rest of the motor cortex controls various other parts of the body's movement. It is not involved with the cognitive aspects of speech production, though it is located near Broca's area and is activated in speech tasks along with Broca's area.

Wernicke's Area

This semantic-processing area is associated with some memory functions, especially the short-term memory involved in speech recognition and production, as well as some hearing function and object identification. Wernicke's area is most often associated with language comprehension or the processing of incoming written or spoken language.

This distinction between speech and language is key to understanding the role of Wernicke's area to in creating language. It does not simply affect spoken language but also affects written and signed language. Wernicke's area works with Broca's area: Wernicke's area handles incoming speech, while Broca's area handles outgoing speech.

Auditory Cortex

The areas of the brain responsible for recognizing and receiving sound are closely linked with language processing. In spoken language tasks, without correct auditory input, language comprehension cannot happen. As people speak or read words aloud, there is evidence that they listen to themselves as they are speaking to make sure they are speaking correctly. Areas around the auditory cortex, near Wernicke's area, are probably also involved in short-term memory; specifically, a loop is created in which language heard is continuously repeated in the brain in order to maintain that language in the memory.

Visual Cortex

The area responsible for vision, which is important in reading words or recognizing objects as an initial step in naming objects. The visual areas of the brain are usually among the first parts of the brain activated in reading and object-naming activities for speech tests in fMRI and PET scans. Other than this primary visual area located in the occipital lobe, another set of areas associated with vision are located in the parietal lobe, above the visual cortex. This parietal lobe region is associated with object naming and word reading and is thought of as supplementary to the primary visual cortex. The visual cortex, along with the auditory cortex, is one possible first step on the path to language comprehension.

Laniazid   See ISONIAZID.

late-onset MS   Diagnosis of multiple sclerosis (MS) after age 50; only about 9.4 percent of those with MS have late-onset cases. Late-onset MS seems to be more common than experts had previously thought.

Because of other medical problems that affect older people, MS may be overlooked, accounting for a large number of misdiagnosed cases. Whether there is a difference in prognosis for those with late-onset MS is still not understood.

Lawry, Sylvia (1915–2001)   Founder and executive director of the National Multiple Sclerosis Society. Sylvia Lawry profoundly influenced research, disease management, and public policy concerning multiple sclerosis (MS).

Born in Brooklyn in 1915, one of four children of Jacob and Sophie Friedman, Lawry was attending Hunter College to become a lawyer when her younger brother Bernard began suffering visual and balance problems. These symptoms were diagnosed as MS, and for several years, the family searched for a cure. In 1945, Lawry placed a small classified ad in the *New York Times,* asking to contact anyone who had recovered from the disease. When she received more than 50 replies from individuals desperate to find encouraging news about MS, Lawry realized the need for an organized effort to stimulate and finance research on the cure, treatment, and cause of this disease. In 1946, Lawry met with 20 of the nation's most prominent research scientists and founded the Association for Advancement of Research in Multiple Sclerosis with the sole purpose of sponsoring MS research. The organization was renamed the National Multiple Sclerosis Society in 1947. That same year, the first two local chapters of the society were chartered in California and Connecticut.

Although her brother Bernard's health continued to weaken and he ultimately died from MS-related causes in 1973, Sylvia Lawry realized that thousands of others like her brother needed help. With the assistance of Senator Charles Tobey of New Hampshire, whose daughter had MS, Lawry persuaded Congress to adopt legislation on August 15, 1950, establishing what is now the National Institute of Neurological Disorders and Stroke.

In 1967, spurred by the fact that almost a third of the society's research funds were being awarded to investigators outside the United States, Lawry founded the Multiple Sclerosis International Federation to help coordinate fund-raising and service efforts of young societies in Canada, Britain, France, Germany, and other European countries modeled on the U.S. original. The federation became a catalyst for the MS movement in Latin America, Japan, Australia, New Zealand, and Eastern Europe. Today there are 38 member societies around the world.

Lawry served as executive director of the National Multiple Sclerosis Society until 1982 and maintained her role as secretary of the International Federation of MS Societies until 1997. She continued to serve as an officer of the national board and devoted her efforts to the society's international programs.

She died February 24, 2001, in New York City at the age of 85.

Leber's hereditary optic neuropathy   A condition that causes central visual loss in both eyes, that may mimic OPTIC NEURITIS (inflammation of the OPTIC NERVE). Optic neuritis is a common condition in multiple sclerosis.

leg brace   Brace worn on the leg that can stabilize a weakened muscle to make walking easier. Weakness of the leg muscles may make it more difficult to maneuver on stairs, get up from a sitting position, or walk. An ankle-foot brace can stabilize the ankle when there is weakness in the foot muscles. This brace fits into an ordinary shoe and prevents the toes from dragging.

leukodystrophy   A group of genetic disorders characterized by the imperfect development or maintenance of MYELIN (the sheath that protects nerve fibers). Diseases in this class include adrenoleukodystrophy, Alexander's disease, Canavan's disease, Krabbe's disease, metachromatic leukodystrophy, Pelizaeus-Merzbacher disease, Refsum's disease, and phenylketonuria.

Leustatin   See CLADRIBINE.

Lhermitte's sign   A brief, stabbing, electric shock–like PAIN that runs from the back of the head down the spine, arms, and sometimes the legs, triggered by bending the neck forward. This type of sensory discomfort is quite common in multiple sclerosis. Medications such as anticonvulsants may be used to prevent the pain, or a soft collar may be used to limit neck flexion.

Lidwina of Schiedam, Saint (1380–1433)   Hers is possibly the earliest known case of multiple sclerosis (MS) to be described. Lidwina lived in 14th-century Holland. Historical texts reveal that she was afflicted with a debilitating disease that sounds a great deal like MS.

St. Lidwina's disease began soon after she fell while skating, at the age of 16. From that time onward, she developed walking difficulties, headaches, and violent pains in her teeth. By the age of 19, both her legs were paralyzed and she had developed vision problems. Over the next 34 years, St. Lidwina's condition slowly deteriorated, although there were periods of remission; eventually, she died at the age of 53.

St. Lidwina's symptoms were consistent with those of MS, as were her age of onset and the length and progression of the disease. Together these factors suggest that a posthumous diagnosis of MS may be plausible.

See also D'ESTE, SIR AUGUSTUS FREDERIC.

life care community   See CONTINUUM OF CARE RETIREMENT COMMUNITIES.

life expectancy and MS   People with multiple sclerosis (MS) typically live between six to seven years less than the general population. The vast majority of people with MS die from the same diseases as everyone else—heart disease, cancer, or stroke.

A fatal MS lesion is extremely unusual. Without adequate medical care, a person with MS might die as a result of a lesion in the part of the brain that regulates breathing or from large areas of DEMYELINATION that interfere with life-supporting systems in the body. Certain complications of ADVANCED MS, such as severe urinary tract infections, pneumonia, or extensive skin breakdown, also can threaten life and may prove fatal even with adequate treatment. Modern antibiotic therapy and sophisticated supportive care strategies make it possible to control these problems in most cases. Severe untreated DEPRESSION is also known to be responsible for the relatively high suicide rate among people with MS.

While severe MS or its complications may be fatal, the likelihood is so rare that MS is not considered to be a fatal disease.

linoleic acid   A dietary supplement and a major component of evening primrose oil, also found in sunflower seeds and safflower oils, made up of polyunsaturated fatty acids. To date, studies have shown that linoleic acid has only a very modest positive effect on multiple sclerosis. Researchers were interested in studying linoleic acid because these fatty acids are an element of MYELIN, the sheath that protects nerve fibers. There does not appear to be any risk of major side effects when using small amounts of this oil.

Lioresal   See BACLOFEN.

living trust   A notarized legal document in which a person states that some or all of his or her property be held in trust by a trustee, simplifying the eventual disposition of the estate and, in some cases, avoiding probate of the estate after the person's death. One of its advantages is that the person's assets move to heirs without having to go through probate—the process by which the state examines a will and declares it valid. That is especially helpful in states such as California and Florida, where probate can drag on for months. If you own property in several states, multiple probate proceedings may be required.

A revocable living trust can be useful if a patient with multiple sclerosis becomes incapable of taking care of personal financial affairs. In this case, the successor trustee—the person who would distribute trust property after the patient's death—can also, in most cases, take over management of the trust property if the patient becomes incapacitated.

A living trust is also private, while probate is a public process. However, living trusts are not for everyone. At $2,000–$3,000 each, they cost more than wills to prepare, and to make them effective, all the person's assets must be transferred into the trust.

living will   A legal document that allows a person to outline what is to be done about specific health care decisions and whether life-sustaining treatment is to be carried out. Most states recognize living wills.

Lofstrand crutches   A type of forearm crutch that provides greater stability than a CANE and does not require the same amount of strength in the upper extremities.

long-term care   A comprehensive range of medical, personal, and social services coordinated to meet the physical, social, and emotional needs of people who are disabled, such as those with severe multiple sclerosis. A nursing home facility may be the best choice for people who require 24-hour medical care and supervision.

Nursing homes can provide two types of care. Basic care includes services needed to maintain a resident's ACTIVITIES OF DAILY LIVING (including personal care, walking, supervision, and safety). Skilled care requires a registered nurse to provide treatments and procedures on a regular basis. Skilled care also includes services provided by specially trained professionals, such as physical and occupational therapy.

The services nursing homes offer vary from facility to facility. Services often include

- room and board
- medication monitoring
- personal care
- 24-hour emergency care
- social and recreational activities

Because finding the right nursing home can take time, the search for a suitable place should begin long before the person will need to be admitted. There are often long waiting periods for available accommodations. Planning ahead can also make the transition of moving into a nursing home much easier.

Before scheduling a visit to prospective nursing homes, the family should ask about vacancies, admission requirements, level of care provided, and participation in government-funded health insurance options.

Financing options should also be considered. Nursing home care can be paid for via Medicare, Medicaid, private insurance, or personal funds. When evaluating nursing homes, asking the administration what payment options they accept is important.

Medicare is a federal health insurance program providing health care benefits to all Americans age 65 and over. Insurance protection intended to cover major hospital care is provided without regard to income, but only restricted benefits are allowed for nursing home care. In addition, Medicare pays for skilled care only in a nursing facility that has a Medicare license.

Medicaid is a joint federal/state health insurance program providing medical care benefits to low-income Americans who meet certain requirements. Nursing-home care is covered through Medicaid, but eligibility requirements and covered services vary widely from state to state.

Private long-term care insurance is a health insurance option that can supplement Medicare coverage. Private long-term care insurance policies vary; each policy has its own eligibility requirements, restrictions, costs, and benefits.

Lou Gehrig's disease   See AMYOTROPHIC LATERAL SCLEROSIS (ALS) VS. MULTIPLE SCLEROSIS.

lumbar puncture   See SPINAL TAP.

Lyme disease   A tick-borne illness whose hallmark symptom is a bull's-eye red rash surrounding the tick bite. If left untreated, Lyme disease can cause arthritis and disorders of the heart and central nervous system. The disease shares some symptoms with multiple sclerosis (MS).

Symptoms and Diagnostic Path

There may be delayed neurologic symptoms similar to those seen in MS, such as weakness; OPTIC NEURITIS, producing blurred vision; sensations of itching, burning, stabbing pain, or "pins and needles"; confusion; and FATIGUE. Lyme disease symptoms also may have a relapsing-remitting course.

Lyme disease occasionally produces similar abnormalities in tests that are used to diagnose MS, including magnetic resonance imaging (MRI) brain scans and analysis of cerebrospinal fluid.

All these similarities in symptoms and test results have led some people with MS to be tested for the presence of antibodies to the Lyme disease bacteria. The distinction is important because Lyme disease, especially when treated early, often responds to antibiotic therapy, whereas MS does not.

Two recent studies have examined the overlap in diagnosis of MS and Lyme disease, conducted in parts of Long Island, New York, an area where Lyme disease is endemic. In the first study, people who had antibodies in their blood and had a variety of neurological symptoms considered "MS-like," were evaluated with MRI, evoked potentials, and cerebrospinal fluid analysis, including a test for the presence of antibodies to the Lyme disease bacteria in the spinal fluid. While those with the MS-like illness had the highest incidence of abnormal MRIs and were the only ones among those studied with abnormal evoked potentials and oligoclonal bands (indicating an abnormal immune response) in the spinal fluid, they did not have any antibodies in their spinal fluid. The researchers concluded that the few individuals with the MS-like symptoms probably had these symptoms due to MS and had also been exposed to the bacteria.

A companion study looked for the presence of antibodies in the blood of 100 people with the diagnosis of possible MS. Of 89 people who, in fact, turned out to have definite MS, only one had Lyme disease bacteria antibodies. Experts conclude that since the bacteria is uncommon in people with MS, it is unlikely that Lyme disease has any significance in the differential diagnosis of MS.

Lyme disease is most commonly contracted in the northeastern coastal states from Maine to Maryland, in the upper Midwest, and on the Pacific coast during the late spring or early summer, when ticks are abundant, although it may occur whenever the temperature is above 40 degrees Fahrenheit for several consecutive days. Most of the time it is easily treated and does not progress to the chronic stages. It probably causes severe long-term effects in fewer than 10 percent of untreated patients.

The spirochete form of the bacteria is transmitted primarily by the deer tick, the tiniest of which is about the size of the period at the end of this sentence. These ticks are found on deer, birds, field mice, and other rodents. The tick must be attached to its victim for between 36–48 hours before an infectious dose of spirochetes are transmitted. For this reason, simply by checking children often for ticks, parents can usually prevent them from becoming infected.

Most patients are diagnosed in the spring, summer, or early fall. In the northern states, about half of all adult *Ixodes scapularis* ticks are infected. In some places, such as Block Island and Nantucket, the numbers are even higher. Even so, in most sections of the northeast, only between 1 percent and 3 percent of patients have contracted Lyme disease.

The tick that transmits Lyme diseases in California relies on intermediate hosts, such as lizards, that are resistant to infection. For this reason, ticks (and consequently, humans) are infected much less often here than in the northeast.

Most patients who do become infected usually display one or more symptoms between three days and a month after becoming infected. About 60 percent of victims will notice a small red spot that expands over a period of days or weeks, forming a circular, triangular, or oval-shaped rash. The reddened area, which usually appears at the bite site, neither itches nor hurts. Sometimes the rash resembles a red raised bull's-eye rash with a clear center. The rash can range in size from that of a dime to the entire width of the body. As the infection spread, several rashes can appear at different places. Without treatment, the rash begins to disappear within days or weeks.

As the spirochetes move through the body via the blood, other symptoms affecting other parts of the body may appear. These may include flu-like symptoms such as headaches, stiff neck, appetite loss, body aches and fatigue. Although these symptoms may resemble those of common viral infections, Lyme disease symptoms tend to persist or may occur intermittently.

About 20 percent of patients may experience early neurological problems, including facial paralysis, meningitis, encephalitis, or numbness or tingling in other parts of the body. Many of these symptoms resemble MS.

After several months of being infected, slightly more than half of those patients not treated with antibiotics develop recurrent attacks of painful and swollen joints that last a few days to a few months. The arthritis can shift from one joint to another; most often, the knee is infected. About 10–20 percent of untreated patients who experience temporary arthritic symptoms will go on to develop chronic Lyme arthritis. In contrast to many other forms of arthritis, Lyme arthritis is typically not symmetrical, thus one side of the body may be more affected than the other.

One out of 100 Lyme patients develop heart problems such as irregular heartbeat for a few days or weeks, generally appearing several weeks after infection. Most patients will not be aware of this problem unless their doctor detects it. Other nervous system complications include memory loss, concentration problems, and changes in mood or sleeping habits. Nervous system abnormalities usually develop several weeks, months, or even years after an untreated infection. These symptoms often last for weeks or months and may recur.

Lyme disease is not easy to diagnose because its symptoms mimic those of many other diseases. Joint pain can be misdiagnosed as inflammatory arthritis, and neurologic signs may be misidentified. Diagnosis includes consideration of exposure to ticks, symptoms, and the result of blood tests to determine whether the patient has antibodies to Lyme bacteria. The tests are most useful in later stages.

Treatment Options and Outlook

Antibiotics (tetracycline or amoxicillin) usually provide a complete recovery if given early enough. Most patients who are treated in later stages of the disease also respond well. Unfortunately, cases that are not diagnosed soon enough may resist antibiotic treatment. In a few people, symptoms of persistent infection may continue, or the disease may recur, so that doctors prescribe repeated long courses of antibiotics. The value of this approach remains debated.

Patients with chronic Lyme disease may exhibit varying degrees of permanent damage to joints or the nervous system. This usually occurs among those who were not diagnosed in the early stages of the disease or for whom early treatment was not successful. Deaths from Lyme disease have been reported only rarely.

However, experts at the Centers for Disease Control and Prevention (CDC) do not recommend automatic treatment with antibiotics after every tick bite.

Risk Factors and Preventive Measures

Experts recommend that it is far better to prevent the disease than to try to treat it.

Lyme vaccine Although a vaccine against Lyme disease (LYMErix) was approved in 1999 for people aged 15–70 years, as of February 25, 2002, the manufacturer announced that the vaccine will no longer be commercially available, citing poor sales. LYMErix had caused controversy in recent years, as patients charged they were sickened by the vaccine and asked the government to restrict sales; some filed lawsuits against maker GlaxoSmithKline. Federal health officials say they have found no evidence that the vaccine was dangerous.

The Food and Drug Administration (FDA) approved the sale of LYMErix in 1998, but the CDC had urged that only people at high risk of Lyme disease be vaccinated because the expensive vaccine did not offer complete protection. Studies showed it was 80 percent effective after people received all three required shots. After vaccinations began, though, some patients reported arthritis, muscle pain, and other symptoms similar to those found with Lyme disease itself. Because 15 percent of the U.S. population has arthritis, scientists found it difficult to determine how symptoms were connected to LYMErix.

When the CDC reexamined 905 possible side effects reported to the government between 1998 and July 2000, their results (published in the journal *Vaccine*) found no signs that Lymerix caused arthritis but did find 22 cases of allergic reaction. Still, at least seven lawsuits are pending over alleged vaccine reactions, and several hundred more people may file. The FDA is continuing to investigate.

magnetic resonance imaging (MRI) A diagnostic test that produces very clear pictures of the human body by using powerful magnetic fields. These fields create resonating signals in the nuclei of hydrogen atoms, found in the water contained in all body tissues and fluids. Computers translate the increased energy of the hydrogen nuclei into cross-sectional images of the body. A contrast agent (GADOLINIUM) can be injected intravenously to enhance the sensitivity of the MRI scan even further.

MRI is the preferred method of imaging to help establish a diagnosis of multiple sclerosis (MS) and is now often used to detect disease progression in seemingly stable patients. It is the most sensitive noninvasive way of imaging the brain, spinal cord, or other areas of the body.

MRI is particularly useful in detecting central nervous system demyelination (destruction of the nerve covering called MYELIN). Demyelination slows or halts nerve impulses and produces the symptoms of MS.

Studies have repeatedly shown that MRI of the brain can reveal areas of demyelination that are not apparent on a computerized axial tomography scan, although about 5 percent of patients with clinically definite MS do not show lesions on MRI and the absence of demyelination on MRI does not rule out MS. Also, since many lesions seen on MRI may be in "silent" areas of the brain, there is not always a correlation between the MRI scan results and a patient's symptoms. In addition, people over the age of 50 often have findings on MRI that resemble MS but are actually related to the aging process and have no clinical significance. In short, although MRI may be useful in helping to confirm a diagnosis of suspected MS, it cannot be used exclusively to diagnose the disease.

Once a positive diagnosis of MS has been established, there is no reason why a patient should have further diagnostic MRI scans. Subsequent scans, however, may prove useful in tracking the progress of the disease or helping to establish the prognosis. For example, some researchers have demonstrated that the degree of COGNITIVE DYSFUNCTION, as demonstrated by neuropsychologic testing, can be correlated with the amount of demyelination seen in certain areas of the brain on MRI.

Procedure

Before undergoing MRI, the patient should remove personal items such as a watch, wallet (including any credit cards with magnetic strips that can be erased by the magnet), and jewelry.

During the test, the patient should experience no unusual sensations. The test takes about 40–80 minutes. During that time, several dozen images may be taken.

Risks and Complications

An MRI poses no risk to the average person if appropriate safety guidelines are followed. People who have had heart surgery can be safely examined with MRI, as can people with the following medical devices:

- artificial joints
- brain shunt tubes for hydrocephalus
- cardiac valve replacements (except the Starr-Edwards metallic ball/cage)
- medication pumps that are disconnected
- staples
- surgical clips or sutures
- vena cava filters

However, some conditions may make an MRI examination inadvisable. A patient should inform the doctor if he or she has any of the following conditions:

- cerebral aneurysm clip
- claustrophobia
- cochlear implant
- gastroesophageal reflux (a common disease that causes heartburn)
- heart pacemaker
- implanted devices: insulin pump (for treatment of diabetes), narcotics pump (for pain medication), nerve stimulators ("TENS"), spine stabilization rods
- inability to lie prone for 30–60 minutes
- lung disease (severe) such as tracheomalacia or bronchopulmonary dysplasia
- metal in the eye or eye socket
- pregnancy
- weight above 300 pounds

magnetic resonance spectroscopy imaging (MRSI)
A noninvasive analytical technique that has been used to study metabolic changes in the brain in order to rule out tumors, strokes, seizure disorders, depression, and other diseases affecting the brain. It has also been used to study the metabolism of other organs.

MRSI is similar to MAGNETIC RESONANCE IMAGING (MRI). However, MRSI depends on the behavior of other chemical elements, such as phosphorus and calcium, to identify the chemical composition of diseased tissue and produce color images of brain function. MRSI uses a continuous band of radio wave frequencies to excite hydrogen atoms in a variety of chemical compounds other than water. These compounds absorb and emit radio energy at characteristic frequencies that can be used to identify them. Generally, a color image is created by assigning a color to each distinctive spectral emission. This makes up the spectroscopy part of MRSI.

MRSI, which is still experimental and is available in only a few research centers, can be conducted as part of a routine MRI, but MRSI and MRI use different software to acquire and mathematically manipulate the radio signal.

Marcus Gunn pupil Another name for afferent pupillary defect, an abnormal reflex response to light that is a sign of nerve fiber damage due to OPTIC NEURITIS (inflammation of the OPTIC NERVE), a symptom of multiple sclerosis.

The pupil (the dark portion of the eye in the center) normally contracts when a light is shined into that eye (direct response) or the other eye (indirect response). In a Marcus Gunn pupil, the pupil becomes larger rather than smaller when light is shown into that eye.

The syndrome is named for Robert Marcus Gunn, a 19th-century Scottish eye surgeon who in 1883 described a 15-year-old girl with a peculiar type of congenital eye problem that included an associated winking motion of the affected eyelid when she moved her jaw.

Marie, Pierre (1853–1940) French neuropathologist and a top student of Jean-Marie CHARCOT, the founder of neurology. Marie believed that multiple sclerosis (MS) was caused by infection and remained convinced that one day a vaccine would be found to protect against the disease.

Born and educated in France, Marie was the son of a wealthy bourgeois family from Paris who started out studying law before deciding to enter medical school. In 1878, he began studying neurology under the guidance of Charcot at the Salpêtrière and Bicêtre hospitals in Paris. Before long, Marie became one of Charcot's most outstanding students, serving as his laboratory and clinic chief and his special assistant.

Throughout his working life, Marie continued in the footsteps of Charcot, seeking an understanding of MS. At the time Marie was studying MS, its pathology was well established and clinical symptoms were recognized. However, the cause of MS remained a mystery. Louis Pasteur's discoveries of microorganisms and immunology prompted Marie to perceive MS in a new light. In 1884, Marie provided the next great step in the search for a cause of MS by suggesting for the first time that the disease might be caused by an infectious agent.

As brilliant a clinician as his teacher Charcot, Marie wrote numerous articles and books and developed an international school of neurology. Marie also identified and described a series of disorders with which his name is linked.

Marie led a quiet, happy, private life with his wife and children, but his happiness was shattered when his daughter Juliette died of appendicitis. After resigning from his chair at the Salpêtrière in 1925 at the age of 72, he spent the winters at Côte d'Azur and the summers at his estate in Normandy. He was further devastated by the death of his wife from erysipelas and his only son from botulism, which he had contracted during studies at the Pasteur Institute. After these losses, Marie became a virtual recluse until his death at the age of 86.

marijuana (*Cannabis sativa*) This hemp plant, when administered as a drug, can ease pain in some patients with multiple sclerosis (MS) and may also reduce SPASTICITY when smoked.

In a 2004 study examining marijuana and MS pain, marijuana showed a modest but relevant reduction in pain according to researchers at the Danish Pain Research Center and Department of Neurology at Aarhus University Hospital in Denmark. This first study assessing marijuana's effectiveness against MS pain was published in the July 2004 issue of the *British Medical Journal.*

MS patients experience many different types of pain, including central pain (discomfort caused by MS lesions that alter chemicals that transmit pain signals or that may change the way signals are transmitted to pain regions in the brain). In the Danish study, 24 MS patients with central pain took placebo capsules or capsules containing dronabinol, a cannabis extract, for three weeks. Those taking the cannabis extract had significantly lower pain intensity and greater pain relief compared with patients taking the placebo. They also had less pressure-related pain and better mental health. The greatest pain relief came during the last week of their treatment. The most common side effects were dizziness, headaches, fatigue, and muscle aches, which lessened over time, indicating that patients had adapted to the drug.

This new finding adds to growing evidence of the painkilling potential of cannabis. Animal research has shown that cannabinoids can decrease pain sensation caused by inflammation, damaged nerves, and cancer. Also, studies have pointed to cannabinoids as helping control pain from muscle spasticity (muscle stiffness and limb rigidity) in patients with MS.

Some pain reduction may have been related to fewer spasms. Despite the lessened pain, however, the underlying disease did not change.

Well known for its mind-altering properties, marijuana is also used medicinally for its antinausea benefits. A number of other clinical trials have been conducted to explore the role marijuana plays in treating tremor and balance control in small numbers of people with MS. Most of these studies have been done with an active ingredient in marijuana called tetrahydrocannabinol (THC). Because THC can be given by mouth, controlling the dose is easier.

Treatment for Spasticity

Studies of THC in the treatment of spasticity have had mixed results. Although some people reported feeling less spastic, this could not always be confirmed by objective testing. Even at best, the effects lasted less than three hours, and side effects (especially at higher doses) included weakness, dry mouth, dizziness, relaxation, confusion, short-term memory impairment, space-time distortions, and lack of coordination.

Treatment for Tremor

A small study administering THC for eight seriously disabled patients with significant tremor and lack of muscle coordination (ATAXIA) noted improvement in tremor in two patients that could be confirmed by an examination by a physician. Another three reported improvement in tremor that could not be confirmed.

All eight patients taking THC experienced a high, and two reported feelings of discomfort and unease.

Treatment for Balance

Smoking marijuana was shown to worsen control of posture and balance in 10 people with MS and 10 who did not have MS according to one study. All 20 study participants reported feeling high.

Marijuana Derivatives

Four different CANNABINOIDS (derivatives of marijuana) temporarily relieved spasticity and/or tremor in mice, according to researchers in the United Kingdom and United States. Researchers believe that similar derivatives of marijuana might be developed for human use. Researchers are not sure whether the psychoactive effects of these cannabinoids can be minimized enough to make their development as a treatment feasible.

Other Studies

A large clinical trial involving 660 people with different forms of MS was conducted in Britain to determine whether taking capsules of marijuana extracts and its component THC could help control spasticity. Subjects reports of improvement could not be confirmed by objective measures.

massage   The most common of all bodywork therapies used to relax muscles, reduce stress, and relieve conditions exacerbated by muscle tension. Many people with multiple sclerosis use massage for relief of various symptoms.

- The friction produced by massage can improve circulation, increasing blood flow through superficial veins through deeper arteries and through veins. It can increase capillary dilation through light stroking. It may be helpful in preventing the development of pressure sores, but should not be used if pressure sores or reddened areas of inflammation are present.

- Massage is useful in any condition in which a reduction in swelling or mobilization of tissues leads to pain relief. It can provide pleasurable stimulation, giving the client a chance to relax and relieve anxiety and fear. If massage is used as an aid for controlling pain, it should be used under the advice of a physician.

- Massage can help relax muscles and enhance range of motion exercises in those experiencing spasticity.

Types of Massage

Several types of massage are commonly practiced in the United States today:

- Acupressure stems from the traditional Chinese practice of acupuncture but uses fingers rather than needles to stimulate specific parts of the body.

- Shiatsu is a Japanese system based on finger pressure, which focuses on prevention rather than healing. Its purpose is to increase circulation and restore energy balance in the body.

- Swedish massage uses the traditional techniques of effleurage (a long, gliding stroke), petrissage (kneading and compression), vibration (a fine, rapid, shaking movement), friction (deep circular movements with thumb pads or fingertips), and tapotement (a series of quick movements using the hands alternatively to strike or tap the muscles).

- German massage combines Swedish movements with therapeutic baths (people with MS who are heat sensitive should avoid hot baths.)

Other Types of Bodywork

- Alexander technique: a movement therapy intended to correct bad habits of posture and movement that lead to muscle and body strain and tension.

- Feldenkrais method: a technique described as "awareness through movement," designed to make patterns of movement easier and more efficient by correcting habits that unduly strain muscles and joints.

- Rolfing or Aston variations: an effort to correct body alignment by applying deep pressure to the fascia, the tissues that cover muscles and internal organs.

- Trager method (Tragerwork): a method in which gentle, rhythmic touch is combined with exercises to release tension in posture and movement.

MBP   See MYELIN BASIC PROTEIN.

McDonald Diagnostic Criteria for MS   The traditional, standard diagnostic criteria for multiple sclerosis (MS) using clinical and laboratory findings as supportive evidence and requiring two attacks of disease separated in space and time. The criteria were developed in April 2001 during an international panel in association with the National MS Society, which recommended revised diagnostic criteria for MS. These revised criteria are known as the McDonald criteria after their lead author, W. I. McDonald.

measles virus   One of more than a dozen viruses and bacteria, (including canine distemper, human herpesvirus 6, and *Chlamydia pneumonia*) that have been investigated to determine if they are involved in the development of multiple sclerosis (MS). As yet, none has been definitively proven to trigger MS.

mechanical aids for spasticity ASSISTIVE DEVICES that can help a person with multiple sclerosis manage SPASTICITY and prevent contractures. These mechanical aids include toe spreaders and finger spreaders, which help to reduce stiffness in hands and feet and help in mobility, and orthoses for ankles-feet, which take the stress off the knee and align the foot with the ankle at a desired angle.

Medicaid A state program that may provide payment for nursing home care, adult day care, or at-home nursing care for people, including those with multiple sclerosis, if the person meets the financial need requirements. Medicaid also covers hospitalization, some medications, physical exams, and more. Patients usually become eligible for Medicaid only when their own money has been depleted to the point where they are below the federal poverty level. Eligibility is calculated not just based on the patient's income but also on the spouse's situation, if the patient is married.

In order to prepare for accessing Medicaid, it is possible to transfer assets from a patient's name to another person (such as an adult child). However, this transfer must take place at least 30 months before the patient applies for Medicaid coverage.

Each state has different Medicaid rules and regulations. In some states, adult children and spouses are not legally required to spend their own money to support family members in nursing homes. In other states, "relative responsibility laws" require a family to support the patient financially.

medical history A detailed assessment of a person's illnesses and health in the past, including a past record of signs and symptoms as well as current health status. The type of symptoms that have occurred over a long period of time may suggest multiple sclerosis, but only a full physical examination and medical tests can confirm the diagnosis.

Medicare A federal social security program that provides money for health care for people 65 or older or for those who are disabled at any age. If a participant with severe multiple sclerosis gets sick, Medicare should cover the temporary illness, although maximum coverage is just 150 days and involves a co-payment.

If the following services are deemed reasonable and necessary, Medicare will cover:

- evaluation and management visits by physicians or other health care providers
- physical, occupational, and speech therapy
- psychotherapy or other behavior management therapy provided by a mental health provider
- home health care if the individual is homebound and requires a skilled service—such as nursing services—or physical, occupational, or speech therapy, even if the patient attends adult day care
- medically necessary services, such as physical, occupational, and speech therapy or hospice care

Medicare does not cover one of the greatest expenses incurred by Medicare beneficiaries: long-term care. Funding for long-term care is provided only through Medicaid once patients spend their remaining assets. Long-term care specifically includes room and board in an assisted living facility; custodial care in a nursing home; and 24-hour personal care in the home. Medicare also will not cover adult day care.

medulla One of three parts of the BRAIN STEM, the medulla looks like a thickened extension of the spinal cord and contains the nuclei of the ninth through the 12th cranial nerves. It is here that the brain receives and relays taste sensations from the tongue and sends signals to speech, tongue and neck muscles. The medulla also contains the groups of nerve cells that control the automatic activities of the heartbeat, breathing, blood pressure, and digestion, sending and receiving information about these automatic functions via the vagus nerve. It is also responsible for coughing, sneezing, and gagging.

melatonin A hormone, released into the blood by the pineal gland, that follows a 24-hour rhythm; blood levels of melatonin may rise to up to 10 times higher at night. The hormone seems to stop a number of endocrine gland functions. During relapses, people with multiple sclerosis have abnormally low levels of melatonin, according to some research. Melatonin has also been associated with the worsening of some autoimmune diseases. Its use in multiple sclerosis is controversial.

memory A biological phenomenon, rooted in the senses, that begins with perception and that actively utilizes many areas of the brain to reassemble a thought into a coherent whole. When a person rides a bike, for example, the memory of how to ride the bike comes from one set of brain cells; the memory of how to get from here to the end of the block comes from another; the memory of rules for biking safety comes from still another. Yet people are never aware of these separate mental experiences or that they are coming from different parts of the brain because they all work together so well. In fact, experts say there is no firm distinction between how a person *remembers* and how a person *thinks*.

Multiple sclerosis may affect memory as a result of physical damage to both myelin (the sheath surrounding nerve cells) and the nerve cells within the frontal and temporal lobes of the brain. This can affect white matter connections and short-circuit message conduction. In fact, magnetic resonance imaging studies have indicated that the extent of demyelination in the brain can be directly related to the severity of memory problems.

Still, scientists still do not fully understand exactly how a person remembers or what occurs during recall. The search for how the brain organizes memories and where those memories are acquired and stored has been a never-ending quest among brain researchers.

Still, enough information is known to make some educated guesses. The process of memory begins with encoding and then proceeds to storing and then retrieval.

Encoding

Encoding is the first step in creating memory. Each sensation travels to the part of the brain called the hippocampus, which integrates these perceptions into one single experience as they occur. The hippocampus, experts believe, consolidates information for storage as permanent memory in another part of the brain (probably the cortex).

To encode a memory properly, a person must first be paying attention, which is why most of what occurs every day is simply filtered out and only a few stimuli pass into conscious awareness. If a person remembered every single thing, memory would soon become bogged down and overloaded. What scientists are not sure about, however, is whether stimuli are screened out during sensory input or after the brain processes their significance. Scientists do know that how someone pays attention to information may be the most important factor in how much is remembered.

A memory begins with perception, yet it is encoded and stored using the language of electricity and chemicals. Nerve cells connect with other cells at a point called a synapse, where all the action in the brain occurs as electrical pulses that carry messages leap across gaps between cells. The electrical firing of a pulse across the gap triggers the release of chemical messengers called neurotransmitters. These neurotransmitters diffuse across the spaces between cells, attaching themselves to neighboring cells. Each brain cell can form thousands of links like this, giving a typical brain about 100 trillion synapses. The parts of the brain cells that receive these electric impulses are called dendrites, feathery tips of brain cells that connect to the neighboring cell.

The connections between brain cells can change all the time. Brain cells work together in a network, organizing themselves into groups that specialize in different kinds of information processing. As one brain cell sends signals to another, the synapse between the two gets stronger. The more active the two brain cells are, the stronger the connection between them grows. Thus with each new experience, the brain slightly rewires its physical structure. In fact, how people use their brain helps determine how the brain is organized. It is this flexibility, which scientists call plasticity, that can help a brain rewire itself if it is ever damaged.

As a person learns and experiences the world, changes occur at the synapses and dendrites as more connections in the brain are created. The brain organizes and reorganizes itself in response to experiences. It forms memories triggered by the effects of outside input prompted by experience, education, or training. These changes are reinforced with use. As a person learns and practices new information, intricate circuits of knowledge and memory are created in the brain. If a musician plays a piece of music over and over, for example, the repeated firing of certain cells in a certain order in the brain makes it easier to repeat this firing later on. As a result, the person gets better at playing the music and is able to play it faster with fewer mistakes. If practiced long enough, the musician can play it perfectly. Yet if practicing stops for several weeks, the person will probably notice that the result is no longer perfect. The brain has already begun to "forget" what it once knew so well.

Storing

Once a memory is created, it must be stored. Many experts think that memories can be stored in three ways: as sensory input, in short-term memory, and ultimately, as long-term memory. Because there is no need to maintain everything in the brain, the different stages of human memory function as a sort of filter that helps to protect people from the flood of daily information.

As previously mentioned, the creation of a memory begins with its perception. The registration of this information during perception occurs in the brief sensory storage that usually lasts only a fraction of a second. A person's sensory memory allows a perception such as a visual pattern, a sound, or a touch to linger for a brief moment after the stimulation is over.

After that first flicker, the sensation is stored in short-term memory, a fairly limited cache that lasts for just 20 or 30 seconds before being replaced with other material (unless the sensation is constantly repeated). Most people find it impossible to remember a phone number or word after using it the first time—because it is stored in only the ultra-short-term memory. However, after using or thinking about something more frequently, the

information will then become part of short-term and later part of the long-term memory. Important information is eventually transferred from short-term memory into long-term memory (in a process called retaining). Long-term memory has an unlimited capacity store. Unlike sensory and short-term memory, which decay rapidly, long-term memory can store information indefinitely.

People tend to store material on subjects they already know something about, since the information has more meaning to them. This is why someone with a normal memory may be able to remember in depth more information about one particular subject.

Most people think of long-term memory when they think of memory itself. However, most experts believe information must first pass through sensory and short-term memory before it can be stored as a long-term memory. When a person wants to remember something, it is first retrieved on an unconscious level and then brought into the conscious mind at will.

Retrieval

There are four types of remembering:

- *recall:* the active, unaided remembering of something from the past

- *recollection:* the reconstruction of events or facts on the basis of partial cues that serve as reminders

- *recognition:* the ability to identify previously encountered stimuli correctly—such as when someone sees an old girlfriend's face across the room and recognizes who she is

- *relearning:* the evidence of the effects of memory—material that is familiar is often easier to learn a second time

Although most people think they either have a "bad" or a "good" memory, in fact most people are fairly good at remembering some things and not so good at remembering others. If someone has trouble remembering something (assuming the person is healthy), it is usually not the fault of the entire memory system but an inefficient component of one part of the memory system.

That assembly process of memory first begins with the onset of sexual maturity and tends to get worse as people reach middle age. This age-dependent loss of function appears in many animals.

As a person learns and remembers, the connections between new cells are reinforced and made stronger. With age, though, these synapses begin to falter. This begins to affect how easily a person can retrieve memories.

Studies also have shown that many of the memory problems experienced by older people can be improved—or even reversed. Studies of nursing home populations show that patients were able to make significant improvements in memory when given rewards and challenges. Physical exercise and mental stimulation can also improve mental function.

Evidence from animal studies suggests that stimulating the brain can stop cells from shrinking and can even increase brain size in some cases. For example, studies show that rats living in enriched environments with lots of toys and challenges have larger outer brains with larger, healthier brain cells. Animals given lots of mental exercise have more dendrites, which allow their cells to communicate with each other. Research has shown that with age, a stimulating environment encourages the growth of these dendrites and a dull environment impedes that growth.

memory loss　About half of all people with multiple sclerosis (MS) will develop some degree of MEMORY loss, but only 5–10 percent of those individuals develop problems that are severe enough to interfere in a significant way with everyday activities. Many other people with MS experience no problems with memory at all; rarely, memory problems may become so serious that the person can no longer be cared for at home.

MS may affect memory as a result of physical damage to both MYELIN (the sheath surrounding nerve cells) and the nerve cells within the frontal and temporal lobes of the brain. This can affect white matter connections and short-circuit message conduction. In fact, MAGNETIC RESONANCE IMAGING studies have indicated that the extent of DEMYELINATION in the brain can be directly related to the severity of memory problems.

However, MS can also affect memory indirectly, because MS is often associated with DEPRESSION, anxiety, stress, and fatigue. All of these may compromise cognitive functioning because of their effects on concentration. Anyone who cannot concentrate is going to have memory problems, regardless of whether the person has MS. Fatigue can be particularly hard on the ability to sustain any type of challenging mental task.

Although memory loss is more common among people who have had the disease for a long time, it can be seen early in the disease—even as the first symptom. This memory loss most often seems to affect recent memories—such as those of recent conversations, events, or content of reading material or TV programs.

Symptoms and Diagnostic Path
Three areas of function have been implicated in memory impairments in MS: retrieval, slowed processing speed, and acquisition. Retrieval problems occur when information that has been learned cannot be remembered. Slowed information-processing speed means that thinking, reasoning, and problem solving occur more slowly. Slowed acquisition of new information means that the person takes longer to learn new material.

Since the essence of learning involves the acquisition and subsequent recall of new information, the importance of assessing the impact of MS on these processes cannot be overestimated.

Just as the physical symptoms of MS can vary considerably from person to person, so can cognitive changes differ from one to the next. Moreover, it is common for certain functions to remain largely intact while others are more severely affected.

One of the most vexing memory deficits seen in people with MS is word-finding difficulty—the experience of having a word on the tip of the tongue but not being able to remember it. Other problems related to memory loss include difficulty with attention and concentration and problems in putting thoughts into words.

The first signs of memory loss may be subtle. The person may have difficulty in finding the right words to say or trouble remembering what to do on the job or during daily routines at home. Decisions that were once easy may now be carried out with poor judgment. Often the family becomes aware of the problem first, noticing changes in behavior or personal habits.

People with MS and their families should seek medical help if they are concerned about memory loss. Even early in the disease, memory problems can have an impact on performance at home and at work. In fact, research has shown that memory problems and fatigue are two primary reasons for ending a career. Since memory also can be affected by aging or medications, a careful evaluation is necessary to determine the cause of these mental changes.

To evaluate a person with MS for memory problems, a trained health professional (such as a NEUROPSYCHOLOGIST, SPEECH-LANGUAGE PATHOLOGIST, or OCCUPATIONAL THERAPIST) administers a battery of tests. Based on these tests, the person's memory deficits and strengths can be determined.

Treatment Options and Outlook

Many people find that coming up with strategies to cope with areas of memory loss is helpful (called "cognitive neurorehabilitation"). Studies have explored the benefits of rehabilitation for memory loss. Thus far, the greatest promise seems to be straightforward compensatory techniques such as using notebooks, computers, filing systems, tape recorders, and so on. Some people find that working on organizational skills, putting things back there they belong, and immediately writing notes of things to remember is helpful.

People whose memory problems appear to be related to FATIGUE may find that medications used to treat fatigue (such as amantadine or Modafinil) can help improve memory. However, these medications are not usually helpful if the problem is not fatigue related.

During the last few years, numerous studies have been conducted about ways to slow down or at least stabilize memory loss. Results thus far have been mixed, with INTERFERON beta-1a showing the most potential. However, since the disease-modifying agents have all been shown to reduce the accumulation of new demyelinating lesions, it is likely that over time they should all help to stabilize memory loss. Some studies also have examined possible treatments that may temporarily improve memory function without altering its long-term course. Thus

far the most successful has been DONEPEZIL, which has been shown to improve verbal memory modestly in patients with MS.

Studies currently under way are investigating the natural history of memory loss along with better ways of diagnosing and treating problems seen in people with MS. Experts hope that in the future, people with MS will have access to a combination of disease-modifying therapies, symptomatic treatments, and rehabilitation that will significantly modify the course and impact of the memory loss seen in MS.

menopause and MS   Some women with multiple sclerosis (MS) say that their symptoms become worse with menopause. In one study of 19 postmenopausal women, 54 percent reported that their symptoms became worse with menopause, and 75 percent of those who had tried HORMONE REPLACEMENT THERAPY (HRT) reported it helped reduce their symptoms. Researchers suggest that the results of the small study support the possibility that the drop in estrogen levels that accompanies menopause may have an adverse effect on the MS disease process. Therefore, HRT may improve MS symptoms. Further research is needed, especially given the recent findings from the Women's Health Study that the overall risks of HRT (higher risks of heart disease, stroke, and breast cancer) may outweigh the benefits for all women.

menstrual cycle   Although it is not entirely clear what effects hormonal changes have on neurologic symptoms in multiple sclerosis (MS), symptom worsening premenstrually has been reported.

In one study, 70 percent reported that their MS symptoms seemed to change at a regular time in their cycle. Most of those who reported a change indicated that the change, usually involving a worsening of their symptoms, occurred within one week of the onset of menses. WEAKNESS, imbalance, FATIGUE, and DEPRESSION were the symptoms most frequently reported to worsen.

In other studies, MAGNETIC RESONANCE IMAGING scans of women at different times of the menstrual cycle indicated that disease activity may vary according to differing hormonal levels. These findings have all come from small, uncontrolled studies.

Much more research is needed to characterize the relationship between MS and the menstrual cycle.

Mental Health Inventory (MHI) Assessment A test of several areas of mental health, including anxiety, DEPRESSION, behavioral control, positive affect, and general distress. The full-length MHI consists of 18 items; there is also a shorter version with five items. The MHI, one of the components of the MULTIPLE SCLEROSIS QUALITY OF LIFE INVENTORY, is a self-report questionnaire that takes less than 10 minutes to administer.

mental status testing A diagnostic tool used by a doctor to help determine the extent of behavioral and thinking problems in people with multiple sclerosis (MS). In such an exam, the person is asked questions such as, "What is today's date?" and "Who is the president of the United States?" Individuals might be asked to draw a clock face in an empty circle, count backward by sevens from 100, or put a stamp onto an envelope in the correct place. A numerical score is given at the end of the test that can be compared with the average scores of people at different levels of impairment.

A range of other tests have been designed to assess the degree of impairment in people with MS, including thinking problems and functional impairment. Some of these tests include the MINI-MENTAL STATUS EXAMINATION, the Hamilton Rating Scale for Depression, and the Present State Examination, which can assess depression, anxiety, delusions, and hallucinations.

mercury A heavy metal that some claim can leak from AMALGAM DENTAL FILLINGS, damaging the immune system and causing a broad range of diseases, including multiple sclerosis (MS), by contributing to the demyelinating process. (DEMYELINATION destroys the MYELIN sheath that surrounds and protects nerve fibers.)

However, MS experts say that no scientific evidence connects the development of MS with dental fillings containing mercury. Although poisoning with heavy metals such as MERCURY, lead, or manganese can damage the nervous system and produce symptoms such as tremor and WEAKNESS, the

damage is inflicted in a different way and the course of the disorder is also different.

methotrexate A synthetic IMMUNOSUPPRESSANT drug that in theory could reduce relapse rates and delay disease progression in multiple sclerosis (MS) by blocking certain functions of the immune system. It is highly effective in the short term against EXPERIMENTAL AUTOIMMUNE ENCEPHALOMYELITIS, the animal model for MS.

In some people, low doses of the immunosuppressant methotrexate may slow the course of CHRONIC-PROGRESSIVE MS, particularly in those with SECONDARY PROGRESSIVE MS.

To date, studies have found beneficial effects on only the upper body. A study of methotrexate in the 1970s did not show benefit to people with MS. However, interest in the drug has renewed since a recent controlled trial showed the drug had some benefit in MS patients. In this trial, 30 people with primary or secondary progressive MS who were still able to walk received weekly low-dose methotrexate. Arm function deterioration slowed down compared with the function of those receiving placebo, but there was no difference in worsening of leg function or in overall disability.

Just as with all immunosuppressants, this drug can have toxic side effects. However, it may be taken in low enough doses for MS that side effects are generally minimal.

methylprednisolone A steroidal, anti-inflammatory medication used to decrease the number of inflammatory cells and swelling, often administered for acute flare-ups of multiple sclerosis to shorten the exacerbation and improve symptoms.

See also CORTICOSTEROIDS.

minimal assessment of cognitive function in MS A psychological assessment for people with multiple sclerosis (MS) using a 90-minute battery of seven neuropsychological tests developed by an expert MS panel in 2001. This test includes assessments of speed/working memory, learning and memory, executive function, visual-spatial processing, and word retrieval.

minimal record of disability (MRD) A standardized method for assessing the clinical status of a person with multiple sclerosis (MS). The MRD is designed to help health professionals plan and coordinate care, and to provide a standardized way of recording repeated clinical evaluations of individuals for research purposes. The MRD includes five parts:

- demographic information
- the neurological functional systems developed by John Kurtzke, which assign scores to clinical findings for each of the various neurologic systems in the brain and spinal cord (pyramidal, cerebellar, brain stem, sensory, visual, mental, bowel, and bladder)
- the disability status scale (developed by John Kurtzke), which gives a single composite score for the person's disease
- the incapacity status scale, which is an inventory of functional disabilities relating to activities of daily living
- the environmental status scale, which provides an assessment of social handicap resulting from chronic illness

mini-mental status examination (MMSE) A test of orientation and simple thinking ability that can be used for a quick clinical assessment of people with multiple sclerosis. The MMSE includes assessments of orientation, memory, attention and calculation, language, ability to follow commands, reading comprehension, ability to write a sentence, and ability to copy a drawing. It is used in clinical settings because it tends to take less time to administer than some of the longer, more involved assessments.

However, a person's education, job, and cultural and background factors can strongly influence MMSE scores. The test may falsely indicate dementia in normal but poorly educated people or may indicate that a mildly demented person is normal. This is why the dividing line between "normal" and "demented" should be used only in context with the person's history and overall condition. Cultural, educational, and social factors must also be considered when attempting a diagnosis.

misdiagnosis of MS Although there have been many advances in the diagnosis of multiple sclerosis (MS), it is still possible to confuse MS symptoms with those of other diseases. As a result, a diagnosis may result in a "false negative" (no diagnosis of MS when it exists) or a "false positive" (a diagnosis of MS when the problem is really something else).

Doctors may reach a false negative if a person has symptoms but no abnormal findings upon examination. Sometimes doctors confuse the DIZZINESS of MS as Ménière's syndrome (a disorder of the inner ear), confuse the NUMBNESS or WEAKNESS of MS as a slipped disk or pinched nerve or misdiagnose DOUBLE VISION as being caused by a stroke.

It is also possible to diagnose MS when symptoms are actually caused by something else. Studies suggest between 9 and 12 percent of people who are diagnosed with MS have other diseases; another 5 percent diagnosed with MS do not have the disease; instead, their symptoms are of unknown origin.

Many diseases can mimic the symptoms of MS, including stroke, tumors, infection, neuritis, and MONONUCLEOSIS. Alcoholism can cause slurred speech and BALANCE PROBLEMS.

A misdiagnosis may be suspected if

- the patient is diagnosed with MS after age 50 or before age 10
- the symptom is hemianopic field defects (half the visual field is impaired in both eyes—which is only very rarely caused by MS)
- geographical background not conducive to MS (such as in Asia or the tropics)
- pain as the main symptom

mitoxantrone (Novantrone) A chemotherapy drug approved in 2000 by the U.S. Food and Drug Administration (FDA) to reduce neurologic disability and/or the frequency of clinical relapses in people with secondary progressive, progressive-relapsing, or worsening RELAPSING-REMITTING MS. In addition to being the first drug approved in the United States for SECONDARY PROGRESSIVE MS, it offers new treatment options for others experiencing worsening of the disease.

Mitoxantrone appears to be safe and well tolerated, according to short-term studies with 603 individuals with MS. Among the more common side effects seen in the two major controlled studies were nausea, hair loss, urinary and upper respiratory tract infections, and menstrual disorders.

However, the longer-term safety of Novantrone for people with MS may be more troublesome. In larger doses, the drug may negatively affect the heart, primarily in cancer patients. Although no clinically significant cardiac problems were seen in the relatively short MS trials, the FDA recommends that Novantrone be used only by those with normal heart function and only until the maximum cumulative dose is reached. Cardiac monitoring is required.

See also DISEASE-MODIFYING AGENTS.

mobility impairment   Problems in walking and getting around independently are a major consideration among people with multiple sclerosis (MS), which can profoundly affect a person's quality of life. Most commonly, people with MS find they must restrict activities due to SPASTICITY, impaired balance, coordination difficulties, tremor, and WEAKNESS. The ultimate effect of these problems can lead to atrophy, contracted muscles, and poor conditioning.

Proper exercise and effective strategies to cope with impaired mobility tailored for the individual are essential to break the cycle that can occur when weakness, FATIGUE, DEPRESSION, and HEAT intolerance lead to reduced exercise and further impaired mobility.

See also EXERCISE.

modafinil (Provigil)   A prescription medication used to treat excessive daytime sleepiness; it is prescribed for patients with multiple sclerosis to ease FATIGUE. The most frequent mild-to-moderate side effects include headache, nausea, nervousness, rhinitis, diarrhea, back pain, anxiety, insomnia, DIZZINESS, and indigestion.

models of care   A multifaceted concept that broadly defines the way health services are delivered. Among people with multiple sclerosis (MS), the goals of care are to stabilize disease, maintain wellness, maximize function and independence, and maintain productivity and a meaningful place in society. However, the many different ways that MS can affect individuals requires a wide array of professional services throughout the lifetime of a person with the disease. Many types of health professionals, care centers, health services and community organizations are involved, and these must continue to develop and maintain quality healthcare services that meet identified needs. The challenge is to sustain a level of support to meet individual and family needs throughout a lifetime.

modified fatigue impact scale (MFIS)   A modified form of the FATIGUE IMPACT SCALE that assesses the effects of fatigue in terms of physical, cognitive, and psychosocial functioning of individuals with multiple sclerosis (MS). The assessment is based on interviews with individuals with MS about how fatigue impacts their lives.

monoclonal antibodies   An antibody produced artificially. An antibody is an infection-fighting protein produced by the B cells in a person's immune system in response to a foreign invader. The monoclonal antibody is a synthetic version of this antibody, first produced in the lab in 1975 by combining a mouse's B cells with tumor cells (because these reproduce rapidly). When this fused mouse cell is cloned, the result is a monoclonal antibody.

Monoclonal antibodies can be designed to attack a specific cell while preserving the rest of the immune system. In multiple sclerosis (MS), monoclonal antibodies can be designed to attack just those cells that target myelin, leaving the rest of the person's immune cells alone. Monoclonal antibodies have been shown to be effective in treating the animal model for MS. In addition, researchers have demonstrated that monoclonal antibodies directed against specific T lymphocytes that are involved in the autoimmune process in people with MS can down-regulate the activity of these T cells.

One of the monoclonal antibodies, NATALIZUMAB (Tysabri), was approved in 2004 but was suspended after one drug-related death.

Monoclonal antibodies that react with and stop the activity of immune cells can be used as IMMUNOSUPRESSANTS. These would be helpful in treating MS since an abnormal immune response is believed to cause the destruction of myelin. This destruction slows or halts nerve impulses, producing the symptoms of MS.

Although monoclonal antibodies do not cause toxic side effects common in other types of immunosuppressant treatments, they can trigger allergic reactions in some people, since the antibodies are made from mouse cells. A combination mouse-human cell called a hybrid antibody is expected to reduce reactions in the future.

See also EXPERIMENTAL AUTOIMMUNE ENCEPHALO-MYELITIS.

mood swings   Swings between cheerfulness and sadness or irritation, also called emotional lability, are common in people with multiple sclerosis (MS). Some people have lesions in the brain that cause mood swings. Others may be taking medications that contribute to mood swings, such as high-dose steroids. Mood swings may also stem from emotional distress in the face of the day-to-day challenges of MS.

In some cases, severe, persistent mood swings may indicate an underlying mental illness called bipolar disorder. Since the right diagnosis is important, mood swings should be discussed with a doctor. Depending on the cause, this condition may respond to antidepressant medications, mood-stabilizing medications, changes in the dosage of steroid medication (or the use of lithium or Depakote with it), psychotherapy, and family counseling.

motor cortex   Part of the CEREBRAL CORTEX that extends from ear to ear across the roof of the brain and affects movement and coordination. It lies just in front of the sensory cortex. Each hemisphere's motor cortex controls the muscles on the opposite side of the body. A variety of regions in the central nervous system send input to the motor cortex: the sensory cortex, the premotor and supplementary motor areas, the basal ganglia, and the cerebellum.

The corticospinal tract connects the motor cortex to the motor neurons in the spinal cord and brain stem; this descending tract also branches out

to other structures important in motor activity. Damage to this tract can cause a loss of voluntary movement below the damaged area, although reflex activity will persist because reflex resides segmentally in the spinal cord.

motorized scooters   Scooters powered by electricity or gas are one type of mobility device that, while not intended for all-day use, can help those who are still able to walk to some degree. Adequate sitting balance and the use of the arms and hands are also essential. A PHYSICAL THERAPIST must be involved when choosing a motorized scooter, to ensure safety.

motor nerve   A nerve devoted to carrying impulses outward from the CENTRAL NERVOUS SYSTEM to activate a muscle or gland. Motor nerves cause muscle contractions and stimulate glands to secrete hormones.

motor neuron   The final neuron in the brain-to-muscle pathway that carries nerve impulses to muscles, controlling muscular activity.

See also MOTOR NEURON DISEASE.

motor neuron disease   A progressive, degenerative disease of the nerves that control muscles that at first may appear similar to multiple sclerosis. The condition usually begins in middle age, causing muscle weakness and wasting of the tongue, hands, and other parts of the body. Patients may also experience speech or swallowing problems.

Motor neuron disease primarily affects the motor cells of the spinal cord, the motor nuclei in the BRAIN STEM, and the corticospinal fibers. The three distinct forms of motor neuron disease include amyotrophic lateral sclerosis (ALS or Lou Gehrig's disease), progressive muscular atrophy, and progressive bulbar palsy. Although the latter two conditions start with patterns of muscle weakness different from ALS, these conditions usually develop into that disease.

Symptoms and Diagnostic Path
Two types of motor neuron disease (usually inherited) affect much younger patients. Infantile

progressive spinal muscular atrophy (Werdnig-Hoffmann paralysis) affects infants at birth or shortly after, with weakness progressing to death in several months to several years. A milder form (chronic spinal muscular dystrophy) begins at some point in childhood or adolescence, triggering progressive WEAKNESS that may never lead to serious problems. The cause is unknown.

Treatment Options and Outlook

Weakness usually spreads to the muscles needed for breathing within four years, but exceptions do occur. Some people have lived more than 20 years after the initial diagnosis. Although scientists have no way to slow the degeneration of the nerves, they may be able to lessen the resulting disability.

motor symptoms   Problems in walking may occur quite early in multiple sclerosis, especially in people who have many different symptoms. Motor symptoms may include WEAKNESS in an affected arm or leg progressing to SPASTICITY, hyperreflexia, CLONUS, extensor plantar responses, and muscle contractures. Spasticity is very common; although spasticity may help some people to walk, it can be painful and interfere with personal hygiene and daily activities.

MS certified specialist   A voluntary certification for health care experts, offered by the Consortium of MS Centers, that reflects knowledge in the specialization of multiple sclerosis (MS) care. This certification reflects the knowledge necessary to provide optimal care to those individuals and families living with MS. Certification establishes a basic knowledge required for practice and encourages continuous learning so that those in MS care sustain a basic level of knowledge about the disease and its implications.

All licensed health professionals with one year of experience caring for people with MS are eligible to take the certification examination. Those who successfully pass the examination will be called a multiple sclerosis certified specialist. Professionals who may want to pursue certification include rehabilitation professionals, licensed nursing professionals, social workers, psychologists, NEUROPSYCHOLOGISTS, and other licensed personnel.

MS 150 Bike Tour   The country's largest organized cycling series, sponsored by the National Multiple Sclerosis Society to raise money for the society. The bike tour includes more than 100 bike rides coast to coast from April through November. Proceeds support multiple sclerosis (MS) research and chapter programs for people with MS and their families. Information is available by calling 800-FIGHT-MS.

MS Walk   A national fund-raising event, held every spring at more than 200 sites around the country, in which people walk to raise money for the National Multiple Sclerosis Society. All walks have an accessible route so people of all abilities can take part. Funds raised support multiple sclerosis (MS) research and chapter programs for people with MS and their families. For information about local MS Walks, call 800-FIGHT-MS.

multifocal demyelinating process   A process in which MYELIN (a protective nerve coating) is damaged or destroyed in more than one area. The disease process of multiple sclerosis is a multifocal demyelinating process.

multiple sclerosis (MS)   A chronic, unpredictable neurological disease that affects the BRAIN, SPINAL CORD, and OPTIC NERVE (the CENTRAL NERVOUS SYSTEM [CNS]). It damages the fatty tissue (MYELIN) that surrounds and protects nerve fibers and interferes with the transmission of electrical impulses. As myelin is lost in areas throughout the central nervous system, it leaves areas of scar tissue (sclerosis). These damaged areas are also known as plaques or lesions. Sometimes the disease process damages or destroys the nerve fiber itself. When myelin or the nerve fiber is damaged, it disrupts the ability of the nerves to conduct electrical impulses to and from the brain, which produces the symptoms of MS. Most experts believe MS is an autoimmune disorder, which means the person's own immune system attacks healthy tissue.

Most people are diagnosed between the ages of 20 and 50, although the disease can occur in young children and older adults. MS is not contagious, is not directly inherited, and is not considered a fatal disease. In fact, most people with MS do not become severely disabled. In very rare cases, MS is so malignantly progressive that it results in early death, but most people with MS have a normal or near-normal life expectancy.

About 400,000 Americans are living with a diagnosis of MS, and every week another 200 people are diagnosed. However, because doctors are not required to report cases of MS to the government, and because someone can have MS without symptoms, actual numbers can only be estimated. About 2.5 million people in the world have MS. Women outnumber men with the disease by 50 percent (that is, three women have the condition for every two men).

About two-thirds of people with MS are not severely affected by the disease. They live normal and productive lives, and they remain able to walk. However, most will need an aid such as a cane or crutches, and some will use a scooter or wheelchair because of fatigue, weakness, or balance problems.

Experts still do not know exactly what causes MS. However, they suspect that the condition is probably triggered by a combination of several factors, including immunologic, genetic, and environmental ones.

Immune related Scientists now generally accept that MS involves an autoimmune process— an abnormal immune response directed against the central nervous system. The exact antigen, or target that the immune cells are sensitized to attack, remains unknown. In recent years, however, researchers have been able to identify which immune cells are mounting the attack, some of the factors that cause them to attack, and some of the sites, or receptors, on the attacking cells that appear to be attracted to the myelin to begin the destructive process. The destruction of myelin, as well as damage to the nerve fibers themselves, slows or halts nerve impulses, producing MS symptoms. Researchers are looking for highly specific, immune-modulating therapies to stop this abnormal immune response without harming normal immune functions.

Environmental Migration patterns and epidemiologic studies have shown that people who are born in a part of the world where people are at low risk for MS and then move to an area with a higher risk before the age of 15 acquire the higher risk of their new home. Such data suggest that exposure to some environmental agent that occurs before puberty may affect a person's risk of later developing MS. Some researchers theorize that MS develops because a person is born with a genetic predisposition to react to some environmental agent that, upon exposure, triggers an autoimmune response. Sophisticated new techniques for identifying genes may help answer questions about the role of genes in the development of MS.

Infections Since all children are exposed to numerous viruses and bacteria, some experts believe that a virus or other infectious agent may possibly trigger MS. Although many infectious microorganisms have been investigated, no one agent has emerged as a proven trigger. However, there are a number of reasons for the persistent belief in a link between viruses and MS.

First, the disease has a distinct geographical distribution, which suggests there could be a contagious aspect to the condition. That is, a virus may be related to the inflammation that in some people may trigger MS. The number of MS cases increases the farther away a person travels from the equator in either direction. Second, MS clusters also occur in certain areas, such as the clusters that occurred between 1943 and 1989 in the FAEROE ISLANDS, which lie northwest of Scotland. During World War II, this region was occupied by British troops. The incidence of MS rose each year for 20 years after the war, leading some researchers to think that the troops might have brought with them some disease-causing agent.

The third reason to suspect a viral basis for MS is that some viruses are strikingly similar to the myelin protein and may therefore cause confusion in the immune system, causing the T cells to continue to attack their own protein rather than the viral antigen. More than one antigen may be involved; some may trigger the disease, and others may keep the process going.

Different MS patients may possibly be affected by different organisms, and infections may cause some, but not all, cases of MS. Organisms that are at the top of the suspect list are those that can affect the central nervous system. More than a dozen viruses and bacteria, including measles, hepatitis B, and canine distemper, are being investigated to determine if they are involved in the development of MS. The top three suspects are HERPESVIRUS 6, CHLAMYDIA PNEUMONIAE, and EPSTEIN-BARR VIRUS. So far, however, no germ has been definitively linked to MS.

Genes   Although MS is not hereditary in a strict sense, having a parent or sibling with the condition increases an individual's risk of developing the disease. The average person in the United States has about a two in 1,000 chance of developing MS. Children or siblings of a person with MS, however, have double that chance of developing the disease if they are female, while their chances remain the same if they are male.

Genes are pieces of the DNA molecule, located along the chromosomes in the nuclei of cells. Most of the cells in a person's body have two complete sets of genes—one inherited from the mother and one from the father. Each set, numbering from 30,000–40,000 genes, contains all the instructions needed to build all human proteins. The complete set is known as the human genome.

Some studies suggest that certain genes have a higher prevalence in populations with higher rates of MS. Common genetic factors have also been found in some families where more than one person has MS. However, no single gene has been found that is responsible for the disease. Scientists believe that a person is susceptible to developing MS only if he or she inherits an unlucky combination of several genes. Today, advances in molecular genetics and the identification of families in which several members have MS (multiplex MS families) increase the likelihood that MS genes may be discovered.

In the early 1990s, three large whole-genome screens focusing on the MS markers were performed in the United States, the United Kingdom, and Canada. By 1996, investigators had found up to 20 locations in the genome that might contain genes linked to MS susceptibility. However, no single gene was found to have a major influence on MS susceptibility. Although the genes themselves appear normal, scientists believe that susceptibility is probably related to the combination of genes.

When the susceptibility genes are eventually identified, scientists will have to figure out how those genes influence the immunological and neurological aspects of MS. Because the immune system is involved in producing symptoms, many scientists think that at least some of the susceptibility genes will be related to the immune system. Indeed, reports have already linked immune system genes, including those for the immunoglobulins and for the major histocompatibility complex (MHC), to MS. Results reported to date have confirmed that the MHC region holds one or more genes that seem likely to be related to MS susceptibility.

Race   MS occurs more often among people with northern European ancestry. However, people of African, Asian, and Hispanic backgrounds are not immune.

Other triggers   Some conditions do not cause MS, including exposure to excessive HEAT or STRESS, but may worsen symptoms.

Emotional tension that may cause poor concentration, MEMORY LOSS, ANXIETY, or poor problem solving—or a host of physical problems—is often a concern for people with MS. People often report having relapses after experiencing a severe emotional trauma, such as the death of a close relative or the breakup of a relationship. Even if stress does not cause a relapse, it may make the patient feel worse, which can lead to the patient's belief that stress is causing a relapse.

Although exercise could be considered somewhat stressful, research suggests that moderate exercise boosts patients' feelings of well-being and modestly increases strength and conditioning.

Avoiding stress is a good idea for anyone, but it is not always possible. Learning how to handle the normal stress of daily life does make sense for patients with MS. Relaxation techniques, such as meditation, controlled breathing, and listening to soothing music, can be helpful. Other people find a lukewarm bath or watching TV can ease stress. If stress continues to be a problem, people may want to consult a mental health expert for counseling.

Symptoms and Diagnostic Path

No single lab test or diagnostic method can, by itself, determine if a person has MS, although MAGNETIC RESONANCE IMAGING (MRI) is a great help in reaching a definitive diagnosis. Moreover, in early MS, symptoms that might indicate any number of possible disorders can come and go. As a result, a diagnosis can be made only by carefully ruling out all other possibilities.

Nevertheless, it is important to diagnose MS as quickly as possible so patients can begin to adjust to the condition. In addition, appropriate treatments can be started as early in the disease process as possible, which is important since permanent neurologic damage can occur even in the earliest stages of MS.

When trying to determine if a patient has MS, a doctor will first conduct a complete physical examination, discuss the patient's medical history, and review past or current symptoms. Next the physician will perform a variety of tests to evaluate mental, emotional, and language functions; movement and coordination; vision; balance; and the senses. However, no tests are specific for MS, and no single test can be considered 100 percent conclusive.

A diagnosis of MS requires objective evidence of two attacks (also known as exacerbations, flares, or relapses)—the sudden appearance or worsening of an MS symptom that lasts at least 24 hours. The two attacks must have occurred at least one month apart in different areas of the CNS, and there can be no other explanation for these attacks or symptoms.

Magnetic resonance imaging   MRI is the preferred method of imaging the brain to detect the presence of plaques or scarring caused by MS. The MRI can detect lesions in different parts of the central nervous system and tell the difference between old and new lesions. An MRI is a painless, noninvasive scan that can reveal detailed pictures of the brain and spinal cord. These images are able to show scarred areas of the brain.

Still, the diagnosis of MS is not made on the basis of an MRI alone, since other diseases create lesions in the brain that look like those caused by MS. Moreover, some lesions are found in healthy individuals (especially older people) that are not caused by any disease.

On the other hand, a normal MRI cannot rule out a diagnosis of MS since about 5 percent of patients who have confirmed MS on the basis of other symptoms do not show any lesions with an MRI. Instead, these people may have lesions in the spinal cord or lesions that cannot be detected by MRI. Eventually, however, brain or spinal lesions in most people with MS will appear on MRI.

Nevertheless, the longer the MRI remains negative, the more questionable the diagnosis becomes. If the MRI findings continue to be negative more than a year or two after the initial diagnosis is made, every effort should be made to identify another possible cause for the symptoms.

Other tests   Not every patient requires every possible test. However, if a clear-cut diagnosis cannot be made based on the symptoms and the initial tests outlined above, other evaluations may be needed. These may include assessments of visual EVOKED POTENTIALS, cerebrospinal fluid, and blood.

- *Evoked potential tests* are electrical diagnostic studies that measure the conduction of messages to the brain. They can reveal slowing of nerve transmissions, often providing evidence of scars along nerve pathways that is not apparent on a neurologic exam. Evoked potential tests are painless and noninvasive. In visual EP, small electrodes are placed onto the patient's head to monitor brain waves and the response to visual stimuli. The time the brain takes to receive and interpret messages is a clue to the patient's condition.
- *Cerebrospinal fluid* obtained by a spinal tap is tested for levels of certain immune system proteins and for the presence of substances that detect an immune response within the central nervous system. These substances are found in the spinal fluid of about 90–95 percent of people with MS, but they are also present in other diseases. Therefore, they cannot be exclusively relied upon as positive proof of MS.
- Although no definitive blood test is available for MS, blood tests can rule out other causes for various neurologic symptoms, such as Lyme disease, collagen-vascular diseases, certain rare hereditary disorders, and AIDS.

MS varies so greatly in each individual that predicting the course the disease might take is hard. However, some studies show that people who have few attacks in the first five years after a diagnosis of MS, long intervals between attacks, complete recoveries, and sensory-only attacks generally have a less debilitating form of the disease.

On the other hand, people whose early symptoms include tremors, lack of coordination, or frequent attacks with incomplete recoveries generally have a more progressive form of MS. These early symptoms indicate that more myelin has been damaged.

A diagnosis of MS usually specifies one of four different types: relapsing-remitting, secondary progressive, primary progressive, or progressive-relapsing.

Relapsing-remitting MS   The most common form of MS, relapsing-remitting MS is characterized by periods of exacerbation in which new symptoms may appear and previous ones may worsen. The attacks are followed by periods of remission, when disease activity subsides and may be unnoticeable. A remission may last for months or even years. About 85 percent of MS cases begin as relapsing-remitting.

Secondary progressive MS   Within 10 years of the initial diagnosis, more than half of patients with relapsing-remitting MS begin to experience a gradual worsening of symptoms with or without occasional flare-ups, minor remissions, or plateaus. This form of MS is called secondary progressive; 90 percent of people with relapse-remitting MS transition to a secondary progressive disease course within 25 years. However, those figures may shrink substantially as a result of the introduction of what are known as DISEASE-MODIFYING AGENTS.

Primary progressive MS   This type of MS is characterized by a nearly continuous worsening of the disease from the very beginning, with no distinct relapses or remissions. There may be temporary plateaus with minor relief from symptoms but no long-lasting relief. About 10 percent of people with MS have primary progressive MS.

Progressive-relapsing MS   This form of the disease is quite rare and takes a progressive course from the onset with obvious acute attacks, with or without recovery along the way. In contrast to relapsing-remitting MS, the periods between relapses are characterized by continuing disease progression. About 5 percent of people with MS have progressive-relapsing MS.

The primary symptoms of MS vary a great deal from one person to the next. They depend on what part of the nervous system has been affected by the inflammatory, demyelinating process in the CNS. Although the symptoms tend to wax and wane over the course of the disease, some people experience symptoms that slowly worsen and never improve.

The most common symptoms include WEAKNESS, fatigue, BOWEL DYSFUNCTION, BLADDER DYSFUNCTION, changes in mental function (including problems with memory, attention, and problem solving), emotional problems, DEPRESSION, DIZZINESS, NUMBNESS or PINS AND NEEDLES, PAIN, sensitivity to heat, SEXUAL PROBLEMS, SPASTICITY TREMOR, and VISUAL PROBLEMS (including OPTIC NEURITIS and blurry or DOUBLE VISION). Less common symptoms include HEADACHES, HEARING LOSS, ITCHING, SEIZURES, speech problems, and SWALLOWING PROBLEMS.

All of these are considered primary symptoms of MS because they are a direct result of the destruction of myelin and of damage to the nerve fibers themselves. Demyelination and nerve damage impair function by interfering with the transmission of nerve impulses to muscles and other organs. Many of the following symptoms can be managed effectively with medication, rehabilitation, and other management strategies.

Weakness   One of the most disabling symptoms of MS is a feeling of weakness in the arms, legs, or face either on one entire side of the body or in only one leg or one arm. The weakness can range from a slight loss of strength to total paralysis. It may appear gradually over a number of years, or it may appear quite suddenly over a period of hours. Often, weakness may be caused by damaged nerves that interfere with nerve signals, preventing instructions from reaching the arms and legs. This type of weakness is not caused by any type of loss in muscle strength. Weakness may also be caused by fatigue or by simple disuse. Typically, weakness may affect one leg, making it hard to lift, especially at the end of the day. Some people experience weakness in both legs. Such weakness may be particularly evident when stepping up onto a stair or curb. Although less common, some patients may experience similar sensations of heaviness or clumsiness in one or both of their arms and hands, which may affect the ability to grip, push, or lift.

Fatigue Up to 80 percent of patients report feeling extremely tired, which can significantly interfere with the ability to function. Fatigue is the most common reason why people have to quit their jobs. The cause of MS-related fatigue is not known. However, it usually occurs every day and may appear early in the morning even after a restful night's sleep. It tends to get worse as the day progresses and may be aggravated by heat and humidity. However, MS-related fatigue does not appear to be directly linked with either depression or the degree of physical impairment. Although fatigue is common in people with any type of nervous system disorder, not every person with MS experiences the symptom. In many others, fatigue comes and goes without apparent cause.

Bowel dysfunction CONSTIPATION is a special concern among people with MS, although diarrhea, incontinence, and other problems of the stomach and bowels can also occur. Patients may experience constipation because they do not drink enough or get enough exercise or because food moves more slowly through the intestinal tract. In addition, certain medications, such as antidepressants or bladder control drugs, may cause constipation. Loss of bowel control in patients with MS may be related to constipation or directly caused by MS and should be evaluated by a health care provider.

Bladder dysfunction Urinary and bladder problems are common symptoms that appear in about 80 percent of patients with spinal cord damage from MS. They occur when the disease blocks or delays transmission of nerve signals in areas of the CNS that control the bladder and urinary sphincter. (The sphincter is the muscle surrounding the opening of the bladder that either keeps urine in or allows it to flow out.) Just like other MS symptoms, bladder problems may only occasionally be an issue—at least in the beginning. With severe forms of the disease, the bladder problems may progress to a chronic condition. If left untreated, bladder dysfunction may cause emotional and personal hygiene problems that can interfere with normal life.

Cognitive problems Between 50 and 60 percent of all patients with MS will develop some degree of slowed ability to think, reason, concentrate, or remember. However, only 5–10 percent develop problems severe enough to interfere with everyday activities significantly. Although these problems are more common among people who have had the disease for a long time, cognitive problems may also be seen early in the disease, even presenting as the first symptom.

Cognitive problems are caused by both physical brain changes and emotional difficulties of having a chronic illness. For example, MS is associated with depression, anxiety, stress, and fatigue, all of which can slow down cognitive function. Fatigue can be particularly challenging to a patient's ability to think clearly. Just as the physical symptoms of MS can vary considerably from person to person, cognitive changes can vary in the same way. Moreover, it is common for certain functions to be largely intact while others are more severely affected.

MEMORY loss is the most common cognitive problem that MS patients experience. Other cognitive functions frequently affected in MS include the speed of information processing, planning and prioritizing, impairment in visual perception and constructional abilities, word-finding ability, abstract reasoning and problem solving, and attention and concentration (especially sustained attention and the ability to divide attention between separate tasks).

Depression A persistent low mood is a common problem for patients with MS. In most cases, it can be effectively treated with a combination of antidepressant medications and psychotherapy. Depression is the logical result of a difficult chronic condition with the potential of permanent disability; it also can be a side effect of some drugs (such as steroids) prescribed to treat MS. Some evidence indicates that INTERFERON medications in particular may trigger or worsen depression in susceptible individuals. Depression may also be caused by the disease process itself if MS damages the myelin and nerve fibers in areas of the brain involved in emotional expression and control. Depression may also be associated with disease-related changes in the immune or neuroendocrine systems.

Dizziness The sensation of feeling off balance or lightheaded is a common symptom during MS flares. Dizziness is caused by damaged areas in the complex neural pathways that coordinate visual, spatial, and other input to the brain needed to produce and maintain equilibrium.

Numbness One of the most common symptoms of MS—often the first symptom—is a numbness that may range from mild to so severe that it interferes with the ability to use the affected body part. For example, a person with very numb feet may have difficulty walking. Numb hands may prevent writing, dressing, or holding objects safely. Because of the decrease in feeling, patients should be careful to protect the area from cuts, bumps, bruises, burns, or other injury.

Pain Several types of painful symptoms are common in MS; as many as 70 percent of patients in one study reported experiencing some kind of pain. Age at onset, length of time with MS, or degree of disability do not appear to have any link to whether a person will have pain, although twice as many women experience the problem. MS pain often affects several areas of the body and changes over time, waxing and waning for no apparent reason. Patients often have trouble describing the pain, which can be dull or burning or simply feel like pressure. The pain is caused in MS patients by overactive nerves that send pain signals for no good reason.

Heat In many cases, high temperatures tend to worsen MS symptoms temporarily and cause significant weakness as the higher temperature causes damaged nerves to function less efficiently than usual. Overheating may occur when the weather is very hot or humid or if the patient has a fever, sunbathes, gets overheated from exercise, or takes very hot showers or baths.

Sexual problems Sexual arousal begins in the CNS as the brain sends messages to the sexual organs along nerves running through the spinal cord. If MS damages these pathways, sexual response (including arousal and orgasm) may be directly affected. Sexual problems may also be linked to MS symptoms such as fatigue or spasticity as well as psychological factors relating to self-esteem and mood. In fact, 63 percent of people with MS report that their sexual activity declined after their diagnosis. Other surveys of persons with MS suggest that as many as 91 percent of men and 72 percent of women may be affected by sexual problems.

Visual problems Visual impairment is a quite common symptom in patients with MS. It is related to an inflammation of the OPTIC NERVE (the nerve connecting the eye to the brain) in a condition known as optic neuritis. Patients usually notice visual loss in the center of the visual field in one eye, often along with an aching pain. Other patients may complain of blurred or foggy vision. Visual change typical of MS lasts for days to weeks at a time; symptoms of fogginess or visual problems that last for less time are probably not related to this disease.

Tremor These rhythmic, involuntary muscular contractions are characterized by to-and-fro movements of a part of the body and can affect the hands, head, vocal cords, trunk, and legs. Most tremors, however, affect the hands. The types of tremors in MS vary markedly. An intention tremor can range from mild to quite disabling. Some people have such severe tremors in their arms and hands that they cannot perform the simplest manual tasks; other patients experience transient movements of the head or body that are rarely noticed.

There are several types of tremors:

- *Intention tremors* occur only during physical movement; there is no shaking when a person is at rest. The tremor develops and becomes more pronounced as the person tries to grasp or reach for something or move a hand or foot to a precise spot. This is the most common and generally most disabling form of tremor that occurs in people with MS.

- *Postural tremors* occur when a limb or the whole body is being supported against gravity. For example, a person who has a postural tremor will shake while sitting or standing but not while lying down.

- *Nystagmus* is a tremor that produces jumpy eye movements.

Tremors occur because there are plaque-damaged areas along the complex nerve pathways that are responsible for coordination of movements. People with MS who have tremors may also have associated symptoms, such as difficulty in speaking (dysarthria) or difficulty in swallowing (dysphagia).

These activities are governed many of the same pathways involved in coordinating movement.

Tremor is considered to be one of the most difficult symptoms to treat, and to date, there have been no reports of consistently effective drug therapies. Varying degrees of success have been reported with such drugs as the anti-tuberculosis agent isoniazid, the antihistimines Vistaril and Atarax, the beta-blocker propranolol (Inderal), the anticonvulsive medication primidone (Mysoline), a diuretic acetazolamide (Diamox), and anti-anxiety drugs buspirone (Buspar) and clonazepam (Klonapin).

Weights and other devices can be attached to a limb to inhibit or compensate for tremors. An occupational therapist is the health professional who can best advise about assistive devices to aid in the management of tremor.

Tremor can have significant emotional and social impact, especially when people choose to keep to themselves rather than be embarrassed by tremor. Isolation can lead to depression and further psychological problems. A psychologist, social worker, or counselor may be able to help a person with MS deal with these issues and become more comfortable in public.

Controversy continues over the role of alcohol or tetrahydro-cannabinol (THC), the active ingredient in marijuana, in treating tremor. Only small studies have been done, characterized by conflicting results. Marijuana remains a controlled substance under current policies of the U.S. Drug Enforcement Agency,

In the most severe types of tremor, surgical procedures are sometimes used. A thalamic implant, originally developed for Parkinson's disease, is being tried in MS. While relief of tremor using this method has been seen in some individuals, the outcomes are not always predictable, and their role in severe tremor is still being determined. In the meantime, thalamic implants are considered "experimental" and may not be covered by most insurance policies.

Secondary symptoms In addition to the common primary symptoms, complications can arise as a result of the primary symptoms; these are called secondary symptoms. For example, bladder dysfunction can cause repeated URINARY TRACT INFECTIONS. Inactivity can impair muscle tone and cause a range of problems, including disuse weakness (not related to demyelination), poor bone density, and shallow, inefficient breathing. Immobility can also lead to BEDSORES. Although secondary symptoms can be treated, it is better to avoid them by treating primary symptoms.

Tertiary symptoms Tertiary symptoms of MS are the social, vocational, and emotional complications associated with the primary and secondary symptoms. The diagnosis of a chronic illness can be damaging to self-esteem and self-image. A person who becomes unable to walk or drive may no longer be able to work. The strain of dealing with a chronic neurologic illness may affect personal relationships. People with MS frequently experience emotional changes as well; mood swings and depression can occur as primary, secondary, or tertiary symptoms of the disease. Professional help from mental health professionals, physical therapists, and occupational therapists may help patients manage many of these issues.

It is important to remember that not every person with MS experiences all of these symptoms. Some people may experience only one or two of them over the course of the disease, while others experience quite a few. Symptoms can come and go quite unpredictably, and no two people experience them in exactly the same way. Most of the symptoms of MS can be effectively managed, and complications can be avoided with regular care.

Treatment Options and Outlook
Treatment of MS includes

- treating acute exacerbations
- slowing down the disease using DISEASE-MODIFYING AGENTS
- managing symptoms with medication and rehabilitation

Treating acute exacerbations The most common treatment for an acute MS attack is a three- to five-day course of high-dose intravenous corticosteroids, which provides maximum benefit with fewest side effects. These drugs, the first agents to successfully treat MS, include methylprednisolone (Solu-Medrol) and dexamethasone (Decadron). Both courses may require hospitalization, although it is possible to have IV treatment on an outpatient basis. Depending on the physician's preference, the patient's condition, and the length of the treatment, the IV steroids may be followed by a one- to two-week tapering dose of oral steroids.

However, long-term use of steroids is not recommended, since there is no evidence to suggest that continuous steroid administration slows progression of MS or improves symptoms over a long period of time. However, several studies have found that monthly one-day pulses of IV methylprednisolone may help treat patients with progressive MS. These studies are still preliminary and require larger numbers of patients before making definitive recommendations.

The side effects of long-term continuous steroid use are serious and well-documented, including stomach ulcers, weight gain, acne, cataracts, osteoporosis, deterioration of the top of the thigh bone, and diabetes.

Disease-modifying agents Other medications have been proven to reduce attack rates and severity of attacks; these treatments need to be administered for years. Most users of a disease-modifying drug have fewer and less severe MS attacks. In individual clinical trials using a drug versus an inactive placebo treatment, MS attacks were reduced by 28 to 66 percent. Most users had fewer or smaller lesions (some had no new lesions at all) within the central nervous system.

These drugs are an important weapon in the fight against MS because permanent damage to nerve fibers occurs early in MS in association with the destruction of myelin. Overall brain shrinkage also occurs early in the disease, and damage is ongoing even when the person has no symptoms. For this reason, MS specialists advise the early use of a drug that limits lesion formation and brain shrinkage. Limiting lesions may reduce future permanent disability for many people with MS.

There are now five disease-modifying medications approved for use in relapsing forms of MS by the U.S. Food and Drug Administration (FDA). While all of these have proven records of partial success, none is a cure for MS, nor will any prevent pre-existing recurring symptoms, such as fatigue or numbness, which typically come and go in an hour or a day.

- *Immunomodulators:* Betaseron (beta interferon 1b), Avonex (beta interferon 1a—intramuscular), Rebif (beta interferon 1a—subcutaneous), Copaxone glatiramer acetate (Copaxone)

- *Immunosuppressant:* (Novantrone) mitoxantrone

Betaseron is given every other day by injection under the skin. Side effects may include flu-like symptoms following injection, which lessen over time for many, and injection site reactions, about 5 percent of which need medical attention. Less common side effects include allergic reactions, depression, elevated liver enzymes, and low white blood cell counts. Avonex is given once a week by injection into the muscle. Possible side effects include flu-like symptoms following injection, which lessen over time for many. Less common side effects are depression, mild anemia, elevated liver enzymes, allergic reactions, and heart problems. Copaxone is given every day by injection under the skin. Side effects include injection site reactions and (less commonly) dilation of blood vessels; chest pain; a reaction immediately after injection, which includes anxiety, chest pain, palpitations, shortness of breath, and flushing. This reaction may last 15 to 30 minutes, passes without treatment, and has no known long-term effects. Rebif is given three times a week by injection under the skin. Side effects include flu-like symptoms following injection, which lessen over time for many, and injection site reactions. Less common side effects include liver abnormalities, depression, allergic reactions, and low red or white blood cell counts.

Novantrone is given four times a year by IV infusion in a medical facility. There is a lifetime limit of 8 to 12 doses. Side effects include blue-green urine 24 hours after administration; infections; bone marrow suppression resulting in fatigue, bruising, and low blood cell counts; nausea; hair thinning; bladder infections; and mouth sores. Novantrone is a chemotherapeutic drug originally developed for certain forms of cancer. The total lifetime dose is limited in order to avoid possible heart damage. People taking Novantrone should have regular tests of their heart function. It cannot be used in people with pre-existing heart problems, liver disease, and certain blood disorders.

Managing side effects of Avonex, Betaseron, Rebif, Copaxone The flu-like side effects of the interferon products Avonex, Betaseron, and Rebif usually can be minimized, or a doctor may stop one medication and prescribe another of these immunomodulators. All the injectable drugs, including Copaxone, may cause injection site reactions, including bumps, bruises, pain, and infections. Good injection techniques can minimize problems. Auto-injecting devices may be helpful.

Women who are pregnant or plan to become pregnant should discuss disease-modifier use with their physicians. None of these medications is approved for use during pregnancy or breast-feeding. Most women will be advised to avoid using these medications during pregnancy.

Many factors will influence the physician's assessment of the best medication choice. One of them will be lifestyle issues that could affect a person's ability to keep taking a treatment for a long period of time.

The annual expense of these drugs is significant. Many private insurance plans do not cover prescription drugs at all. Those that do cover procedures such as IV infusions in a medical facility may have a list (a "formulary") of specific drugs covered by the plan. For example, Medicare Part B covers Avonex, but only when administered by a physician. Novantrone, which must be given in a medical facility, is also covered by Medicare Part B. Until January 1, 2006, Medicare will not cover self-administered prescription drugs (including Avonex) if given away from a doctor's office, except for participants in the limited Medicare Demonstration Project.

Medicaid includes prescription drug coverage, but Medicaid lists of covered drugs are under state control and vary from state to state.

Each of the drug companies runs a program designed to help people apply for and use all the state and federal programs for which they are eligible. They also help some people who are uninsured or underinsured through patient assistance programs. Means-testing usually includes offsets for high medical costs, so many middle-income people are eligible.

Chemotherapy (immunosuppressants) Chemotherapy drugs generally refer to the use of potent cytotoxic (cell-killing) agents prescribed for some forms of cancer. These drugs not only kill tumor cells but can destroy normal cells as well. The cells that are most vulnerable to cytotoxic agents are those that grow and divide rapidly, such as cancer cells, hair and intestinal cells, red blood cells, and the white blood cells that make up the immune system.

The rationale for using chemotherapy to treat MS stems from the fact that MS is considered to be an autoimmune disease: an abnormal immune response by certain white blood cells mounts an attack on the myelin of the central nervous system. Destruction of myelin slows or halts nerve impulses and produces the symptoms of MS.

Since chemotherapy drugs lowers the number of white blood cells, it should theoretically slow down or halt this autoimmune destruction. Some of the many chemotherapeutic agents that have been used to treat MS are described below. The results of many clinical trials have not conclusively shown them to be of definite value, and their use in treating MS remains controversial.

Azathioprine (Imuran) The usc of this drug as a treatment for MS remains controversial. A drug that suppresses the immune system, AZA-THIOPRINE is commonly used to treat autoimmune diseases such as rheumatoid arthritis, and as part of chemotherapy for some cancers. Over the past 20 years, azathioprine has been the subject of numerous clinical trials both in the United States and abroad to see if it is useful as a treatment for MS. The results (using different patient populations, different doses, and different protocols) have been mixed. Some benefit, in the form of slowed progression or fewer relapses, was noted in 60 percent of the trials. There was no apparent benefit in the other trials. Some patients have not been able to take azathioprine because of severe nausea.

Other potential side effects of azathioprine include severe anemia or leukopenia (shortage of white blood cells), liver damage, and a long-term increased risk of developing cancers such as leukemia or lymphoma. The decision to use azathioprine is a complicated one, and should be made by the physician and the patient together, after a discussion of the potential risks and benefits.

Cladribine (Leustatin)   Recent studies have shown no benefit in MS. Side effects have included infections and bone marrow suppression with reduced platelet counts.

Cyclophosphamide (Cytoxan)   This potent immunosuppressive drug is usually given to treat cancer. It has been used for treating MS for many years, mostly in uncontrolled studies, where it was often but not always reported to improve the condition of people with primary or secondary progressive MS. More recent studies have shown that, at best, there is only a modest benefit from cyclophosphamide.

A study in people with rapidly progressive disease is currently under way. The drug is currently used only in selected situations. Its use should be discussed with a neurologist and decisions reached on an individual basis. The side effects of short-term treatment with high doses are hair loss, nausea, occasional bladder injury, and risk of infection. Long-term side effects include sterility, mutations, and the increased risk of cancer.

Cyclosporin A   This drug significantly reduced rejection rates in organ transplantation, but experts have concluded that the risks of cyclosporine outweigh the benefits for treatment of MS and do not justify its use under most circumstances. It is rarely used today.

Unlike most immune-suppressing drugs, it appears to have a specific action primarily against one type of white blood cell (the helper T cells). Since there is some evidence that these cells are abnormally active during acute exacerbations of MS, and since it has been shown to be effective in treating other autoimmune diseases in humans and EAE (the animal model of MS), cyclosporine was tried in a double-blind, placebo-controlled trial in patients with progressive MS. In this study of almost 600 men and women, those patients who received cyclosporine had a slightly (but statistically significant) slower rate of disease progression than the placebo group over two years. There were no significant differences in ability to perform activities of daily living and no change in MRI or spinal fluid test results. There were serious side effects associated with cyclosporine use, namely kidney damage and high blood pressure.

Another study done in Germany compared cyclosporine to another immunosuppressive agent (azathioprine). More than 80 patients in each treatment group completed a two-year double blind protocol. No significant differences between the two groups were apparent at the end of the study, but the cyclosporine group had twice as many side effects as the azathioprine-treated patients.

Methotrexate   This synthetic immunosuppressive drug is highly effective in the short term against rheumatoid arthritis (an autoimmune disease). It also effectively prevents EAE, the animal model for MS. Although a clinical trial of methotrexate in the 1970s did not show benefit to MS patients, there has been renewed interest in the drug, and a recent controlled trial showed the drug had modest benefit. In this trial, 30 people with primary or secondary progressive MS who were still able to walk received weekly low-dose methotrexate. Deterioration of arm function was slowed, compared to the arm function of those receiving a placebo, but there was no difference in worsening of leg function, or in overall disability.

Complementary and alternative medicines (CAMs)   Alternative medicine is widely used in the community and more frequently by people with MS. Alternative medicine includes everything from drugs and diet to food supplements, mental exercises, and lifestyle changes. These therapies come from many different disciplines and traditions—yoga, hypnosis, guided imagery, relaxation techniques, traditional herbal healing, Chinese medicine, macrobiotics, naturopathy, and many others.

Managing symptoms   Rehabilitation is an integral part in the treatment of MS symptoms. Rehabilitation stresses improvement and maintenance of function, particularly treating problems related to activities of daily living such as walking, dressing and personal care, using mobility aids (such as a cane or wheelchair), or performing tasks at work. It also addresses speech and memory problems, sexual difficulties, bladder and bowel needs, and overall fitness.

PHYSICAL THERAPY (PT) can help strengthen weakened or uncoordinated muscles and improve balance. PT might include range-of-motion exercises, stretching, strengthening, assistance with walking, and the best ways to be fitted for and to use canes, walkers, or other assistive devices. PT can also include exercises to increase overall function and stamina and transfer training (for example, learning how to move safely from wheelchairs to cars).

OCCUPATIONAL THERAPY focuses on improving independence in daily living. An occupational therapist (OT) is a specialist in energy conservation to combat fatigue. OTs teach techniques for dressing, grooming, eating, and driving and exercises for coordination and strength. An OT can recommend equipment and ways to adapt the home or workplace.

SPEECH THERAPY improves communication for those who may have difficulty speaking or swallowing due to weakness or poor coordination. Techniques used by speech therapists (also called speech pathologists) might include exercise, voice training, or the use of special devices. Speech therapists provide treatment for DYSPHAGIA, which may involve dietary changes, exercises, and/or stimulation designed to improve swallowing. In very severe cases that do not respond to these measures, feeding tubes may be inserted directly into the stomach to provide the necessary fluids and nutrition.

COGNITIVE REHABILITATION offers exercises and strategies to improve memory, attention, information processing, and reasoning, which may become slowed due to loss of myelin in the brain. Cognitive rehab sessions with a neuropsychologist, speech pathologist, or OT might focus on exercises to improve particular cognitive skills. Or these sessions might teach ways to compensate for problems, including time management, organization methods, and use of computers.

VOCATIONAL REHABILITATION specialists focus on retraining or use of adaptations and accommodations on the job. They may work independently or in consultation with an OT.

Bowel and bladder care Training in bowel and bladder care may be needed to prevent or compensate for incontinence. If the urge to urinate becomes great before the bladder is full, some drugs may be helpful, including propantheline bromide (Probanthine), oxybutynin chloride (Ditropan), or imipramine (Tofranil). BACLOFEN (Lioresal) may relax the sphincter muscle, allowing full emptying. Intermittent catheterization is effective in controlling bladder dysfunction. In this technique, a catheter is used to periodically empty the bladder.

Spasticity There are two major antispasticity drugs with good safety records: baclofen (Lioresal) and TIZANIDINE (Zanaflex). While no drug can cure spasticity, they may be especially helpful for people confined to a wheelchair who are having trouble with leg or arm stiffness, or whose leg spasms are particularly painful.

Baclofen is a muscle relaxant, the most common drug used to treat spasticity. It can dramatically decrease spasms, while improving muscle tone and posture, and acts on the lower spinal cord and its descending motor pathways where MS lesions are often found. Researchers believe the drug affects the reflex involved in maintaining muscle tone, relaxing the main muscle groups in the arms, legs, and trunk. This has an overall inhibiting effect on spasms. Therefore, if the person has a GAIT PROBLEM, walking will almost always get better after Baclofen is administered. Fluidity of movement, range of joint motion, and quickness of movement also improves. People with spasticity in the legs typically improve more than those whose arms are spastic.

Unfortunately, strength and coordination are not improved with this drug. Physicians typically start off with a low dose and slowly increase it until maximum benefit is reached. (Taking too high a dose at first can trigger fatigue and weakness.) People with MS often take this drug in the morning, when it is usually difficult to get out of bed. Baclofen can be taken as needed, and an individual usually can regulate the dosage themselves after an initial discussion with the doctor.

Usually administered orally, Baclofen has few serious side effects other than fatigue or weakness, although it may interact dangerously with alcohol and other drugs. It can cause seizures and hallucinations if stopped suddenly. Baclofen should be used cautiously in women with MS who are pregnant, and by alcoholics, diabetics, or those with kidney disease. People taking other medications such as central nervous system depressants, muscle relaxants, and the insomnia drug Ethinamate should be particularly careful about using Baclofen. Some research also suggests that smoking may interfere with the absorption of Baclofen, especially if the person smokes more than a pack a day.

Baclofen also can be given by an implanted pump (intrathecal baclofen), which is placed under the skin of the abdomen and connected directly to the lower half of the spinal cord. Because the implant is technically difficult to place and involves higher risks and costs, intrathecal baclofen is used only for severe spasticity that cannot be managed with oral medication. It can, however, produce dramatic improvement when the oral medication was ineffective.

Tizanidine (Zanaflex) is a short-acting drug used to treat the increased muscle tone associated with spasticity. While it does not provide a cure for the problem, it is designed to relieve the spasms, cramping, and tightness of muscles. In order to minimize unwanted side effects with this medication, the physician typically starts the person on a low dose and gradually increases it until a well-tolerated and effective level is reached. Because peak effectiveness occurs one to two hours after dosing and ends between three to six hours after dosing, a physician will prescribe a dosing schedule that provides the most relief during activities and periods of time when it is most important that the patient have symptom relief.

Common side effects that should be reported to the doctor as soon as possible include burning, prickling, or tingling sensations; diarrhea; fainting; fever; loss of appetite; nausea; nervousness; pain or burning during urination; skin sores; stomach pain or vomiting; yellow eyes or skin; and blurred vision. Since it may be difficult to tell the difference between common symptoms of MS and some side effects of tizanidine, a doctor should be consulted if a symptom suddenly appears while a patient is on this drug. Treatment also includes regular stretching exercises.

Pain Pain syndromes are not uncommon in MS. In one study, 55 percent of the people studied had what is called "clinically significant pain" at some time during the course of a lifetime with MS. Almost half (48 percent) were troubled by chronic pain. This study suggested that factors such as age at onset, length of time with MS, or degree of disability played no part in distinguishing the people with pain from the people who were pain free. There are several types of pain and treatments in MS.

Trigeminal neuralgia is a stabbing pain in the face that can occur as an initial symptom of MS. While it can be confused with dental pain, this pain is neurologic in origin and can usually be treated successfully with medications such as CARBAMAZEPINE (Tegretol) or PHENYTOIN (Dilantin).

Lhermitte's sign is a brief, stabbing, electric-shock-like sensation that runs from the back of the head down the spine, brought on by bending the neck forward. A soft collar may be used to limit neck flexion.

Dysesthesias are often treated with the anticonvulsant medication GABAPENTIN (Neurontin). Dysesthesias may also be treated with an antidepressant such as AMITRIPTYLINE (Elavil), which modifies how the central nervous system reacts to pain.

Back and musculoskeletal pain can have many causes, including spasticity; treatment of spasticity may also help with pain control. Pressure on the body caused by immobility, incorrect use of mobility aids, or the struggle to compensate for gait and balance problems may all contribute. An evaluation to pinpoint the source of the pain is essential. Treatments may include heat, massage, ultrasound, physical therapy, and treatment for spasticity.

Chronic disabling pain may require referral to a multidisciplinary pain clinic where medication, physical therapy, counseling, and other therapies may be used.

Other treatments Fatigue may be partially avoidable by changing the daily routine to allow more frequent rests. Amantadine (Symmetrel) and PEMOLINE (Cylert) may improve alertness and lessen fatigue. Visual disturbances often respond to corticosteroids. Other symptoms that may be treated with drugs include seizures, vertigo, and tremor.

multiple sclerosis quality of life-54 instrument (MSQOL-54) A health-related quality-of-life measure that combines both generic and MS-specific items into a single test, to assess MS-specific issues such as fatigue, cognitive function, and role limitations. The MSQOL-54 is a structured, self-report questionnaire that the person can generally complete with little or no assistance in less than ten minutes.

multiple sclerosis quality of life inventory (MSQLI) assessment An assessment measuring quality of life that is both generic and MS-specific. The MSQLI consists of a set of 10 self-report questionnaires that the person with MS can generally complete in less than an hour with little or no intervention from an interviewer. However, people with visual or upper extremity impairments may need to have the MSQLI administered as an interview. The MSQLI addresses the concerns most relevant to the MS population.

multiplex MS families Large families in which many members have been diagnosed with multiple sclerosis (MS). In families in which MS occurs in many relatives, the risks of getting MS for any given individual are significantly higher than they are for an individual who has no family members with MS.

muscle tone A characteristic of a muscle that describes its resistance to stretching. Abnormal muscle tone can be defined as hypertonic (increased muscle tone, as in SPASTICITY), hypotonic (reduced muscle tone), flaccid (paralysis), or atonic (loss of muscle tone). Muscle tone is evaluated as part of the standard neurological exam in patients suspected of having multiple sclerosis.

musculoskeletal pain A type of pain experienced by some people with multiple sclerosis (MS) that can have many causes, including SPASTICITY. Pressure on the body caused by immobility, incorrect use of mobility aids, or the struggle to compensate for gait and balance problems may all contribute to the discomfort. In order to treat this pain properly, the patient must undergo an evaluation to pinpoint the source of the pain. Treatments for musculoskeletal pain related to MS may include heat,

MASSAGE, ultrasound, PHYSICAL THERAPY, or treatment for spasticity.

myalgia Tenderness and PAIN in the muscle.

myelin The white matter rich in protein and lipids (fatty substances) that insulates the nerves, enabling them to conduct impulses between the brain and other parts of the body.

Myelin consists of a layer of proteins packed between two layers of lipids. An abnormal autoimmune reaction in multiple sclerosis (MS) is believed to initiate an attack on the myelin, resulting in bare spots and scarred areas along the nerve. This destruction of myelin is known as DEMYELINATION. When demyelination occurs, nerve fiber conduction slows down and sometimes stops altogether. Impaired bodily functions or altered sensations associated with those demyelinated nerve fibers are identified as symptoms of MS.

Although myelin is found in both the central nervous system (CNS) and the peripheral nervous system (PNS), only the destruction of CNS myelin produces the symptoms of MS.

CNS myelin is produced by special cells called OLIGODENDROCYTES, whereas PNS myelin is produced by Schwann cells. Although the two types of myelin are chemically different, they both promote efficient transmission of nerve impulses along the axon (the threadlike extensions of neurons that make up nerve fibers). Each oligodendrocyte can myelinate several axons.

The myelin layer is segmented, and small areas or nodes are naturally unmyelinated. As chemical ions pass in and out of the axons, the electrical current they generate is conducted down the nerve and jumps from node to node. Myelin prevents the current from leaking out of the nerve at inappropriate points and decreases the electrical resistance of the nerve. This helps make sure the nerve impulse is conducted efficiently.

Researchers are concentrating on trying to understand how myelin-producing cells function, how they form myelin, and how they might form new myelin after disease. Understanding how these cells might form new myelin is the best hope for recovery of function and is an important and growing area of MS research.

myelin basic protein (MBP) A major component of MYELIN that can often be found in abnormally high levels in the patient's cerebrospinal fluid if the myelin is damaged, as happens in multiple sclerosis (MS). This substance becomes elevated as axonal damage occurs when the disease progresses.

myelin oligodendrocyte glycoprotein (MOG) A component of MYELIN that is being studied for its potential role as an autoantigen in multiple sclerosis within the central nervous system.

myelin repair Myelin is the protective sheath that covers nerve fibers. An abnormal autoimmune reaction in multiple sclerosis (MS) is believed to initiate an attack on the myelin, resulting in bare spots and scarred areas along the nerve. Healing damaged myelin is the only way to reverse the damage caused by MS and restore function. This will not be possible, however, until experts find a way to stop the immune system from damaging the central nervous system tissue in the first place.

Scientists have discovered that the body heals some lesions naturally. This occurs by stimulating OLIGODENDROCYTES (myelin-producing cells) in the area or recruiting young oligodendrocytes from further away to begin making new myelin at the damaged site. Researchers are now working to identify the molecular signals that are used by the body to activate the oligodendrocytes so that those signals can be mimicked to stimulate additional repair. Scientists are also studying certain proteins known as growth factors in order to identify their potential role in myelin repair.

As scientists work to stimulate myelin repair, they are also focusing their attention on several properties of myelin that work to interfere with this repair process. Eventually, treatments may be developed to stop these components of myelin from inhibiting the repair process.

Scientists are investigating several different strategies for stimulating the repair of myelin. Antibodies (immune proteins that attach to specific molecules) have been successfully used to stimulate myelin repair in rodents with an MS-like disease. Based on the outcomes from this research, the antibodies will undergo preliminary testing for safety in people with MS.

Efforts are also being made to replace damaged oligodendrocytes and nerve cells surgically. Scientists are working to identify potential sources of replacement cells for those that are damaged by MS, such as skin-derived cells, bone marrow and umbilical cord blood cells, fetal cells, adult brain cells, and Schwann cells. The usefulness of these replacement cells will depend on finding or creating the signals needed to stimulate their transformation and growth into healthy new cells.

myelitis An inflammatory condition of the spinal cord in which the spinal cord loses the ability to transmit impulses. In transverse myelitis, the inflammation spreads across the tissue of the spinal cord, causing a loss of normal ability to transmit nerve impulses up and down, as though the spinal cord had been severed. It may appear along with multiple sclerosis.

myelography An X-ray examination of the brain and spinal cord to check for lesions typical of multiple sclerosis (MS). The technique begins with a SPINAL TAP (lumbar puncture) and injection of a special X-ray contrast material into the spinal canal. The patient is tilted while a series of X-rays are taken at different angles, after which most of the contrast fluid is removed. The study is performed to see if excess myelin is in the cerebrospinal fluid, which can indicate DEMYELINATION (lesions that indicate the destruction of myelin).

Noninvasive tests such as CT SCANS or MAGNETIC RESONANCE IMAGING provide good resolution for diagnosing MS. Myelography is rarely used; but if performed, fluid obtained during the procedure may provide additional information about inflammation and evidence of infection.

Side Effects

This procedure may be uncomfortable. Common side effects include nausea and vomiting, flushing, pressure, headache, and some pain (especially when the fluid is removed). Although serious side effects are rare, they may include infection and allergy to the contrast dye.

Myobloc   See BOTULINUM TOXIN.

myoclonus   Spasm or twitching of a muscle or a group of muscles that occurs in various brain disorders such as multiple sclerosis.

natalizumab See DISEASE-MODIFYING AGENTS.

necrosis The death or decay of tissue, which is the result of the loss of blood supply, burning, and other severe injuries. Necrosis can also be caused by some medications commonly used to treat multiple sclerosis flares.

Neosar See CYCLOPHOSPHAMIDE.

nerve A bundle of nerve fibers (axons) that are either afferent (leading toward the brain and helping to perceive sensory stimuli of the skin, joints, muscles, and inner organs) or efferent (leading away from the brain and influencing contractions of muscles or organs).

nerve block A procedure used to relieve otherwise intractable SPASTICITY, including painful FLEXOR SPASMS. An injection of phenol into the affected nerve interferes with the function of that nerve for up to three months, potentially increasing a person's comfort and ability to move.

nerve cell See NEURON.

nerve growth factors (NGFs) One of several naturally occurring proteins in the brain that promotes nerve cell growth and survival. Experiments on rats have shown that NGFs promote growth of new connections between synapses in the brain, which could help restore memory loss. Scientists have shown that NGFs stimulate the growth of tiny projections of a growing nerve cell that carry information between cells. NGFs have the potential to repair or protect the adult brain. They were first discovered in the 1950s by developmental biologist Rita Levi-Montalcini, who won a Nobel Prize in 1986 for that work.

NGFs are one of the human growth factors currently being studied for their potential to restore nerve function. At least eight different varieties of growth factors are currently being studied. Each has a different target cell in the body, and each has a possible role in protecting the body's nerve cells against damage from disease.

In a variety of learning and memory tests, California researchers have shown that infusions of NGF into the brain could improve learning capacity and increase the size of brain cells that had previously shrunk. In a study in the mid-1980s, scientists took several rats with memory impairment and gave them NGF. The rats' ability to negotiate the maze improved, coming close to the ability seen in older rats with no impairment.

In 1999, scientists at the University of California at San Diego showed that brain cells in aging monkeys were restored to near-normal size and quantity after surgical implants of cells genetically altered to produce NGF.

The federal government approved human trials for NGF in 1999 after a team of researchers showed the protein reversed deterioration in the brains of aging monkeys.

Working with these factors is not easy, however. Most of these protein molecules are large and hard to handle. They must be pumped directly into the brain, because they will not cross the blood-brain barrier.

nervous system A vast network of cells that carries information coded as nerve impulses to and from all parts of the body. The system is divided into the CENTRAL NERVOUS SYSTEM (the brain and spinal cord) and the peripheral nervous system (the nervous tissue outside the cranium and verte-bral column). In the average adult human, the brain weighs about three pounds and contains about 100 billion nerve cells and trillions of sup-port cells called glia.

neuralgia Nerve PAIN that can be severe. It appears along the length of a nerve and arises within the nerve itself, not in the tissue from which the sensation seems to arise.

neurasthenia FATIGUE or exhaustion, often greater than what would seem to be appropriate from purely physical causes.

neurectomy A surgical procedure designed to treat severe spasms that do not respond to other interventions by cutting the affected nerve.

neurogenic bladder Bladder problems associated with difficulties in the spinal cord and character-ized by a failure to empty urine, a failure to store urine, or a combination of the two. This is a condi-tion that may occur in people with multiple sclero-sis (MS). Although many people do not experience bladder problems at the beginning of the disease, the likelihood of developing these problems increases over time.

At some point, about 75 percent of all people with MS will experience some type of bladder problem, most often frequency and urgency. In addition to these symptoms caused by a neuro-genic bladder, other problems include urinary hes-itancy, NOCTURIA, and incontinence.

Treatment Options and Outlook
People with neurogenic bladder must cope with two problems—the social and psychological aspects of having a bladder problem and the medical com-plications that may result from this disorder.

Often the first type of treatment that many peo-ple select is to wear absorbent, padded briefs dur-ing the day to cope with dribbling or incontinence. Some patients enthusiastically embrace the chance to wear these special undergarments instead of having to deal with medications, their side effects, or catheterization. Others find having to wear pro-tective pants to be psychologically devastating. For these patients, medication or INTERMITTENT SELF-CATHETERIZATION is the only possible choice to deal with neurogenic bladder problems. However, psy-chological issues are only one aspect. Urinary tract complications can be life threatening when appro-priate management is not implemented.

See also BLADDER DYSFUNCTION; BLADDER INCON-TINENCE.

neuroglial cells Special cells that are packed around and between the neurons, helping to sup-port the delicate nervous tissue. The neuroglial cells make up about half the volume of the brain. In addition to providing support for neurons, they regulate the ionic environment outside neurons. Ionic balance is critical to electrical function.

neurological examination Tests of movement and coordination, reflexes, vision, balance, sensa-tion, mental ability, and emotions used in diagnos-ing multiple sclerosis (MS) and other neurological conditions. During the examination, the doctor will look for injury to the 12 pairs of nerves in the head (CRANIAL NERVES) that relate to the senses of smell and taste, vision, eye movement, face and scalp sensations, face and neck muscle coordina-tion, hearing and balance, swallowing and the gag reflex, and movement of the tongue.

Certain signs and symptoms are more indicative of MS than others. In the beginning, though, the most definitive diagnosis a neurologist will proba-bly make, even if MS is suggested, is "probable MS." Whatever the results of the neurological exam, diagnosing definite MS from a single episode is not possible. This is because there are a number of other conditions of unknown cause that, like MS, are demyelinating, but unlike MS strike only once. In order to diagnose MS, at least two episodes must be separated by at least one month and the location of the lesions must be in at least two distinct sites in the central nervous system, or one episode plus evidence of demyelination on MRI.

The following tests may all be part of the neu-rological exam.

Babinski's sign In this test, which checks for signs of disease process in the motor neurons of the PYRAMIDAL TRACT, the doctor draws a semisharp object along the bottom of the foot. The normal response in adults and children is for the toes to reflex downward (flexor response). In babies and people with neurological problems of the corticospinal tract, the big toe moves upward (extensor response).

Optic neuritis This condition of the eye is caused by inflammation and DEMYELINATION of the OPTIC NERVE and causes one of the most common symptoms in MS. In this test, the patient reads letters from a board and takes a test for color vision using a color chart. An examination with an ophthalmoscope will reveal pallor of the optic nerve if there are old optic neurites.

Reflexes Reflexes are checked with both ends of the hammer. The reflexes can be normal, brisk (too easily evoked), or absent.

Romberg's sign This test checks for uncoordination or clumsiness of movement that is not the result of muscular weakness (ATAXIA). It requires the patient to stand with his or her feet together and eyes closed. People with ataxia have great difficulty standing still under these conditions.

Sensory This test is done with tuning forks and pins, and it tests the level of sensory perception in certain parts of the body. Patients are examined for the ability to feel pain (a pinprick), a light touch, temperature, and vibration (a tuning fork); for sense of the position of the arms or legs; and for reflexes.

Chaddock's sign In this test, similar to that for Babinski's sign, the neurologist touches the skin at the outside of the ankle. A positive (pathological) response is upward fanning of the big toe, as with Babinski's sign.

Hoffmann's sign This test for problems in the corticospinal tract is similar to that for Babinski's sign but checks the hands rather than the feet. In this test, the neurologist taps a nail on the third or fourth finger. A positive response is seen in flexion of the last section of the thumb.

Doll's eye sign In this test, the neurologist is looking for dissociation between movement of the eyes and of the head. A positive response is indicated by the eyes moving up when the head moves down.

Emotional condition The doctor can usually judge a patient's emotional condition during the exam by paying attention to a patient's actions and statements.

Gait and coordination The neurologist evaluates ataxia in various parts of the body by observing the patient walking normally, walking heel to toe, and using a FINGER-TO-NOSE TEST. In addition to ataxia, the neurologist will also be looking for INTENTION TREMOR (shaking when performing small motor movements).

Hearing loss This test is done by lightly clicking the fingers next to each ear and asking the patient near which ear the click was made.

Heel-shin test This is a test for ataxia and dysfunction in the CEREBELLUM. In this test, while lying down, the person brings the ball of the heel onto the knee of the other leg and then moves it down the shin to the ankle. The test assesses coordination of movements by noting how well the person can complete the movement.

Lhermitte's sign This test can reveal lesions on the spinal cord in the neck. The neurologist will ask the patient to lower the head toward the chest. A positive Lhermitte's sign will generate buzzing, tingling, or electrical shock sensations in one or more parts of the body during this activity.

Mental ability The neurologist will assess mental ability by asking the patient to repeat a series of numbers or answer simple questions about dates, places, and current events. If there is a suggestion of mental problems caused by MS, the doctor may order tests designed to identify more subtle changes than the ones that may be evident from the brief mental section of the neurological examination.

Muscle strength In this test, the neurologist assesses various muscle groups by having the patient push with arms and legs against the doctor's hand. Dexterity, muscle tone, and muscle control are also tested. Differences in strength between the left and right sides are easier to evaluate than symmetrical loss unless the weakness is severe.

See also NEUROLOGIC SIGN.

neurologic sign An objective physical problem or abnormality identified by a doctor during the NEUROLOGICAL EXAMINATION. Neurologic signs may differ significantly from the symptoms reported by the patient because they are identified only with specific tests and may cause no noticeable symptoms.

neurologist A physician who specializes in the diagnosis and treatment of conditions related to the nervous system, such as multiple sclerosis (MS). Neurologists conduct examinations of a person's nerves, reflexes, motor and sensory functions, and muscles to determine the cause of MS symptoms. A neurologist can perform detailed exams of all the neurological structures in the body, including the nerves of the head and neck, muscular strength and movement, sensation, balance, and reflexes. In some cases, detailed questions about memory, speech and language, and other cognitive functions are part of the examination.

Neurologists are often confused with neurosurgeons, who perform operations on the nervous system. Neurologists do not perform surgery but limit their practice to using medical treatments. Because MS is a disease of the nervous system and almost never involves surgery, neurologists are the specialists who normally manage this condition.

Neurologists also use other common tests, including computerized axial tomography and MAGNETIC RESONANCE IMAGING to provide detailed pictures of the brain, spinal structures, and blood vessels. A neurologist can also perform a SPINAL TAP (lumbar puncture) to obtain a sample of cerebrospinal fluid for analysis.

To become a neurologist, a student must complete a four-year premedical university degree, followed by four years of medical school and at least three years of specialty training in an accredited neurology residency program. After residency training, neurologists may choose to enroll in a one- or two-year fellowship program, which offers the opportunity to focus on a subspecialty of neurology, such as movement disorders.

After completing these educational requirements, neurologists may seek certification from the American Board of Psychiatry and Neurology. To be eligible for certification, an applicant must be a licensed physician with the required years of residency and have passed both a written and oral exam administered by the board.

See also CT SCAN.

neurometrics A method for diagnosing brain disorders by comparing auditory EVOKED POTENTIALS from several different regions of the brain with tracings taken from normal human beings.

neuromyelitis optica See DEVIC'S DISEASE.

neuron Another name for nerve cell, the basic functional unit of the nervous system. In the brain, the neurons are responsible for information processing by converting chemical signals to electrical signals and then back to chemical signals again.

About 50 million neurons are in the cerebral cortex, 40 billion more are in the cerebellum, and another 10 billion are in the rest of the brain and spinal cord. The average number of neurons varies dramatically from one person to the next and seems to have nothing to do with general intelligence (some animals have more neurons than humans do). Apparently, quantity is less important than the quality of the connections between the neurons.

There are two kinds of neurons—motor and sensory. Motor neurons are concerned with movement. Sensory neurons receive impulses from receptors in the eyes, skin, muscles, joints, and organs.

A neuron consists of a compact cell body made up of the nucleus, many long-branched extensions called dendrites, and a long fiber called the axon, with twiglike extensions at its end. Neurons are the major type of cell that make up the brain and nervous system, carrying signals to and from the brain and performing all of the brain's work. Each neuron receives electrical impulses through dendrites, which next to one another in a gigantic web whose tiny branches direct signals toward the body of the nerve cell.

If enough arriving signals stimulate the neuron, the neuron fires, sending this electrical pulse down its axon. The axon connects through synapses into the dendrites of another cell.

Information is carried inside a neuron by electrical pulses. However, once the signal reaches the end of the axon, it must be carried across the synaptic gap by chemicals called neurotransmitters. On the other side of the synapse is another dendrite, containing receptors that recognize these transmitting molecules. In a series of complicated steps, the receptor biochemically opens a channel to let charged ions pass through. The movement of ions generates an electrical current that changes the voltage of the postsynaptic neuron. If the shift is positive enough, this neuron will fire an action potential of its own. At the same time, the first neuron emits enzymes into the cleft that terminate the transmission and reabsorb any excess transmitter chemicals left in the synapse.

A single neuron can receive signals from thousands of other neurons, and its axon can branch repeatedly, sending signals to thousands more. The amazing ability of brain cells to make just the right connections may have been gained at the expense of their ability to reproduce. Almost all other cells in the body can regenerate. When these body cells die, they are replaced by others. Only in the brain are cells irreplaceable. Humans are born with almost all of the brain cells they will ever have. Those that die (about 18 million a year between ages 20 and 70) are lost forever.

The more connections, the more myelination, the stronger the brain structure becomes. Demyelination therefore serves to weaken the neuron's ability to communicate, resulting in the wide panoply of symptoms typical of multiple sclerosis.

Neurontin   See GABAPENTIN.

neuro-ophthalmologic evaluation   A comprehensive eye examination that includes analysis of the patient's current problem plus the person's entire medical history, including previous hospitalizations, operations, serious illnesses, family history, and medication allergies. The evaluation includes a complete eye examination with testing of peripheral vision (visual field test). In addition, the patient may have a partial or complete NEURO-LOGICAL EXAMINATION to test strength, sensation, and coordination.

In addition, the NEURO-OPHTHALMOLOGIST will review the records and scans from previous evaluations, if applicable. After the examination, the neuro-ophthalmologist will discuss the diagnosis, the need for any additional testing, and possible treatment.

neuro-ophthalmologist   A doctor who specializes in the diagnosis and treatment of neurological disorders such as multiple sclerosis that affect the eye and visual function. Neuro-ophthalmologists take care of visual problems that are related to the nervous system and not the eyes themselves.

Humans use almost half the brain for vision-related activities, including sight and eye movements. Neuro-ophthalmology, a subspecialty of both neurology and ophthalmology, requires specialized training and expertise in problems of the eye, brain, nerves, and muscles. Neuro-ophthalmologists complete at least five years of clinical training after medical school and are usually board certified in neurology, ophthalmology, or both.

Neuro-ophthalmologists have unique abilities to evaluate patients from a neurologic, ophthalmologic, and medical standpoint. This means that costly medical testing is often avoided.

Some of the common problems evaluated by neuro-ophthalmologists include optic nerve problems (such as OPTIC NEURITIS and ischemic optic neuropathy), visual field loss, unexplained visual loss, transient visual loss, visual disturbances, DOUBLE VISION, and abnormal eye movements.

See also NEURO-OPHTHALMOLOGIC EVALUATION.

neuropathology   A neurology specialty concerned with the causes and effects of neurological conditions instead of their diagnosis and treatment. Neuropathology is usually determined by a NEUROLOGIST or neurosurgeon.

neuropathy   Disease or damage to the peripheral nerves (in the upper and lower extremities). Neuropathy is characterized by numbness and weakness, pain, or tingling, depending on which nerves are affected. Most neuropathies occur from damage or irritation to the axons (the conducting fibers that make up nerves) or to the fatty substance called MYELIN that insulates the axons.

Precise symptoms depend on whether the affected nerve fibers are sensory or motor nerves. Sensory nerve damage may cause sensations of cold, NUMBNESS, and tingling, whereas motor damage may lead to muscle wasting and WEAKNESS.

neurophysiology   The fundamental workings of nerve cells and how they become damaged at different stages of multiple sclerosis.

neuropsychological tests   Assessments that can evaluate the extent of MEMORY loss or BRAIN damage in people with suspected multiple sclerosis. This kind of testing was first used as a way to distinguish between those whose abnormal behavior was caused by brain dysfunction and those whose problems were caused by psychological factors.

neuropsychologist   A psychologist with specialized training in neurology and the evaluation and treatment of cognitive function, and intensive training in psychological assessment. The relationship of neuropsychology to other neurosciences is an evolving one. It may include not only diagnosing brain problems such as multiple sclerosis (MS) but assessing treatment programs and a person's progress as well as planning rehabilitation programs.

Neuropsychologists use a battery of standardized tests to assess specific cognitive functions and identify areas of cognitive impairment. They also provide treatment for individuals with cognitive impairment related to MS.

A clinical neuropsychologist may enter private practice and offer various forms of psychotherapy and cognitive rehabilitation to individuals, families, or groups. They can administer standardized psychological and neuropsychological tests and both interpret and report on the results. Neuropsychologists may furnish legally recognized clinical and diagnostic opinions. They may conduct diagnostic interviews about the presence, scope, and treatment of cognitive or neuropsychological disorders.

A neuropsychologist and NEUROLOGIST differ in several ways. A neurologist is a physician who deals with the structural and physiological consequences of MS, among other disorders. The neuropsychologist is a Ph.D. who investigates the cognitive and behavioral impact of MS.

neurotrophic factor   A protein, such as NERVE GROWTH FACTOR, that promotes nerve cell growth and survival. Growth factors elsewhere in the body support cell division. Although nerve cells cannot divide, they can regenerate after injury. Neurotrophic factors help in this regeneration. They also promote the growth of axons and dendrites, the neuron branches that form connections with other neurons.

neutralizing antibodies (NABs)   A type of antibody produced in response to INTERFERON beta, a treatment for multiple sclerosis. The biological effects of NABs is uncertain, but it is possible that their presence may be associated with a reduced effectiveness of interferon beta treatment.

Nine Hole Peg Test (9-HPT)   A brief standardized test of upper extremity function that is the second component of the MS Functional Composite test administered at each doctor visit. In this test, both the dominant and nondominant hands are tested twice. The patient is seated at a table with a small shallow container holding nine pegs and a wood or plastic block containing nine empty holes. At the start of the clock, the patient picks up the nine pegs one at a time as quickly as possible and places them in the nine holes. Once they are in the holes, the patient removes them again as quickly as possible, one at a time, replacing them into the shallow container. The total time to complete the task is recorded.

In recent years, experts have realized it is useful to measure arm and hand function, especially in people with severe disability. In the last few years, the 9-HPT has been one of the most frequently used measures of upper extremity function in people with multiple sclerosis.

nocturia   The need to urinate at night, which is one of the symptoms of multiple sclerosis.

See also BLADDER DYSFUNCTION.

Novantrone   See MITOXANTRONE.

numbness   A reduced sensitivity to touch. Numbness is one of the most common symptoms of multiple sclerosis and is often the first symptom. The numbness may range from mild to so severe that it interferes with the ability to use the affected body part. For example, a person with very numb feet may have difficulty walking. Numb hands may prevent writing, dressing, or holding objects safely. Because of the decrease in feeling, people should be careful to protect the area from cuts, bumps, bruises, burns, or other injury.

Treatment Options and Outlook

No medications can ease numbness. However, most cases of numbness are not disabling and tend to improve on their own. Self-help measures may include

- exercise to maintain muscle tone
- rest and relaxation techniques for improved energy levels
- avoidance of temperature extremes

In very severe cases, a NEUROLOGIST may prescribe corticosteroids, which are often useful in temporarily restoring sensation.

nystagmus   Uncontrolled horizontal or vertical eye movements, a common symptom of multiple sclerosis (MS). Nystagmus may be mild, occurring only when a person looks to the side, or it may be severe enough to impair vision.

In people with MS, nystagmus is often associated with internuclear ophthalmoplegia (a loss of coordination between the two eyes) caused by a lesion in an area of the brain called the medial longitudinal fasciculus. Nystagmus may also be caused by lesions in the CEREBELLUM, the area of the BRAIN STEM where the vestibular cranial nerve begins, or further along the vestibular pathways. The condition reduces vision in a number of ways, including oscillopsia—a sense that the world is wiggling, which may occur in one eye, or both. It typically causes general poor vision and often loss of balance.

Symptoms and Diagnostic Path

The most common symptom of nystagmus is DIZZINESS. Other symptoms include jerky eye movements, loss of balance, or a sense that the world is wiggling.

A low-vision specialist can analyze the extent of loss and recommend aids and strategies to help the MS patient make the most of his or her existing vision. Low-vision specialists are licensed doctors of ophthalmology or optometry who will assess how the patient's eyesight functions in everyday life—not just how well the person can read an eye chart. The specialist may ask questions about glare, contrast, sensitivity to light, and color perception, using special charts to measure other aspects of vision. A typical session with a low-vision specialist lasts two to three times longer than a standard eye exam, since the specialist needs as much information as possible on the patient's medical and vision history as well as his or her individual needs.

Treatment Options and Outlook

The low-vision specialist may be able to prescribe or recommend an optical device, such as microscopic or telescopic eyewear, a magnifier, a filter, or a closed circuit television system. (The closed circuit television [CCTV] can magnify items such as photographs, letters, book pages, and even the labels on medicine bottles onto a television screen. Some CCTVs are freestanding; others plug into the patient's TV and use its screen.)

Some drugs and special prisms have been reported to be successful in treating the visual deficits caused by nystagmus and a related eye movement disorder, OPSOCLONUS, which causes jumping vision. However, the existing medications for nystagmus, such as anticonvulsants and muscle relaxants, may not work well. The antiseizure drug GABAPENTIN (Neurontin) may be helpful.

Surgery is not usually recommended for nystagmus, but new research is focusing on optical devices to stabilize the jiggling visual environment of people with nystagmus. As difficult as this disorder may be, nystagmus often goes away spontaneously. In any case, the brain eventually learns to ignore the wiggling, restoring more normal vision.

occipital lobe   One of four major pairs of lobes of the CEREBRAL CORTEX that includes the center of the visual perception system. This part of the BRAIN may be affected by multiple sclerosis.

The occipital lobe is involved in visuospatial processing, discrimination of movement, and color discrimination. Light reaches the sight centers in the occipital lobe through a complex pathway. After light hits the retina, the information is transmitted to the lateral geniculate nucleus in the thalamus. At this stage, the brain interprets the light that the eye receives. From there the axons show the image in the visual association cortex that identifies what the eyes are seeing. ·

When one side of the occipital lobe is damaged, sight is lost in both eyes. Lesions in the occipital lobe can cause unusual side effects, such as blindsight. A person with blindsight claims to have no vision at all, but when asked, the person can point to or identify objects at a distance unconsciously. Other lesions in the occipital lobe have been known to cause an inability to identify faces, known as prospagnosia ("face blindness"). Lesions can also cause writing impairments and an inability to recognize words (alexia). Disorders of the occipital lobe may cause illusions and hallucinations that can cause objects to appear larger or smaller than they really are or make an object appear to be a different color. Lesions in the parietal-temporal-occipital association area can cause word blindness (alexia) and loss of the ability to write (agraphia). Once damaged, the occipital lobe is hard to repair.

occupational therapist   A health care professional whose role is to help people with disabilities, such as those with multiple sclerosis (MS), and other disabling conditions maintain everyday skills that are essential for independent living and that allow for productivity at home and at work. Occupational therapists can analyze how MS affects the way a person performs daily tasks and help the person learn new ways to carry out familiar activities.

Occupational therapists offer individualized treatment using appropriate exercise and adaptive equipment. The four major areas targeted by the occupational therapist include upper-body strength, movement, and coordination; the use of assistive technology to enhance accessibility and independent living; fatigue management through energy conservation, work simplification, and stress management; and compensatory strategies for impairment in thinking, sensation, and vision.

Therapists also offer ongoing evaluation and treatments to maintain the range of motion and muscle strength of a person's arms and hands. This can help successfully complete activities of daily living, such as dressing, eating, toileting, and bathing.

occupational therapy   Occupational therapy can help people with disabilities, such as those with multiple sclerosis (MS), stay active by improving their ability to carry out specific ACTIVITIES OF DAILY LIVING that primarily involve the arms and hands. Such activities include grooming, dressing, eating, handwriting, and driving.

A physician can provide a referral to an OCCUPATIONAL THERAPIST, whose services are usually covered by insurance. Occupational therapists can prescribe exercises designed to develop fine coordination or compensate for tremor or WEAKNESS. They can suggest ASSISTIVE DEVICES such as button hooks and dressing aids. Occupational therapists may also evaluate WHEELCHAIRS, room arrangements, or other living or working conditions and recommend adjustments for a more efficient and safe environment.

For patients with MS, occupational therapy generally provides assessment, treatment, and recommendations in the following areas:

- arm and hand therapy
- handwriting aids
- home modification
- driver evaluation and vehicle modification
- cooking and homemaking adaptations
- eating and dinnerware adaptations
- computer modifications
- workplace or work equipment modifications
- leisure skills
- manual or electric wheelchair use
- bathtub and toilet equipment use
- dressing and grooming aids

ocular dysmetria The constant undershooting or overshooting of the eyes when a patient tries to fix his or her gaze on something. A form of DYSMETRIA, this symptom can trigger a sense of nausea. Ocular dysmetria suggests the presence of lesions in the CEREBELLUM (the brain region responsible for coordinating movement). It is a symptom of several neurological conditions, including multiple sclerosis.

See also VISUAL PROBLEMS.

ocular inflammation Inflammation of the iris or other parts of the eye is reported in about 10 percent of people with multiple sclerosis. The symptoms may be mild or severe; complications depend on the extent of the inflammation.

oligoclonal bands A diagnostic sign that indicates an abnormal level of certain antibodies in the CEREBROSPINAL FLUID. Oligoclonal bands are seen in about 90 percent of people with multiple sclerosis (MS). However, oligoclonal bands are not specific to MS.

oligodendrocyte implants An experimental, minimally invasive method to transplant modified MYELIN-producing OLIGODENDROCYTE cells directly into the brain to stimulate nerve and axon growth. If feasible, this approach might help people whose multiple sclerosis is not caused by an autoimmune response (in which the new cells would be attacked, just as the person's own cells had been).

oligodendrocytes Special cells of the central nervous system that produce MYELIN.

See also OLIGODENDROCYTE IMPLANTS.

ophthalmoplegia See INTERNUCLEAR OPHTHALMOPLEGIA.

optic atrophy Wasting of the OPTIC DISC caused by partial or complete degeneration of OPTIC NERVE fibers. Optic atrophy is associated with a loss of visual acuity. This finding may occur in people with multiple sclerosis.

See also VISUAL PROBLEMS.

optic disc A small blind spot on the surface of the retina where cells of the retina converge to form the OPTIC NERVE. It is the only part of the retina that is insensitive to light.

See also VISUAL PROBLEMS.

optic nerve The nerve that carries impulses from the eyes to the brain, also known as the second cranial nerve. Inflammation of the optic nerve may occur as a sign of a neurologic disease affecting nerves in various parts of the body, such as multiple sclerosis (MS).

A person can see because the small nerves of the retina (the inner surface at the back of the eye) sense light and transmit impulses to the optic nerve, which carries them to the brain. VISUAL PROBLEMS occur if there is a problem anywhere along the optic nerve and its branches or if there is any damage to the areas at the back of the brain that sense visual stimuli.

The optic nerve follows an unusual route from the eyes to the back of the brain. Each nerve splits, and half of its fibers cross over to the other side at the optic chiasm. Because of this arrangement, damage along the optic nerve pathway causes peculiar patterns of vision loss. Inflammation of the optic nerve is characterized by sudden blurry vision. As the nerve tissue becomes swollen and red, the nerve fibers stop working properly. If many of the nerve fibers are involved, the vision may be very poor. However, if the OPTIC NEURITIS is mild, the vision will be nearly normal. If the optic nerve is damaged between the eyeball and the optic chiasm, vision may be lost in that eye. However, if the problem lies further back in the optic nerve pathway, vision may be lost in only half the visual field of both eyes. If both eyes lose peripheral vision, the cause may be damage at the optic chiasm.

Studies with up to 10 years of follow-up have demonstrated that 50–60 percent of people with isolated optic neuritis go on to develop MS. More recent studies reported that those persons with optic neuritis who also had abnormalities in their cerebrospinal fluid or on MAGNETIC RESONANCE IMAGING were more likely to develop MS.

Since the optic nerve enters the back of the eye where it appears as a small disk, an ophthalmologist can examine it by looking in the eye with an ophthalmoscope. Swelling of the optic nerve may or may not be visible depending on whether the optic neuritis is affecting the optic nerve near the eyeball. Since optic neuritis can be confused with many other causes of poor vision, an accurate medical diagnosis is important. If a cause can be found and treated, further damage may be prevented. Tests may include ultrasound, computerized axial tomography imaging (CT SCANS), or visual brain wave recordings. Other tests may include assessments of color vision, side vision, and pupil reactions to light.

optic neuritis Inflammation or DEMYELINATION of the OPTIC NERVE (the nerve that transmits light and visual images from the retina to the brain) that cannot be seen during an eye examination. Because the nerve is located behind (retro) the eye, the condition is also known as retrobulbar neuritis. It is one of the most common beginning symptoms of multiple sclerosis (MS). However, it can also be caused by an isolated neurological lesion, with full recovery of vision and without progression to clinically definite MS.

Between 50 and 60 percent of people with isolated optic neuritis go on to develop MS. About 20 percent of people with this condition develop MS within two years after the onset of optic neuritis. About 17 percent of people experience impaired eye movement.

Other studies suggest that people with optic neuritis who also have abnormalities in their cerebrospinal fluid or on BRAIN SCANS are more likely to develop MS. Although other disease processes can cause optic neuritis, MS is the most likely cause in a young, otherwise healthy individual.

Symptoms and Diagnostic Path

Optic neuritis typically begins abruptly with blurring, graying, or loss of vision—with or without pain—most often in only one eye. Only rarely will both eyes be affected at the same time. Loss of vision is usually worst within the first few days and generally improves within one to three months without treatment. There may be pain in the eye socket, especially when moving the eyes. Vision may temporarily get worse after exercising or after a hot bath.

Since the optic nerve enters the back of the eye where it appears as a small disk, an ophthalmologist can examine it by looking in the eye with an ophthalmoscope. Swelling of the optic nerve may or may not be visible depending on whether the optic neuritis is affecting the optic nerve near the eyeball. Since optic neuritis can be confused with many other causes of poor vision, an accurate medical diagnosis is important. If a cause can be found and treated, further damage may be prevented.

Tests may include ultrasound, computerized axial tomography (CT) scans, or visual brain wave recordings. Other tests may include assessments of color vision, side vision, and pupil reactions to light.

Treatment Options and Outlook

Although this condition usually improves without treatment, recent research suggests that a short course of intravenous methylprednisolone, sometimes followed by a tapered course of oral steroids, may reduce the inflammation and restore vision more quickly. However, no definitive evidence shows that treatment with steroids produces a more complete recovery than that which would have happened without treatment.

A person with MS can have inflammation and/or demyelination of the optic nerve without any symptoms. In these subclinical cases, an electrical diagnostic test called visual EVOKED POTENTIALS will be able to reveal lesions along the optic pathways. For this reason, visual evoked potentials are often used as part of the diagnostic workup for MS, since a positive finding can provide evidence of a second demyelinating event even without symptoms.

Although optic neuritis is often the first sign of MS, not everyone who has an episode of optic neuritis develops MS. The 10-year risk of developing clinically definite MS after a single episode of optic neuritis was 38 percent, according to one recent study; the 12-year risk was 40 percent. Most of those patients who developed MS did so within the first five years after the initial episode of optic neuritis. The presence of brain lesions revealed by magnetic resonance imaging (MRI) when the optic neuritis was first noticed was the strongest predictor of MS. Within the study group, people with at least one brain lesion on MRI at the time of the optic neuritis episode had a 56 percent risk of developing MS within 10 years, while those with no brain lesions had only a 22 percent risk of developing MS within 10 years.

See also VISUAL PROBLEMS.

orthotics   A support for weak or ineffective joints, such as lightweight inserts that are worn inside shoes to increase stability and decrease FATIGUE. Often prescribed for patients with multiple sclerosis (MS), orthotics can help with SPASTICITY in the foot and can help brace the foot if the patient is experiencing FOOT DROP (a condition in which the toe of the shoe scrapes the ground during walking). Certain types of orthotics also help support the ankle, thus stabilizing the entire leg.

Although a wide range of positioning aids, braces, splints, and ambulatory aids are available in drugstores and orthopedic catalogs, health experts believe it can be dangerous for patients to self-prescribe orthotics. The wide variety of styles, sizes, and types of orthotics makes selecting the best type and fit for the individual especially difficult. An incorrectly fitted orthotic may cause blisters or pain, cut off circulation, or even cause the patient to trip. Instead, a PHYSICAL THERAPIST should fit people for orthotics.

Some people adjust well to orthotics, while others find they cause additional problems. Orthotics can add ounces to the weight of the leg, and they can be hot in the summer. They can also require a lot of energy to put on and take off each day. Patients with MS who already struggle with pain or swelling in their feet or legs and who have trouble tolerating shoes or socks may find orthotics to be particularly uncomfortable.

See also ORTHOTIST.

orthotist   A person skilled in making mechanical appliances (ORTHOTICS) such as braces or splints that help to support functioning of the leg.

oscillopsia   Continuous, involuntary, and chaotic eye movements that result in a visual disturbance in which objects appear to be jumping or bouncing. Oscillopsia is a symptom of multiple sclerosis.

See also NYSTAGMUS; OPTIC NEURITIS; VISUAL PROBLEMS.

Osmond, Alan (1949–   )   Eldest performer of the singing group the Osmond Brothers, who was diagnosed with primary progressive multiple sclerosis (MS) in 1986. This form of the illness differs from the more common relapsing-remitting MS in that it does not typically get better for substantial periods of time but instead worsens steadily.

The husband of Suzanne and the father of eight sons, Osmond first noticed a problem when his fingers could not move on his trumpet as fast as they normally could. This was following by gait problems and FOOT DROP. Once he was properly diagnosed, Osmond tried to keep the illness a secret because he was embarrassed and worried his fans would be uncomfortable seeing him perform. However, when he learned that a tabloid was going to reveal his secret, he consulted former child actor ANNETTE FUNICELLO, who also suffers from MS. She encouraged him to tell his own story.

Still performing with family, Osmond has enlisted in a clinical trial to determine the effectiveness of glatiramer acetate as a potential medication for MS patients.

See also FAMOUS PEOPLE WITH MS.

osteoporosis   A condition in which the bones begin to thin. Although this problem commonly occurs in older women, there is a higher incidence in people with multiple sclerosis due to inactivity and use of steroids.

other diseases vs. MS   Many diseases share symptoms with multiple sclerosis (MS). Many of them can appear before any brain lesions become visible on a MAGNETIC RESONANCE IMAGING (MRI) scan. MS is a disease that may affect any area of the nervous system, thus causing a wide variety of symptoms such as visual problems, weakness, or numbness.

The most common diagnoses that share symptoms with MS include autoimmune problems such as lupus, inflammatory diseases, and fibromyalgia; infections such as LYME DISEASE; thyroid abnormalities; vitamin deficiencies (specifically B_{12} and folate); and chronic fatigue syndrome. Many other diseases overlap symptoms with MS.

Blood tests can rule out many of the diseases that mimic MS. Sometimes people with MS are initially diagnosed with one or more other diagnoses, only to have the initial diagnosis dropped after they clearly developed MS. Because early intervention is vital in effective treatments for MS, correctly diagnosing the cause of any neurological symptoms is important.

Autoimmune Diseases vs. MS

There are a number of other autoimmune diseases than can be confused with MS, as discussed below.

Acute disseminated encephalomyelitis (ADEM) This demyelinating neurological disease causes brain and spinal cord inflammation. Symptoms may include headache, seizure, stiff neck, ataxia, optic neuritis, vomiting, weight loss, lethargy, delirium, or paralysis of an arm, leg, or one side of the body.

ADEM differs from MS in that it is often triggered by an immunization or a viral infection (such as measles) and because there is only one episode of this disease.

Systemic lupus erythematosus (SLE) This chronic inflammatory disease affects the skin, joints, blood, and kidneys, causing swollen joints, extreme fatigue, anemia, skin rash, sensitivity to

sunlight, hair loss, seizure, and Raynaud's phenomenon (fingers that turn white or blue in the cold).

An antinuclear antibody (ANA) test can help confirm lupus, but there are many false positives and false negatives. MS can also trigger a positive ANA result, and lupus does not always produce positive ANA results. A urinalysis or kidney biopsy may be performed to check for kidney problems. Other tests that may differentiate between MS and SLE may include MRI, computerized axial tomography scan, echocardiography, or X-rays. Sometimes MS lesions on the spinal cord can be a distinguishing factor. First-trimester miscarriages are quite common in women with lupus but are not typical of women with MS.

Sjögren's syndrome This chronic disease is caused by white blood cells that attack the moisture-producing glands, affecting the entire body. Symptoms include dry eyes and mouth, difficulty swallowing and speaking, fatigue, joint pain, decreased sensation, and numbness. Just like MS, Sjögren's can plateau, worsen, improve, and vary in severity from mild to severe.

Nerve conduction velocity tests can help differentiate MS and Sjögren's because nerve damage is central in MS and peripheral in Sjögren's. However, diagnosis may be complicated by the fact that sometimes Sjögren's can also affect the central nervous system, causing cognitive impairment and spinal cord involvement.

Some researchers believe that Sjögren's syndrome is linked to MS, but this is controversial.

Myasthenia gravis (MG) This disease is characterized by weakness that occurs when the nerve impulse responsible for triggering movement fails to reach the muscle cells. Individuals with MG have an increased risk of developing other autoimmune diseases.

MG symptoms tend to fluctuate throughout the day, often worsening at night. They include droopy eyelids, facial weakness, impaired eye coordination, and weak limbs, neck, shoulders, hips, and trunk muscles. Muscle fatigue is common and can be aggravated by heat, overexertion, or increased stress. Young women and older men are most commonly affected, although MG can occur at any age. Unlike patients with MS, those with MG experience no loss of or change in sensation. They do not normally experience generalized fatigue—just localized fatigue in overtired muscles.

A blood test for antibodies to acetylcholine receptors is a very specific test for MG; 80 percent of all patients with MG will have abnormally high blood levels of these antibodies.

Sarcoidosis This condition typically appears between the ages of 20 and 40, appearing briefly and healing naturally. However, between 20 and 30 percent of sarcoidosis patients experience some permanent lung damage. In 10–15 percent of the patients, the disease can become chronic. Symptoms include dry mouth, excessive thirst and fatigue, skin rash, vision abnormalities, chronic arthritis, shortness of breath, enlarged lymph glands, cough, and fever. A chest X-ray is one of the most helpful diagnostic tools.

Infectious Diseases vs. MS

Lyme disease (LD) This infection is caused by *Borrelia burgdorferi,* a bacterium carried by deer ticks. If left untreated, the bacteria travel through the bloodstream, causing severe fatigue; a stiff, aching neck; tingling or numbness in the extremities; and facial palsy. The primary symptom is usually a bright red rash (sometimes with a white center, called a bull's-eye rash) that radiates from the tick bite. Diagnosis should be made primarily on the basis of symptoms and evidence of a tick bite, not just blood tests, since the blood tests can often give false negative results if performed in the first month after infection. Those who live or work in residential areas surrounded by tick-infested woods; who hike, camp, fish, or hunt; or who live in endemic areas are at increased risk for this disease.

Human T cell lymphotrophic virus-1 (HTLV-1) This infection is associated with progressive spinal cord dysfunction, causing spasticity, partial paralysis of the lower limbs, bladder and bowel incontinence, and impotence. HTLV-1 can be ruled out with a type of elevated antibody test.

HTLV-1 affects the spinal cord and mimics primary progressive MS. However, because HTLV-1 primarily occurs in the Caribbean, travel to endemic areas is an important risk factor. Besides the Caribbean, other high-risk areas for HTLV-1 include southern Japan and, less commonly, the Pacific coast of South America, equatorial Africa,

and the southern United States. HTLV-1 is also common among intravenous drug users.

Neurosyphilis The advanced form of syphilis can cause visual problems, cognitive changes, and sensory or motor tract dysfunction. However, testing for the production of antibodies can eliminate syphilis and neurosyphilis from the list of possible diagnoses. Neurosyphilis is not as common as it was in the past because syphilis (the precursor to neurosyphilis) is so easily treatable.

Vascular Diseases vs. MS

Stroke This interruption of blood to the brain can be caused by bleeding in the brain or by blood clots that cut off the blood supply to an area of the brain. Stroke can produce symptoms that mimic MS. These symptoms include sudden trouble with vision in one or both eyes, sudden trouble walking, dizziness, loss of coordination, sudden severe headache, confusion, trouble speaking or understanding, sudden nausea, fever, vomiting, or loss of consciousness. When a stroke occurs, neurons die; a major stroke leads to sudden loss of function that is not usually confused with MS. However, smaller strokes (called transient ischemic attacks or TIAs) can produce changes or loss in function that can be similar to an MS flare. Many people with MS have first been misdiagnosed with these small strokes.

Central nervous system angitis This inflammation of the blood vessels of the brain can produce headache, confusion, and other neurologic deficits that slowly worsen.

Dural arteriovenous fistulas These abnormal structures of blood vessels along the spinal cord can deprive the spinal cord of blood, causing weakness, bladder and bowel changes, and sensory symptoms, all of which can wax and wane much like MS. An MRI of the spinal cord, or spinal angiography, may be needed to confirm a diagnosis.

Binswanger's disease This cerebrovascular disease usually appears in older patients with high blood pressure. Demyelination of the white matter surrounding the brain, similar to white matter lesions seen in MS, can appear with this disease.

Additional Diseases vs. MS

Fibromyalgia This nonspecific condition involves pain and fatigue of the muscles, ligaments, and tendons, including shooting or throbbing muscular pain. Other common symptoms include burning, stiffness, fatigue, face and head pain, cognitive impairment, numbness, tingling, dizziness, and coordination problems. Changes in weather, hormonal fluctuations, stress, or depression can all contribute to flares. Although fibromyalgia does mimic MS, it will not show up on an MRI.

Vitamin B_{12} deficiency   This condition may cause demyelination, numbness, and tingling of the hands and feet; fatigue; weakness; and in extreme cases, change in mental status. Although some people believe that vitamin B_{12} can produce more myelin, vitamin B_{12} is helpful to patients only if they have low levels to start with.

Other   Many other diseases are occasionally confused with MS, including muscular dystrophy, amyotrophic lateral sclerosis Lou Gehrig's disease), migraine, hypothyroidism, high blood pressure, Behçet's disease, Arnold-Chiari deformity, and mitochondrial disorders.

oxygen therapy   See HYPERBARIC OXYGEN TREATMENT.

Paced Auditory Serial Addition Test (PASAT) A measure of cognitive function that assesses auditory information processing speed and flexibility, as well as calculation ability. Single digits are presented every three seconds, and the patient must add each new digit to the one immediately prior to it. The score is the total number correct out of 60 possible answers. The PASAT is a sensitive test of some specific cognitive functions frequently affected in multiple sclerosis. However, it is not intended to be a general measure of overall cognitive dysfunction. It is probably most useful for assessing mild to moderate dysfunction, but less useful when cognitive deficits are severe.

paclitaxel (Taxol) A substance derived from the Pacific yew tree that is the active ingredient in Taxol, a leading ovarian and breast cancer drug. Paclitaxel may also act as an immunosuppressant, preventing white blood cells from damaging MYELIN (the protective covering of nerves). A small, preliminary study suggested that paclitaxel may have some benefits in people with advanced multiple sclerosis (MS). It is used in lower doses for people with MS than for cancer patients, so side effects—such as hair loss or nausea—do not occur or are not as severe. Further research is ongoing.

pain Although most people think that multiple sclerosis (MS) is characterized by SPASTICITY and WEAKNESS but not pain, several types of painful symptoms are in fact common to this condition. In a national survey of more than 7,000 patients with MS, 70 percent of them reported experiencing some kind of pain, and at least half were in pain at the time of the survey. Furthermore, the National Multiple Sclerosis Society reports that

almost half of all people with MS are troubled by chronic pain. Age at onset, length of time with MS, or degree of disability does not appear to have any link to whether a person will have pain, although twice as many women as men experience the problem.

MS pain is different from the type of discomfort generally experienced with headache, a joint injury, or muscle strain. MS pain is often more diffuse, affecting several areas of the body. It also changes over time, waxing and waning for no apparent reason. Patients often have trouble describing the pain, which can be dull or burning or simply feel like pressure.

However the pain may be experienced, it is actually generated by the nervous system as a type of phantom pain. A healthy person's nervous system acts as a defense system, transmitting pain signals as a warning when something harmful happens to the body. However, MS patients have overactive nerves that send pain signals for no good reason.

Some of the most common types of pain experienced by patients with MS include sudden (acute) pain, TRIGEMINAL NEURALGIA, LHERMITTE'S SIGN, or girdling pain.

Acute Pain

Some MS pain is brief, quick, and intense but then goes away suddenly. Patients may describe this type of acute pain as burning, tingling, shooting, or stabbing.

Trigeminal Neuralgia (Tic Douloureux)

This stabbing facial pain can be triggered by almost any facial movement, such as chewing, yawning, sneezing, or by touch, chewing, or even brushing the teeth. It may appear as the first symptom of

MS. Typically patients confuse it with dental pain. It can usually be treated successfully with medications such as carbamazepine (Tegretol) or phenytoin (Dilantin).

Lhermitte's Sign

This pain is felt as a brief, stabbing, electric-shock-like sensation that runs from the back of the head down the spine and is brought on by bending the neck forward. Medications such as anticonvulsants may be used to prevent the pain, or a soft collar may be used to limit neck flexion.

Dysesthesia

Some patients report a burning, aching, or girdling around the body, which is a type of pain doctors call DYSESTHESIA. These pains are often treated with the anticonvulsant medication gabapentin (Neurontin). Dysesthesias may also be treated with an antidepressant such as AMITRIPTYLINE (Elavil), which modifies how the central nervous system reacts to pain. Other treatments include wearing a pressure stocking or glove, which can convert the sensation of pain to one of pressure; warm compresses to the skin, which may convert the sensation of pain to one of warmth; and over-the-counter acetaminophen, which may be taken daily, under a physician's supervision.

Chronic Pain

Some types of pain related to MS are chronic, lasting for more than a month. This includes pain from spasticity that can cause muscle cramps or spasms (called FLEXOR SPASMS), tight and aching joints, and back or musculoskeletal pain. Pressure on the body caused by immobility, the incorrect use of mobility aids, or the struggle to compensate for gait and balance problems may all contribute to these types of pain.

An evaluation to pinpoint the source of the pain is essential. These types of chronic pain can often be relieved by medication with baclofen or tizanidine (Zanaflex), ibuprofen or other prescription anti-inflammatory drugs, massage, physical therapy, and heat.

Treatment Options and Outlook

Generally, acute MS pain cannot be effectively treated with aspirin, ibuprofen, or other common nonprescription pain relievers. This is because most MS pain originates in the central nervous system, making it much more difficult to control than joint or muscle pain. Instead, an anticonvulsant medication such as Neurontin or Tegretol may be effective, although doctors are not quite sure how these drugs work. More than six of these anticonvulsants are available. All of them work a bit differently and cause different side effects.

Although these medications work for most people, they can cause FATIGUE, which is already a problem for many patients with MS. Other side effects can include low blood pressure, seizures, dry mouth, and weight gain. Doctors choose an anticonvulsant based on how the patient will be able to tolerate the side effects of that drug. They first prescribe the lowest possible dose, increasing it until the person feels comfortable or until side effects become intolerable. If one medication does not work, doctors will try another.

Unfortunately, some patients find no relief with any anticonvulsant. One to 2 percent of patients have extremely stubborn pain that does not respond to treatment. For these patients, Botox—best known as the antiwrinkle injections that temporarily paralyze a nerve or muscle—has been used for years by some doctors to manage spasticity and bladder problems. It also appears to improve pain. The drug can be injected only into a limited area. This means that even if it is effective, it will not replace the current MS pain medications and is typically effective only for conditions such as trigeminal neuralgia.

Treatment may also include a variety of self-help strategies, such as regular stretching exercises and balancing water intake with sodium and potassium to prevent muscle cramps. In addition, people who remain active and maintain positive attitudes are often able to reduce the impact of pain on their quality of life.

Because pain is a complex problem that may be aggravated by fear and worry, a patient may require treatment at a multidisciplinary pain clinic, where medication may be used in combination with alternative therapies such as biofeedback, hypnosis, yoga, meditation, or acupuncture.

paraparesis A weakness but not total paralysis of the legs, which often occurs in people with multiple sclerosis.

paraplegia   Paralysis of both legs, which can occur in people with multiple sclerosis.

paresis   Partial or incomplete paralysis of a part of the body, a symptom that can occur in patients with multiple sclerosis.

paresthesias   Spontaneously occurring sensations of burning, prickling, tingling, or creeping on the skin that may or may not be associated with any physical findings on neurological examination. Paresthesias are a symptom of multiple sclerosis.

See also PAIN; PINS AND NEEDLES; SYMPTOMS OF MS.

parietal lobes   One of four major pairs of lobes of the CEREBRAL CORTEX located at the upper middle part of the head above the temporal lobes. The parietal lobes include the sensory cortex and the association areas of the brain, which analyze and interpret sensory impulses and function in reasoning, judgment, emotions, verbalizing ideas, and storing memory involved in processing information about body sensation, touch, and spatial organization. The association areas in the parietal lobes are also involved in secondary language and visual processing. Lesions in association areas in the parietal lobes can cause difficulties in learning tasks that require an understanding of spatial perception and the body's position in space.

paroxysmal spasm   A sudden, uncontrolled limb contraction that occurs intermittently, lasts for a few moments, and then subsides.

See also SPASTICITY.

paroxysmal symptom   Any one of several symptoms, as of multiple sclerosis, that appear suddenly (apparently in response to some kind of movement or sensory stimulation), last for a few moments, and then subside. Paroxysmal symptoms tend to occur often in certain individuals and follow a similar pattern from one episode to the next. Examples include acute episodes of TRIGEMINAL NEURALGIA (sharp facial PAIN), tonic seizures (intense spasm of limb or limbs on one side of the body), DYSARTHRIA (slurred speech often accompa-

nied by loss of balance and coordination), and various PARESTHESIAS (sensory disturbances ranging from tingling to severe pain).

See also SPASTICITY.

pars planitis   An uncommon inflammatory condition of the eye that usually has no detectable cause but is occasionally linked to multiple sclerosis, LYME DISEASE, or syphilis.

Symptoms and Diagnostic Path
Pars planitis affects both eyes in 80 percent of cases, causing floaters or blurry vision but no redness or pain. An examination by an eye doctor will reveal inflammation in the fluid that fills the back part of the eye (the vitreous gel). This inflammation can lead to the development of cataracts or swelling of the central retina, both of which cause the blurring of vision.

Treatment Options and Outlook
If a medical workup reveals a cause of the inflammation, the eye will usually respond to the specific treatment of that condition. However, since most cases of pars planitis do not have a detectable cause, the most common method of treating this condition injecting corticosteroids into the white part of the eye. Corticosteroid eyedrops have not been successful.

If corticosteroid injections cannot control the inflammation, then other immunosuppressive drugs such as cyclosporine, AZATHIOPRINE, METHOTREXATE, and CYCLOPHOSPHAMIDE can be used (although careful monitoring of their effectiveness and potential side effects is crucial).

See also VISUAL PROBLEMS.

pemoline   An amphetamine medication used to combat FATIGUE in people with multiple sclerosis. Pemoline is not addictive, although occasionally there have been reports of liver damage with this drug. It works by releasing brain chemicals such as dopamine and noradrenaline that facilitate communication between neurons.

Researchers have found pemoline to be about as effective as AMANTADINE.

perception   The process through which sensory information (hearing, sight, touch, movement, taste, and smell) is recognized and interpreted. Perception involves both the intake of information through the senses and the processing and making sense of information via cognition. Although sensory experience itself is largely automatic for humans, perception also involves learned behavior and intellectual capacity.

percutaneous rhizotomy An outpatient surgical procedure used to treat severe, intractable TRIGEMINAL NEURALGIA, which may be a symptom of multiple sclerosis.

In this treatment method, the surgeon makes a tiny incision in the side of the person's face and blocks the function of the trigeminal nerve using laser surgery, cryosurgery (freezing), or cauterization. Although this procedure blocks the pain, it also produces facial NUMBNESS in many patients. For this reason, physicians use this method only as a last resort.

See also TREATMENT OF MS.

peripheral neuropathy Damage to the nerves of the peripheral nervous system that can be caused by a number of diseases, such as diabetes, but not multiple sclerosis. Damage can occur either to motor nerves (causing muscle weakness) or to sensory nerves (causing pain or numbness). This condition can develop quickly with intense symptoms or slowly over a long period of time.

The first signs of peripheral neuropathy are often problems in climbing stairs, continual numbness, or PINS AND NEEDLES. In severe cases there may be paralysis.

periventricular The area around the ventricles in the brain; multiple sclerosis lesions are often found in this area.

personal care See ACTIVITIES OF DAILY LIVING.

personal care homes See BOARD-AND-CARE HOMES.

PET scan (positron emission tomography) A type of BRAIN SCAN technique that allows scientists to visualize the activity and interactions of particular brain regions as they are used during cognitive operations such as memorizing, recalling, speaking, reading, learning, and other sorts of information processing.

A PET scan combines computerized axial tomography (CT SCAN) and nuclear scanning as a way of peeking into the living brain to help measure early changes in brain function or structure in people with nervous system disorders such as multiple sclerosis.

During a PET scan, a radioactive substance called a tracer is combined with a chemical (such as glucose) and injected into a vein. The tracer emits tiny positively charged particles (positrons) that produce signals. The chemical substance and radioactive tracer chosen for the test vary according to which area of the body is being studied.

A camera records the tracer's signals as it travels through the body and collects in organs. A computer then converts the signals into three-dimensional images of the examined organ. The three-dimensional views can be produced from any angle and provide a clear view of an abnormality. As compared with CT scans and MAGNETIC RESONANCE IMAGING (MRI), PET scans produce less-detailed pictures of an organ.

A PET scan is done in a hospital's nuclear medicine department or at a special PET center by a radiologist or nuclear medicine specialist and a nuclear medicine technologist. The patient may be given earplugs and a blindfold to wear to reduce external distractions. After that, he or she lies on a flat table connected to a large scanner, a camera, and a computer. A baseline scan may be done first, which takes about 30 minutes. The person may be asked to read, perform letter recognition activities, or recite a familiar quotation or passage, depending on whether speech, reasoning, or memory is being tested. People may also be asked to perform deep-breathing exercises to help reduce anxiety.

The PET scanner, which is shaped like a giant doughnut, rotates around the individual. It detects the radioactive patterns and transforms them into three-dimensional tomographic images on a computer screen. The scans are done over a period of time to provide repeated sequences of three-dimensional images. Holding completely still while each scan is being done is very important; otherwise, repeat scans may be needed. It is also important to avoid other conditions that can interfere with PET scan results. These conditions include recent use (within 24 hours) of caffeine, tobacco, or alcohol; high levels of anxiety; sedatives; and medications that affect metabolism, such as insulin.

During the test, individuals are usually alone in the scanner room. However, the technologist will be observing the procedure through a window, and the person can communicate via an intercom. The entire procedure takes between one to three hours. After the test, patients should drink lots of liquids and urinate frequently for the next 24 hours to help flush the tracer.

Patients may feel nothing at all from the needle puncture when the tracer is injected, or they may feel a brief sting or pinch. The scanning procedure itself is painless. Some patients may feel claustrophobic inside the scanner or may be uncomfortable lying still for an extended period of time during the scans.

The radiologist may discuss preliminary results of the PET scans with the patient right after the test. Complete results are usually available in one to two days.

Risks

There is always a slight risk of damage to cells or tissue from being exposed to any radiation, including the low level of radiation released by the radioactive tracer used for a PET scan. However, the risk of damage from the tracer is usually very low compared with the potential benefits of the test. PET scans are not recommended during pregnancy, however, because the radiation could damage a developing fetus. A woman who is breast-feeding should talk to her health professional about possibly stopping breast-feeding temporarily after undergoing a PET scan, because radiation from the radioactive tracer may be passed to an infant through breast milk.

Most of the tracer used in a PET scan will be eliminated from the patient's body within six to 24 hours. Allergic reactions to the tracer occur very rarely. Occasionally, some soreness or swelling may develop at the site where the radioactive tracer was injected. These symptoms can usually be relieved by applying moist, warm compresses to the patient's arm.

A PET scan is an expensive procedure and is not yet widely available.

physiatrist   A physician who specializes in the rehabilitation of physical impairments.

physical activity   Getting sufficient EXERCISE is important to people with multiple sclerosis (MS) because it enhances fitness levels and quality of life. A lack of physical activity may contribute to constipation in less mobile people and also exacerbate existing weakness due to spasticity and fatigue. However, physical activity should be monitored and regulated to avoid becoming overheated, which increases core body temperature and MS-related fatigue. A PHYSICAL THERAPIST should be part of the health care team who can plan a program suited to the needs of the individual.

See also PHYSICAL THERAPY.

physical therapist   A health care professional whose goal is to evaluate and improve a patient's movement and function, with a particular emphasis on assessing muscle strength, flexibility, coordination, balance, endurance, walking ability, and mobility. As part of the rehabilitative process, physical therapy helps people meet the mobility and functional challenges in their family, work, and social lives while accommodating the physical changes brought about by multiple sclerosis.

Physical therapists specialize in ongoing evaluation and treatments to optimize range of motion; improving function and providing instruction on managing physical disabilities; and recommending appropriate exercises to maintain flexibility while preventing and reducing pain. They can also provide instruction about ASSISTIVE DEVICES, braces, or other mobility aids.

See also OCCUPATIONAL THERAPY; OCCUPATIONAL THERAPIST; PHYSICAL THERAPY.

physical therapy   Treatment designed to restore a patient's movement and function, with a particular emphasis on muscle strength, flexibility, coordination, balance, endurance, walking ability, and mobility.

Physical therapy cannot cure the primary symptoms of multiple sclerosis (MS) such as WEAKNESS, tremor, tingling, NUMBNESS, BALANCE PROBLEMS, VISUAL PROBLEMS, paralysis, BLADDER

DYSFUNCTION, or BOWEL DYSFUNCTION. However, therapy can help people compensate for the changes brought about by MS. These compensatory treatments include learning about new movement techniques, strategies, and equipment. Physical therapy can also help lessen or stop secondary MS symptoms by strengthening and loosening muscles. It can help prevent complications such as frozen joints, contractures (muscles that will not stretch out), or BEDSORES. Physical therapists can prescribe stretching and range of motion exercises, and they can suggest exercises to develop trunk control and upper arm muscles. They can provide help in obtaining appropriate assistive equipment, including ambulatory aids, braces, and WHEELCHAIRS. They also train people in walking and using assistive devices. Physical therapists also teach "transfer training"—that is, how to get from one spot to another, such as from a bed to a wheelchair or from a wheelchair to a car. In addition, physical therapists can provide training in how to fall safely in order to cause the least possible damage.

Physical therapy is usually prescribed and tailored to the individual with MS by a NEUROLOGIST or PHYSIATRIST (a physician who specializes in rehabilitation medicine).

Many hospitals offer outpatient physical therapy services, but people may need a doctor's referral to see a physical therapist. The need for physical therapy intervention varies, depending on the level of disability and the course of the disease. Physical therapy can often be completed in one to three office visits. Most physical therapy programs last a few months with the assumption that follow-up exercise programs will be continued at home. The first appointment includes an evaluation and recommendations for exercises. The following appointments check a person's progress and review and expand a home program.

A physical therapist makes recommendations for physical therapy not just to be performed at home but also at an outpatient facility or at a nursing or rehabilitation facility. Many physical therapists can also perform a functional capacity evaluation to provide more information for disability claims based on physical performance. This functional capacity evaluation can be useful if the Department of Social Security denies disability to a person who is unable to work an eight-hour day.

pins and needles Transitory prickly sensations (called PARESTHESIAS) that are one of the primary symptoms of multiple sclerosis. These sensations are caused by the areas of damage on the MYELIN (the protective covering of the nerves in the central nervous system).

See also DEMYELINATION; PAIN.

plantar reflex A reflex response obtained by drawing a pointed object along the outer border of the sole of the foot from the heel to the little toe. The normal flexor response is a bunching and downward movement of the toes. An upward movement of the big toe is called an extensor response (or BABINSKI REFLEX), which may indicate disease in the BRAIN or spinal cord (such as multiple sclerosis).

plaque An area of inflamed or demyelinated central nervous system tissue. Plaques on nerves may be an indication of multiple sclerosis.

plasmapheresis A procedure in which whole blood is removed from the body so that blood cells can be separated from plasma (the liquid portion of blood) and mixed with replacement plasma. The blood, with all its red and white blood cells, is transfused back into the patient.

This process is a successful method for treating autoimmune diseases such as myasthenia gravis and GUILLAIN-BARRE SYNDROME, because it removes the circulating antibodies that are thought to be responsible for these diseases. It is not clear whether plasmapheresis is of benefit in the short- or long-term treatment of multiple sclerosis (MS), and its use in MS remains controversial. Because MS also may involve an autoimmune process (where the body is attacked by its own immune system) and because demyelinating factors have been found in plasma from people with MS, plasmapheresis has been tried as a treatment for MS.

Mixed Results in Progressive Forms of MS
Studies using plasmapheresis in people with PRIMARY PROGRESSIVE MS and SECONDARY PROGRESSIVE

MS have yielded mixed results. One carefully controlled study among MS people who were also receiving medication that suppresses the immune system suggests that people who received both plasmapheresis and immunosuppressants did better than those receiving immunosuppressants alone.

The apparent advantage of plasmapheresis was most pronounced within the first five months of treatment. The study was placebo-controlled to make sure that responses to treatment were based on therapeutic benefit, rather than a psychological effect of receiving treatment. The study was also double-blind; neither the researchers nor the individual enrolled knew who was receiving active treatment until the study was over. Other studies by other investigators did not find plasmapheresis when combined with chemotherapy to be any more effective than chemotherapy alone.

Minimally Shortened Recovery Time from Exacerbations

A more recent clinical trial studied the effect of plasmapheresis in treating acute exacerbations. An exacerbation (also known as an attack, relapse, or flare) is a sudden worsening of an MS symptom, or the appearance of new symptoms, which lasts at least 24 hours and is separated from a previous exacerbation by at least one month. In this multi-center study, 116 people having an exacerbation received ACTH and immunosuppressant medication, and either plasmapheresis or "sham" plasmapheresis (in which the plasma withdrawn from the patient was returned, instead of being replaced). The results indicated a slightly shortened time to recovery in the plasmapheresis treated group compared to the control group. No long-term benefits were observed after a year.

Plasma Exchange

Plasma exchange might contribute to recovery from an acute attack in people with MS or other inflammatory demyelinating diseases who have not responded to standard steroid treatment, according to a recent study on plasma exchange. Researchers recommend that this treatment only be considered for individuals experiencing a severe, acute attack that is not responding to high-dose steroids. Since 90 percent of people experiencing acute attacks respond well to the standard steroid treatment, plasma exchange would be considered a treatment alternative only for the 10 percent or so who do not. For those 10 percent, however, plasma exchange may offer an important and beneficial treatment option.

Side Effects

Side effects of plasmapheresis therapy include occasional infection and blood clotting problems.

Poser criteria A tool for diagnosing multiple sclerosis (MS) that updated the SCHUMACHER CRITERIA in recognition of the diagnostic benefits of laboratory data. The revised criteria have not changed the fact that MS is still essentially a clinical diagnosis and they have been replaced by even newer criteria that acknowledge the importance of MAGNETIC RESONANCE IMAGING (MRI).

The Poser criteria are as follows:

For clinically definite MS:

- two attacks and clinical evidence of two separate lesions
- two attacks, clinical evidence of one and paraclinical evidence of another separate lesion

For laboratory-supported definite MS:

- two attacks, either clinical or paraclinical evidence of one lesion and cerebrospinal fluid (CSF) immunological abnormalities
- one attack, clinical evidence of two separate lesions and CSF abnormalities
- one attack, clinical evidence of one and paraclinical evidence of another separate lesion, and CSF abnormalities

For clinically probable MS:

- two attacks and clinical evidence of one lesion
- one attack and clinical evidence of two separate lesions
- one attack, clinical evidence of one lesion, and paraclinical evidence of another separate lesion

For laboratory-supported probable MS:

• two attacks and CSF abnormalities

position sense   The ability to tell, with the eyes closed, where one's fingers and toes are in space. Position sense is evaluated during the standard NEUROLOGICAL EXAMINATION to check for multiple sclerosis (MS). Typically the patient is asked to touch his or her finger to the nose with eyes closed. The inability of the patient to complete this task successfully is one indicator of possible MS.

post-partum period   While the incidence of multiple sclerosis (MS) flares is lower during pregnancy, there is an increased risk of an MS exacerbation in the first three months after delivery.

See also PREGNANCY AND MS.

postural tremor   A type of tremor that occurs when an arm, leg, or the whole body is being supported against gravity. For example, a person who has a postural tremor will shake while sitting or standing but not while lying down. These tremors occur in patients with multiple sclerosis because areas along the complex nerve pathways that are responsible for movement coordination are damaged. It remains one of the most difficult symptoms to manage and is associated with a poor outcome in rehabilitation.

postvoid residual test   A simple, effective technique to diagnose BLADDER DYSFUNCTION. When used in people with multiple sclerosis, a catheter is passed into the bladder after urination in order to drain and measure urine left in the bladder. A bladder scan provides the same result.

power grading   A measurement of muscle strength used to evaluate weakness or paralysis as part of the standard NEUROLOGICAL EXAMINATION for multiple sclerosis.

pregnancy and MS   Pregnancy appears to have a relatively protective effect on women with multiple sclerosis (MS). The number of MS flares decreases during pregnancy, especially in the second and third trimesters. In general, pregnancy does not appear to affect the long-term clinical course of MS. Women who have MS and wish to have a family can usually do so successfully with the assistance of their neurologist and obstetrician.

Prior to 1950, most women with MS were advised to avoid pregnancy because of the belief that it might make their MS worse. Over the past 40 years, many studies have been done, in hundreds of women with MS, that have almost uniformly reached the opposite conclusion.

Exacerbation rates may rise in the first three to six months after the baby is born, and the risk of a relapse in the postpartum period is estimated to be between 20 and 40 percent. These relapses do not appear to contribute to increased long-term disability. In studies with long-term follow-up of women with MS who had children, no increased disability as a result of pregnancy was found.

Pregnancy may help protect against MS flares because of the increase in a number of circulating proteins and other factors that are natural immunosuppressants. Additionally, levels of natural corticosteroids are higher in pregnant than nonpregnant women.

Women who are taking any drugs for their MS (Avonex, Betaseron, Rebif, Copaxone or Novantrone) should talk with their prescribing physician about their plan to become pregnant. The drugs are not recommended during breast-feeding because it is not known if they are excreted in breast milk. Before she becomes pregnant, a woman should also review any other medications she is taking in order to identify those that are safe during pregnancy and breast-feeding. Studies have indicated a woman has no increased risk of MS relapse associated with breast-feeding. Women who use steroids for acute MS exacerbations may continue to use them during pregnancy, but the use of prednisone by a breast-feeding woman should be carefully monitored.

Women with MS usually need no special gynecologic care during pregnancy. Labor and delivery are usually the same as in other women. Moreover, general anesthesia and anesthesia injected directly into the epidural space of the spine seem to be well tolerated by women in labor.

Women who have trouble walking may find this gets worse during late pregnancy, as they become heavier and their center of gravity shifts. Increased use of assistive devices to walk or use of a wheelchair may be a good idea. In addition, bladder and bowel problems common to all pregnant women may be worse in women with MS who have preexisting urinary or bowel dysfunction. Women with MS may also be more subject to fatigue.

premotor cortex   A part of the brain found in the frontal lobe, closely associated with the motor cortex. The premotor cortex is responsible for identifying objects in space, choosing strategies of action, and programming movement. It also sends output fibers to those reticular neurons that influence the muscles of the back, hips, shoulders, and thighs. It appears to help regulate posture and stabilize the trunk and limbs during complex movements.

pressure sores   See BEDSORES.

primary-care needs   Although multiple sclerosis (MS) is not yet curable, caring for the general health and well-being of the person with MS will positively affect quality of life. People with MS have the same general medical needs, including routine examinations, as those who don't have MS. Routine examinations are best done by a primary-care physician who is aware of the role of MS in the individual's medical care and maintains a "big picture" of the medical needs of the person with MS. These general health issues are sometimes sidelined when MS is diagnosed in an individual. It is important that other health issues that may arise are not automatically deemed to be related to multiple sclerosis.

primary progressive MS   A type of multiple sclerosis (MS) in which symptoms that occur generally do not remit. A few people with MS—10 percent—are diagnosed with this form. The diagnosis usually needs to be made later, after the person has been living for a period of time with progressive disability but no acute attacks.

pro-Banthine   See PROPANTHELINE.

prognosis   The expected outcome of an illness. The expected outcome of multiple sclerosis (MS) varies a great deal from one patient to the next and in general is unpredictable. Although the disorder is chronic and incurable, life expectancy can be normal. A life span of 35 or more years after diagnosis is common.

The amount of disability and discomfort varies with the severity and frequency of attacks and the part of the central nervous system (CNS) affected by each attack. Commonly, there is initially a return to normal or near-normal function between attacks. As the disorder progresses, progressive loss of function with less improvement between attacks occurs.

Most people with MS continue to walk and function with minimal disability for 20 or more years. The factors that most experts believe best predict a relatively benign course are

- female gender
- young age at onset (less than 30 years)
- infrequent attacks
- long interval between the first and second attack
- RELAPSING-REMITTING MS pattern
- low burden of disease as revealed on brain scans
- symptoms predominantly related to the senses
- low disability at two to five years after diagnosis
- involvement of only one central nervous system area at onset
- complete recovery from the first attack

The factors that most experts believe best predict an aggressive course are

- male gender
- many relapses per year
- incomplete recovery from the first attack
- short interval between the first and second attack
- symptoms predominantly of motor tract involvement
- older age of onset
- significant disability two to five years from the acute onset

- early cerebellar involvement
- involvement of more than one area of the CNS at the time of onset

progressive-relapsing MS   This quite rare type of multiple sclerosis (MS) follows a progressive course from the outset, with obvious, acute attacks along the way. It occurs in only 5 percent of people with MS. Researchers are currently trying to identify more precise indicators of the prognosis or predicted disease activity.

progressive supranuclear palsy (PSP)   A rare BRAIN disorder that causes serious and permanent problems with gait and balance and that may be confused with multiple sclerosis (MS). The most obvious sign of the disease is an inability to aim the eyes properly, caused by lesions in the area of the brain that coordinates eye movement. In fact, all of the symptoms of PSP are caused by a gradual deterioration of brain cells in a few tiny but important places in the brain stem.

Symptoms and Diagnostic Path

PSP is a progressive disease but is not itself life threatening, although patients can have serious problems as a result of SWALLOWING PROBLEMS. The most common complications are choking, pneumonia, and fractures from falls. PSP patients also exhibit changes in mood and behavior, including DEPRESSION and apathy.

PSP is often misdiagnosed because some of its symptoms are so much like those of MS as well as those of Parkinson's disease and Alzheimer's disease. The key to establishing a diagnosis is to identify early gait instability and problems moving the eyes and to rule out other similar disorders.

Treatment Options and Outlook

No effective treatment is available, although scientists are searching for better ways to manage the disease. In some patients, the slowness, stiffness, and balance problems may respond to anti-Parkinsonian drugs such as levodopa. However, the effect is usually temporary. The speech, vision, and swallowing problems usually do not respond to any drug treatment.

Physical therapy has not been proven to help, but certain exercises can help keep the joints limber. A gastrostomy procedure may be required to improve swallowing problems. In this procedure, a tube is surgically placed through the skin of the abdomen and into the intestine so that the patient does not have to eat by mouth.

propanolol (Inderal)   A beta-blocker medication that has been used in the management of tremor in people with MULTIPLE SCLEROSIS.

propantheline (Pro-Banthine)   One of a group of antispasmodic drugs used to relieve cramps in the stomach, intestines and bladder. In people with multiple sclerosis, it is used to treat NEUROGENIC BLADDER symptoms to control urination.

proteolipid protein (PLP)   The most abundant protein in MYELIN in the central nervous system.

Provigil   See MODAFINIL.

Pryor, Richard (1940–)   Grammy Award–winning comedian and actor known for his frequent use of colorful language and characterizations of the dark side of the African-American experience. Pryor was diagnosed in 1986 with multiple sclerosis (MS).

Born in Peoria, Illinois, he endured a difficult childhood (his grandparents ran both a brothel and a pool hall). As a young boy, Pryor was cast in a production of *Rumpelstiltskin* at a local public recreational facility. Impressed by his talents, the boy's supervisor continued to arrange showcases just for the young Pryor.

Eventually Pryor dropped out of high school, joined the army, and performed in amateur shows while enlisted. After being discharged, he returned home and worked as a professional comic in clubs in his hometown and other cities. Inspired by comedian Bill Cosby, Pryor found club work in New York. By 1966, Pryor began appearing on summer television shows such as Rudy Vallee's *On Broadway Tonight* and the *Kraft Summer Music Hall*.

Pryor has also appeared in 40 films. These include *Uptown Saturday Night; Bingo Long and the*

Traveling All Stars; Silver Streak; Stir Crazy; See No Evil, Hear No Evil; and *Another You.*

Pryor has led a sometimes difficult life, with five ex-wives and four children, including daughter actress Rain Pryor. He has suffered two heart attacks and undergone quadruple bypass surgery. In 1980, he was rushed to the Sherman Oaks Hospital and Burn Center with accidental third-degree burns over 50 percent of his body. Since being diagnosed with MS in 1986, Pryor has been confined to a wheelchair. Despite his frailty, he returned to live performing in 1992 at the Comedy Store in West Hollywood. He has since appeared at venues around the country, still making jokes about himself and his afflictions. He made a guest appearance in 1995 on the TV show *Chicago Hope,* portraying a patient with MS. In 1999, Pryor won the inaugural Mark Twain Prize for American Humor.

pseudobulbar affect   Also called affective release. A small percentage of people with multiple sclerosis (MS) experience a more severe form of emotional instability in which there are uncontrollable episodes of laughing or crying that are unpredictable and seem to have little or no relationship to actual events or the individual's true feelings. These changes are thought to result from lesions in emotional pathways in the brain. It is important for family members and caregivers to realize that people with MS may not always be able to control their emotions. Medications such as amitriptyline (Elavil) and valproic acid (Depakote) are used to treat these emotional changes, and studies of other medications are currently under way.

pseudoexacerbation   A temporary aggravation of multiple sclerosis symptoms, resulting from something that stresses the body (such as fever, heat infection, severe FATIGUE, or CONSTIPATION), that disappears once the stress is removed. A pseudoexacerbation triggers a symptom flare-up rather than new disease activity or progression.

pyramidal tracts   Motor nerve pathways in the brain and spinal cord that connect nerve cells in the brain to the motor cells located in the cranial, thoracic, and lumbar parts of the spinal cord. Damage to these tracts, as in multiple sclerosis, causes spastic paralysis or weakness.

quad cane A cane that has a broad base on four short extensions, which provide extra stability. A low-profile quad cane is an adjustable device made of aluminum with a chrome-plated steel base. The four-legged quad cane comes with four legs capped with rubber ends and a padded handgrip. A deluxe lightweight quad cane has special legs that form a wider base than standard four-legged canes. A high-base quad cane has raised legs that concentrate the weight and provide a better center of gravity; however, some patients find this variety more difficult to transport.

Those who have trouble balancing on a cane, or whose legs are no longer strong enough to bear their weight, may find that a WALKER is a good alternative.

See also ASSISTIVE DEVICES; CANES; CRUTCHES; ROLLATOR; WHEELCHAIRS.

quadriplegia Paralysis of both legs and arms. While most individuals with multiple sclerosis do not experience this, some with a much more severe course eventually develop it on an ongoing basis.

race and MS Multiple sclerosis (MS) occurs most often in Caucasians of northern Europe and countries with Caucasians of northern European descent, although it can occur in all racial groups. However, MS is fairly uncommon among Caucasians in some areas of Australia, the southern United States, and South Africa.

MS is rare among Asians, Africans, Inuit, Native Americans, and Laplanders, suggesting that they are somehow genetically protected.

radon and MS Ecological studies in Norway show that there appears to be a significant link between rates of multiple sclerosis (MS) and the amount of radon in indoor air, south of 65 degrees N (Iceland). Based on these data, Norwegian scientists suggest that the amount of radon in inhaled air is a risk factor for MS. This hypothesis agrees with several of the known epidemiological characteristics of MS.

range-of-motion exercises Multidirectional movements held for various lengths of time, used in conjunction with stretching exercises. These special exercises are important in people with multiple sclerosis to maintain mobility and skin integrity.

Rebif See DISEASE-MODIFYING AGENTS; INTERFERON.

reflex The involuntary response of the nervous system to a stimulus. A reflex can be elicited by tapping a tendon with a reflex hammer, causing a muscle to contract. Increased, diminished, or absent reflexes can indicate neurologic damage such as that which occurs with multiple sclerosis.

Therefore, testing of reflexes is included as part of the standard NEUROLOGICAL EXAMINATION.

rehabilitation The restoration of functions essential to daily living in individuals who have lost these capacities through injury or illness, such as with multiple sclerosis (MS). Most rehabilitation programs are comprehensive and may include PHYSICAL THERAPY (PT), OCCUPATIONAL THERAPY, SPEECH THERAPY, and COGNITIVE RETRAINING.

Physical Therapy

Physical therapy is designed to help restore and maintain useful movement or function. Physical therapy may include

- stretching and range-of-motion exercises
- exercises to develop trunk control and upper arm muscles
- help in obtaining appropriate assistive equipment, including ambulatory aids, braces and wheelchairs, and so on
- training in walking and appropriate use of assistive devices, such as ambulatory aids, braces, and wheelchairs
- transfer training (how to get from one spot to another, such as from bed to wheelchair or from wheelchair to car)
- training in how to fall safely in order to cause the least possible damage
- patient and family education

PT is also designed to help prevent complications such as frozen joints, contractures (muscles that won't stretch out), or BEDSORES. PT is usually prescribed and tailored to the individual by a neurologist or a PHYSIATRIST (a physician who specializes in rehabilitation medicine).

The need for physical therapy intervention varies, depending on the level of disability, tolerance for activity, and the course of the disease. Most PT programs last only a few months, with the expectation that follow-up exercise programs will be continued at home. An effective home program should be focused on achieving and maintaining optimal function, with periodic follow-up sessions to revise the home program as symptoms change.

Occupational Therapy

Occupational therapy focuses on specific ACTIVITIES OF DAILY LIVING (ADL) that primarily involve the arms and hands. Examples of ADL include grooming, dressing, eating, writing by hand, and driving.

An occupational therapist can prescribe exercises designed to develop good motor coordination or compensate for tremor or weakness or suggest assistive devices, such as button hooks and other dressing aids. Occupational therapists also may evaluate wheelchairs, room arrangements, or other living or working conditions and recommend adjustments for a more efficient and safe environment.

Speech Therapy

Speech therapy is designed to help improve communication skills in people who have difficulty speaking because of weakness or uncoordinated face and tongue muscles. This is generally accomplished through exercises and the use of ASSISTIVE DEVICES. Speech therapists are also trained to evaluate SWALLOWING PROBLEMS (DYSPHAGIA).

Cognitive Retraining

Cognitive function is a relatively new area of rehabilitation. Some rehabilitation centers have developed innovative programs designed to help people compensate for loss of memory or slowed learning ability. Cognitive testing and retraining are most often performed by NEUROPSYCHOLOGISTS, SPEECH-LANGUAGE PATHOLOGISTS, and OCCUPATIONAL THERAPISTS.

Rehabilitation may be carried out in an inpatient or an outpatient setting. A NEUROLOGIST can advise a person with MS as to the most appropriate facilities.

relapse The reappearance or worsening of neurological symptoms in multiple sclerosis (MS); relapses are also called flares, attacks, or exacerbations. Relapses are common in MS. Although experts once thought each relapse indicated the development of new areas of DEMYELINATION, it is now clear that only one plaque out of 10 produces symptoms. A relapse can occur because a new plaque is created or because an old plaque gets bigger. However, whether or not a plaque causes symptoms probably depends on where it is located. Plaques in the brain stem or spinal cord are more likely to produce relapses. During a relapse, a patient will develop a new symptom about 20 percent of the time and a worsening of an old symptom about 80 percent of the time.

A relapse is not the same thing as a fluctuation, which is simply a slight change in a symptom. Fluctuations can appear in response to FATIGUE, STRESS, or emotional upset. When the fatigue or stress is eliminated, the fluctuation goes away. A fluctuation can vary hour by hour, whereas a relapse lasts at least a day or more.

Predicting Relapses

There are two primary ways to tell that a relapse may be imminent. The first is a sense of fatigue, and the second is an increased feeling of vulnerability; some patients report they feel that something unpleasant is about to happen.

Treating Relapses

A relapse is characterized as mild, moderate, or severe. Mild relapses usually improve without treatment over weeks or months, although typically the symptom does not disappear totally. The longer a patient has had MS, the less likely a symptom will disappear as the relapse improves.

Moderate and severe relapses usually require treatment with corticosteroids, either orally (prednisone, cortisone, or decadron) or intravenously (hydrocortisone or METHYLPREDNISOLONE). ADRENOCORTICOTROPIC HORMONE is an older medication, generally not used any more, that stimulates the release of the stress hormone cortisol. It is not clear which is the best way to administer steroids to treat relapses. In severe cases, many experts try intravenous medication followed by oral doses. Although steroids can help a patient recover more quickly from a relapse, they cannot improve the degree of recovery nor prevent a subsequent attack.

As the years progress, people will be less likely to have a full recovery from a relapse without treatment.

Side Effects of Steroids

Steroids do carry the risk of a number of side effects, including allergic reactions, fluid retention, weight gain, stomach upset, psychiatric disturbance, insomnia, increased appetite, or worsening of acne. However, most people usually tolerate steroids fairly well, and some people feel energetic or exuberant while taking them.

Long-term steroid use is not recommended as an MS treatment because steroids become less effective over time while the risk of serious side effects increases dramatically. These side effects include marked bloating of the face and trunk, high blood pressure, cataracts, hardening of the arteries, diabetes, life-threatening infections, and osteoporosis. Steroids can be used more than once a year to treat relapses. However, the more often they are used, the less effective they become.

relapsing-progressive MS The former name for PROGRESSIVE-RELAPSING MS.

relapsing-remitting MS The most common type of multiple sclerosis (MS), characterized by partial or total recovery after distinct relapses (also called exacerbations, attacks, or flares). No visible worsening of the disease occurs between attacks. Instead, there are stable periods that mask the continuing subclinical disease process. About 85 percent of people with MS initially begin with a relapsing-remitting course. However, in 50 percent of the cases, the disease will progress within 10–15 years. An additional 40 percent will progress within 25 years after onset as the disease evolves into the secondary progressive phase.

relative afferent pupillary defect See MARCUS GUNN PUPIL.

remyelination Repair of damaged MYELIN (the insulation around nerves). Some MYELIN REPAIR

may occur spontaneously in multiple sclerosis but is usually a very slow and uncontrollable process.

respiration problems See BREATHING PROBLEMS AND MS.

respite care Services that provide people with temporary relief from caregiving; these services include in-home assistance, short nursing home stays, and adult day care. Respite care can be used for a variety of reasons, such as a vacation, business travel, a weekend getaway, or a family emergency.

retrobulbar neuritis See OPTIC NEURITIS.

Rindfleisch, Eduard (1836–1908) A 19th-century German pathologist who analyzed postmortem brain samples from people with multiple sclerosis (MS). In 1863, Rindfleisch reported a key finding that paved the way for theories of inflammatory involvement in the etiology of MS. He noticed that in all the specimens, a blood vessel was present at the center of each lesion. Rindfleisch came to believe that a primary state of inflammation was responsible for the demyelination.

risk factors of MS A number of risk factors increase the chances that a person might be diagnosed with multiple sclerosis (MS). Although the average person in the United States has about one chance in 1,000 of developing MS, gender, race, environment, and heredity may increase that risk. However, simple risk estimates are oversimplifications that can easily be misinterpreted. For example, risk estimates can vary greatly depending upon the genetic makeup of a person's family, but risk is also affected in part by a person's ethnic background and other factors that haven't yet been clearly identified.

Gender For reasons that scientists do not yet fully understand, MS affects about twice as many women as men. This incidence appears to be increasing, at least in the United States. Men, however, may be more disabled by the disease than women.

Race Different populations and ethnic groups have a very different prevalence of MS. For example, Caucasians have a higher prevalence rate than other racial groups. African Americans in the United States have about half the risk of MS as do Caucasian Americans. But Africans living in Africa almost never get MS.

Environment   MS is a disease of temperate climates and is especially common in Scotland, Scandinavia, and throughout northern Europe. In both hemispheres, its prevalence increases with distance from the equator. The highest incidence occurs in areas above 40 degrees north latitude (around Denver and Philadelphia) and below 40 degrees south latitude (Auckland, New Zealand).

Although studies show that MS is more common in certain parts of the world, if a person moves from an area with higher risk to one of lower risk, the person acquires the risk of the new home *if the move occurs before adolescence.* Young people in low-risk groups who move into countries with higher MS rates display the risk rates of their new surroundings. In contrast, older migrants retain the risk of their original home country. Such data suggest that exposure to some environmental agent, either protective or harmful, is acquired in early life. The risk of disease later in life reflects the effects of the early environment.

Climate   Climate may be related to latitude; several variables of climate (humidity, altitude, precipitation, sunshine, and temperature) each appears to affect the chance of developing MS. However, no one single variable is more important than another.

Heredity   Although genes are important determinants of a person's risk for MS, they are not the only factor. For example, the fact that identical twins born to people with MS share all the same genes but do not always get MS and that more than 80 percent of people with MS do not have a first-degree relative with MS demonstrate conclusively that MS is not directly inherited and that factors other than genetics must be involved.

The baseline risk of getting MS in North America and northern Europe is one in 1,000 (or 0.1 percent). First-, second-, and third-degree relatives of people with MS are at a higher risk of developing the disease. The magnitude of the risk depends on how close the affected relative is. Siblings or the children of an affected woman have a 2–5 percent risk of developing MS. However, a half sibling of an affected person has only a 1.5 percent risk. The adopted sibling of an affected person has a 0.1 percent (or normal) risk of developing MS.

If one fraternal twin has MS, the other twin has only the typical sibling risk (between 2 and 5 percent) because fraternal twins are not genetically identical. However, if one identical twin develops MS, the other twin has a 30 percent chance of developing MS. The more similar the genes are to a family member who has the disease, the higher the risk that person has of developing the disease.

If a young mother develops MS, the risk of her children developing MS is between 2 and 4 percent per child; daughters have a slightly higher risk of developing the disease than do sons. However, the children of men with MS have a lower risk of developing MS than the children of women with the disease.

Researchers believe that more than one gene makes a person more likely to get MS and that this genetic predisposition causes the person to react to some environmental agent that triggers an autoimmune response. Sophisticated new techniques for identifying genes may help answer questions about the role of genetics in the development of MS. Scientists now believe that a person is susceptible to MS only if he or she inherits an unlucky combination of several genes.

Socioeconomic status   MS appears to be associated more often among middle-to-upper socioeconomic levels and is more common among urban individuals. The apparent link between MS and socioeconomic status may be related to the fact that people in northern climates tend to have a higher socioeconomic status as well.

Smoking   According to a 2003 Norwegian study of more than 20,000 people, women were one and a half times more likely to develop multiple sclerosis if they smoked, and men were almost three times as likely to develop the disease if they smoked. By studying men and women together, the study showed that smoking almost doubled a person's risk. An earlier study conducted in 1992 showed that smoking worsens symptoms in people who already have the disease. The study showed that right after smoking, 76 percent of people with MS had a temporary worsening of motor performance by about 14 percent.

Rokitansky, Carl (1804–1878) One of the most outstanding morphological pathologists of the 19th century, who worked at the Institute of Pathology in Vienna. Rokitansky was one of the first to examine multiple sclerosis (MS) lesions microscopically. He made a particularly important observation in 1857 when he noticed "fatty corpuscles" in the MS lesions. This discovery enhanced the pathological understanding of MS and brought neurologists closer to establishing a major feature of MS: nerve demyelination.

rollator A WALKER with wheels that provides more stable support than a cane or crutch. Because the walker is more stable and can stand by itself, older patients with multiple sclerosis often find this device easier to manage. A rollator includes both three- and four-wheeled models that may also include a folding seat. The brakes may be locked in place so the patient may sit safely and safely stand from the sitting position.

See also ASSISTIVE DEVICES; CANES; CRUTCHES; WHEELCHAIRS.

Romberg's sign Loss of the sense of the body's position, as characterized by the inability to maintain balance. Romberg's sign often appears in people with multiple sclerosis. To test for this sign, the NEUROLOGIST will test a patient's balance by having the person stand with feet together, arms outstretched in front, with eyes first open and then closed.

safety issues   A number of safety issues must be addressed when a person is diagnosed with multiple sclerosis (MS). There are also a number of ways to make adjustments in the household so that a person with MS is more comfortable and can manage daily activities more easily. Such household adjustments will also enhance the patient's safety.

Emergency Precautions

The utility company should be notified that a person in the home has MS and depends on power equipment such as oxygen, environment control units, electric beds, and lifts. The local utility company needs to know of these medical needs before an emergency power outage occurs. The person's doctor must fill out a form indicating the medical problem and the type of equipment used so that in an emergency, the utility company will make every attempt to restore service to this home as soon as possible. However, the patient still has the responsibility of keeping a backup power source, such as a power generator. In addition, the local utility company will tag the meters so that when repairs, meter changes, or routine maintenance require that the power be cut off, the company will notify the patient first so backup arrangements can be made.

It also is important to let the local fire department know if a patient might have trouble escaping from the home in the event of a fire. Fire drills should be practiced at home.

Safer Walking and Navigation

Throw rugs should be removed since walking or wheeling on vinyl, ceramic, or wood floors is easier than walking or wheeling on thick carpet. However, vinyl, ceramic, or wood floors may be slippery when wet. Carpet should be a flat, tightly woven, or tight loop style, not a plush, sculptured,

or shag style, which make walking or wheeling difficult. A high-density or commercial pad should be used under the carpet.

A home can be made easier to navigate by installing ramps, railings, or grab bars. If a door is at the top or bottom of the ramp, a level area should be in front of the door. A platform five feet wide by three feet long is recommended at the top of the ramp because it will enable a person in a wheelchair to unlock and open the door. Railing height above ramps is a matter of personal preference. The average-sized person usually finds that a height of 35 to 36 inches works well, but short people may want to consider a railing 32 to 34 inches high. Railings should be on either side of the ramp. They should be $1\frac{1}{4}$ to $1\frac{1}{2}$ inches in diameter with $1\frac{1}{2}$ inch clearance from any obstruction, such as a wall.

Doorknobs can be hard to handle for people with MS; they can be replaced with lever handles. Alternatively, a rubber lever can fit over any standard doorknob.

If a bathroom doorway is too narrow to accommodate a scooter or wheelchair, the door can be replaced with a tension rod and an opaque (or black) shower curtain for privacy.

To navigate easily around the home in a wheelchair, doorways can be widened by 1/2 inch to 3/4 inch by removing the doorjamb strips on one or both sides of the door. An alternative is to install offset hinges to increase the door opening two to three inches, allowing the door to swing out and away from the doorway opening.

Door hinges should be well oiled. Doors that scrape along a rug can be planed to make them open and close more easily.

To enable people with MS to close doors easily, string or cord can be tied around the doorknob so it can be grabbed as the patient moves through the doorway. The door will shut as the string is pulled. Alternatively, one cup hook can be attached to the door near the knob and a second cup hook to the doorjamb on the hinge side. A string or chain can be tied between the hooks and pulled as the patient goes through the doorway, closing the door.

Grab bars are a real safety plus, especially when installed in bathrooms. Grab bars should be installed with a space the width of a clenched fist between the grab bar and the wall. The bars should be anchored to the studs in the wall so they can withstand the pressure and weight when being used. Vinyl-covered hand grab rails are better for grip and absorb less heat.

Hand railings can be installed on both sides of a stairway to provide support going up and down stairs. Basement stairs will be safer if abrasive rubber treads are placed onto each step. For added safety, the edge of the steps can be painted with luminous paint to make them more visible.

Other Safety, Comfort, and Convenience Issues

Traditional light switches should be replaced with rocker panel switches that require less fine motor control and can be turned on or off by pressing with an arm, elbow, or palm of the hand. They are available at hardware and home-building supply stores. Wall switch extenders can lower a light switch 13 to 15 inches below the actual switch, which makes it easy to turn on and off from a wheelchair. Some extenders mount over a standard single light switch, whereas others replace the existing wall plate using the same screws. The device is easy to attach and will not scratch or damage walls. A flat wooden spatula is good for extending the patient's reach when he or she wants to operate a light switch. Lamps can be made touch sensitive. Lamps can be easier to turn on and off if a lamp converter is installed. The converter bypasses the on-off switch and makes the lamp touch sensitive. The converter fits into the socket so that the lamp will light up when touched. With each successive touch, the light gets brighter and then finally turns off.

Individuals who have separate controls for hot and cold water may want to consider installing wrist blades—wide, wing-type handles that are operated by pushing with the forearm, wrist, or

heel of the hand. They are available at most plumbing supply stores and hardware stores.

The type of furniture may also impact how comfortable a patient with MS might be. The best type of chair typically has an armrest; a firm, shallow seat; and a relatively straight back, and it is sturdy and stable. Low, overstuffed sofas and chairs should be avoided because they are difficult to sit down in and stand up from. To make getting up from a chair or sofa easier, furniture should be about 17 inches off the ground. The height of furniture can be adjusted by removing casters or putting measured blocks of wood under each leg until the desired height is achieved.

scanning speech   A type of speech characterized by staccato-like articulation that sounds clipped because the person unintentionally pauses between syllables and skips some of the sounds. A symptom of multiple sclerosis.

Schilder's disease   A rare, progressive, and often fatal DEMYELINATING DISEASE that usually begins in childhood. It features widespread destruction of the MYELIN sheath of the NEURONS in the cerebral hemispheres of the brain. The disorder is a variant of multiple sclerosis (MS).

As with MS, the course and prognosis of Schilder's disease are unpredictable. Some patients experience a progressive, unremitting course, while others may experience significant improvement and even remission. Most patients die within a few months of onset.

Symptoms

This condition may cause dementia, aphasia, seizures, personality changes, poor attention, tremors, balance instability, INCONTINENCE, WEAKNESS, headaches, vomiting, VISUAL PROBLEMS, and SPEECH PROBLEMS.

Treatment

Treatment for the disorder is similar to that of standard multiple sclerosis therapy. It includes corticosteroids, beta INTERFERON or immunosuppressive therapy, and symptomatic treatment.

Schumacher criteria   An outdated checklist formerly used by neurologists to confirm a diagnosis of multiple sclerosis (MS). Although these criteria are less commonly used, they still form the basis for later revised criteria. They have been superseded by the POSER CRITERIA. The Schumacher criteria are

- neurological examination reveals objective abnormalities of central nervous system (CNS) function
- involvement of two or more parts of CNS
- CNS disease predominantly affects the white matter
- person 10–50 years of age at onset
- signs and symptoms cannot be better explained by other disease process
- the CNS involvement follows one of two patterns: two or more episodes, each lasting at least 24 hours and at least one month apart; or slow or stepwise progression of signs and symptoms over at least six months

scintillating scotoma A VISUAL PROBLEM characterized by a combination of a blind area in the visual field with a glittering or shimmering area. This problem may occur in patients with multiple sclerosis.

sclerosis Literally, this term means "scar"—the hardening of tissue. In the condition of multiple sclerosis, "sclerosis" refers to the body's production of scar tissue in areas of lost MYELIN around axons.

Scofield, James (b. 1941) This Pulitzer Prize–nominated poet was diagnosed with multiple sclerosis in addition to depression and congenital liver disease. Also an essayist, Scofield's work has been published in the United States, England, Canada, and India.

His mother died at a young age of a liver disease he has inherited. His father abandoned Scofield and his several siblings. It was not until he was serving as a clerk-typist at a Grand Forks, North Dakota, air base that he read his first poetry, *18 Poems*, by Dylan Thomas.

He has been writing for more than 30 years. When he first began crafting poems, he wrote each day for six years, producing only 26 poems, all of which he destroyed. In the seventh year he produced "Festival," which was published by Bellowing Ark of Seattle, Washington. His first book, *30 Poems*, was published in 1999 and nominated for the Pulitzer.

See also FAMOUS PEOPLE WITH MS.

Scotland The country with the highest per capita incidence of multiple sclerosis (MS) in the world. In Scotland, more than 10,500 people have MS. Genetic susceptibility and environmental factors may explain the unusually high incidence of MS in Scotland. Clusters in this country with a particularly high incidence of MS are currently being investigated.

scotoma A gap or blind spot in the visual field. This dark spot may be related to inflammation of the optic nerve (called OPTIC NEURITIS), which is not uncommon among people with multiple sclerosis. This problem may resolve on its own. Studies suggest that for optic neuritis, treatment with intravenous METHYLPREDNISOLONE, followed by a tapered course of oral steroids, may be useful.

secondary progressive MS A type of multiple sclerosis (MS) that begins with the RELAPSING-REMITTING pattern and that becomes steadily progressive as time passes. Attacks and partial recoveries may continue to occur. Of the 85 percent who begin with relapsing-remitting disease, more than 50 percent will develop secondary progressive MS within 10 years; 90 percent will develop this form within 25 years.

seizures Sudden, violent changes in sensation, awareness, or behavior caused by a brief, abnormal electrical discharge in an injured area of the brain. This is one of the more uncommon symptoms that affects only about 5–10 percent of people with multiple sclerosis (MS). Although some published studies have suggested that seizures are common in people with MS, most experts do not agree.

Several types of seizures may occur. All of these forms result from sudden changes in the transmission of electrical signals from one cell to another.

- Generalized tonic-clonic seizures are brief episodes of unconsciousness with uncontrollable jerking movements of the extremities.

- Generalized absence seizures are momentary lapses of consciousness without abnormal movements.

- Partial complex seizures are periods of stereotyped repetitive activity. The person appears to be awake but does not respond to external stimuli.

Note that paroxysmal symptoms in MS are brief, sudden attacks of abnormal posturing of the extremities, loss of tone in the legs (drop attacks), or other manifestations that may appear similar to an epileptic seizure but are of different origin. Examples of paroxysmal symptoms include paroxysmal pain (such as TRIGEMINAL NEURALGIA); prolonged muscular contractions (tonic spasms) of an arm or leg; LHERMITTE'S SIGN (electric shock–like sensation down the spine when the neck is flexed); and UHTHOFF'S SIGN (transient blurring of vision associated with exertion and higher body temperature).

Seizures are usually diagnosed by the clinical history and an electroencephalogram (a recording of electrical activity in the brain).

Treatment Options and Outlook

Most seizures can be well controlled by use of the appropriate anticonvulsant medication, such as CARBAMAZEPINE (Tegretol), diphenylhydantoin (Dilantin), GABAPENTIN (Neurontin), divalproex sodium (Depakote), and others. Whether or not the incidence of seizures is eventually found to be higher in people with MS, the management strategies are exactly the same. The incidence is low enough that no preventive treatment is recommended.

sensory ataxia　Some people with multiple sclerosis have such severe NUMBNESS in their feet that they cannot feel the floor or know where their feet are, which may lead to a loss of dexterity or clumsiness, even though there may be no symptoms of WEAKNESS involved.

sensory symptoms　A group of symptoms in multiple sclerosis related to bodily sensations such as PAIN, smell, taste, temperature, hearing, which can be impaired due to the destruction of MYELIN (deyelination). Common complaints also include tingling, burning, difficulty in ascertaining joint position, and tightness—described as a constricting feeling such as caused by a girdle, band, or glove. LHERMITTE'S SIGN is another common symptom, characterized by a sudden painful electric sensation radiating down the neck as it is flexed.

See also SAFETY ISSUES.

service dogs　Dogs (usually a larger breed, such as labradors and golden retrievers) that are trained to work with physically disabled individuals, including people with multiple sclerosis. Service dogs can help pull wheelchairs up ramps. When braced in place, the dogs steady and support people as they transfer to and from a wheelchair or rise from a seated position. The dogs can provide balance by walking beside people with unsteady gait and help people get up from falls. With their acute sense of smell, dogs can locate objects, places, and people.

Just like the more familiar seeing eye dog, service dogs are allowed in public places that otherwise ban pets. The Americans with Disabilities Act guarantees this for service dogs, even if state law specifies "guide dogs." Theoretically, service dog users do not have to show anyone documentation of their disability or the dog's training, but carrying a dog's training certificate can be helpful. Sometimes a special harness or leash will make it easier for the public to identify a dog as a working animal.

State laws about service animals sometimes differ from federal regulations (some states give them more privileges). Therefore patients interested in getting a service dog should investigate their state's legislation. However, no one has to accommodate a service dog if it is disruptive or appears to be dangerous.

Finding and training a dog to match a person's specific needs may take from six months to two years. Because of the extensive training required, service dogs usually cost thousands of dollars. However, some nonprofit organizations charge nothing, while others have fees from $150 to $300. Sometimes sponsors can defray the organization's additional costs.

For contact information for service dog training centers, see Appendix I.

sexual problems and MS   Sexual problems are often experienced by people with multiple sclerosis (MS). This is because sexual arousal begins in the vulnerable central nervous system as the brain sends messages to the sexual organs along nerves running through the spinal cord. If MS damages these nerve pathways, sexual response, including arousal and orgasm, can be directly affected. Sexual problems may also be linked to MS symptoms such as FATIGUE or SPASTICITY as well as psychological factors related to self-esteem and mood changes.

In fact, 63 percent of people with MS report that their sexual activity declines after their diagnosis. Other surveys of persons with MS suggest that as many as 91 percent of men and 72 percent of women may be affected by sexual problems.

Unfortunately, although ignoring these problems may interfere with a person's daily life, patients and health care professionals are often reluctant to bring up the subject.

Symptoms and Diagnostic Path

Women may experience fewer or painfully intensified sensations in the vaginal/clitoral area, vaginal dryness, trouble achieving orgasm, and loss of libido. Men may notice problems in achieving or maintaining an erection (ERECTILE DYSFUNCTION), reduced penile sensations, difficulty achieving orgasm and/or ejaculation, and loss of libido.

Some MS symptoms cause problems in both sexes. For example, spasticity can cause cramping or uncontrollable spasms in the legs, causing them to pull together or making them difficult to separate—either of which can make positioning difficult or uncomfortable. Pain or embarrassment can interfere with pleasure, and weakness and fatigue may interfere with libido and function.

Treatment Options and Outlook

A number of treatments are available to treat sexual dysfunction. For men, erectile dysfunction may be treated with SILDENAFIL (Viagra); injectable medications such as papaverine and phentolamine that increase blood flow in the penis; a small penis suppository; inflatable devices; or implants.

Women can ease vaginal dryness by generously applying nonprescription liquid or jellied water-soluble personal lubricants. (Petroleum jelly should not be used because it is not water soluble and may cause infection.)

Both men and women with MS and their partners often benefit from sexual therapy to learn about alternative means of sexual stimulation (such as a vibrator) to overcome slow arousal and impaired sensation. Abnormal sensations and spasms can often be controlled through the use of medication. Techniques such as intermittent catheterization or medication can control urinary leakage during sex.

Sexual problems may lead to other problems such as loss of self-esteem, DEPRESSION, ANXIETY, or anger. Counseling by a mental health professional or trained sexual therapist can address both physiologic and psychological issues. This therapy should involve both partners.

SF-36 Health Status Questionnaire   See HEALTH STATUS QUESTIONNAIRE.

sharpness sensation test   A type of sensory awareness test that may be part of a NEUROLOGICAL EXAMINATION used to help diagnose multiple sclerosis. In this test, a doctor uses a pin or other sharp object to jab a patient's skin lightly. Patients with sensory deficits will not feel the jab equally in all parts of the body and may not feel the pinprick at all in certain areas.

signs and symptoms of MS   See CLINICAL SIGNS AND SYMPTOMS.

sildenafil (Viagra)   Medication used to treat impotence and help improve a man's ability to have an erection in response to stimulation. Sildenafil can be helpful in alleviating SEXUAL PROBLEMS for some people with multiple sclerosis. Unlike local medications that act directly on the penis, this pill circulates throughout the entire body.

The drug was originally designed to improve blood flow in the heart's blood vessels. However, research subjects soon began to report that the drug triggered a remarkable improvement in their ability to achieve and maintain an erection. Further studies were completed. On March 27, 1998, the medication was approved by the U.S. Food and Drug Administration for the treatment of impotence.

About 30–60 minutes after ingestion, the drug is absorbed in the bloodstream, where it inhibits an enzyme found primarily in the penis. Blocking this enzyme allows the smooth muscle in the penis to remain relaxed, boosting blood flow into the penis and generating an erection. Viagra is unique in that it simply enhances a naturally occurring process, which is why erection occurs only as the result of sexual stimulation. In one study, 83 percent of participants reported a better erection after taking Viagra, compared with 12 percent who took a dummy pill. Viagra is eliminated from the body in a few hours.

Side Effects

Viagra produces relatively few side effects. Those that do occur are usually short lived. However, some individuals have reported congestion; diarrhea; facial flushing; headaches; URINARY TRACT INFECTIONS; mild, temporary visual changes in blue/green colors; or increased sensitivity to light. Viagra may also cause headaches or a drop in blood pressure. It should not be used by men with a history of coronary problems or by anyone in combination with nitroglycerin or any other blood pressure drug. Because there is also a potential for heart attack during sexual activity in patients with preexisting heart disease, Viagra should not be used by men for whom sexual activity is inadvisable because of their underlying heart problems.

Viagra and Prostate Cancer

Despite its popularity, there was some initial concern that Viagra has certain chemical effects that could help prostate cancers grow. However, in a 2003 Chinese study in mice that had human prostate cancer cells injected into their prostate glands, scientists found that no evidence that Viagra causes the growth or spread of prostate cancer.

simvastatin (Zocor)   One of a group of common cholesterol-lowering medications. Preliminary studies suggest that such medications also may be helpful in improving symptoms in patients with RELAPSING-REMITTING multiple sclerosis (MS).

Statins help block production of immune factors involved in MS that lead to disability. Their ability to promote an anti-inflammatory response from the immune system suggests a potential treatment for MS.

In a small clinical trial of Zocor in 28 individuals with relapsing-remitting MS, Zocor appeared to reduce the number and volume of GADOLINIUM-ENHANCING LESIONS in the brain (generally interpreted to be new lesions) over the six-month treatment period, according to research published in the May 15, 2004, issue of the *The Lancet*. Previous studies have suggested that this and other statin drugs can alter immune responses in a way that may be beneficial for treating MS. However, larger, controlled trials are needed to determine the drug's safety and effectiveness against MS.

In earlier studies of cells taken from individuals with MS, different forms of statins were capable of inhibiting several immune responses and markers of inflammation typically involved in MS. However, in those studies, statins stimulated the release of some messenger proteins known to increase inflammation as well, making their ultimate value in treating MS uncertain. Additional studies on statins have been published that reported that atorvastatin (Lipitor) prevented or reversed the MS-like disease EXPERIMENTAL AUTOIMMUNE ENCEPHALOMYELITIS (EAE) in mice. The mechanism underlying the drug's ability to treat EAE appears to be immune system modulation rather than a cholesterol-lowering mechanism.

Because standard MS drug treatments are expensive and only partly effective, scientists are always looking for newer, better medications. New research is needed to determine more precisely the clinical effects and best dose, therapeutic window, and potency of statins and to evaluate whether using a combination of drugs might be more effective than using one drug alone. The most significant advantage of statins over existing MS therapies is that statins can be administered by mouth.

sixth nerve palsy   Also called cranial nerve palsy or abducens nerve palsy, this condition is characterized by two conditions: horizontal DOUBLE VISION (diplopia) and an eye that cannot move properly in all directions. Both are caused by damage to the nerve controlling the muscle responsible for side-to-side eye movements. Sixth nerve palsy is often the presenting sign for multiple sclerosis (MS).

Symptoms and Diagnostic Path

Normally, the left muscle pulls the left eye outward and the right pulls the right eye outward. Therefore, if the left sixth cranial nerve is damaged (as in MS), it causes double vision when the patient looks left. If the right sixth cranial nerve is affected, it causes double vision when looking right. The double vision goes away when one eye is closed.

The diagnosis is usually easily confirmed by an ophthalmologist who will observe the eye movements in all fields of gaze. The affected eye will be unable to turn outward beyond the midline (abduct). A magnetic resonance imaging scan can often identify the nerve lesions characteristic of MS.

Treatment Options and Outlook

Patients may help eliminate the double vision by wearing an eye patch or press-on prisms for spectacles. If the condition fails to improve, strabismus surgery may be considered.

skilled nursing care A level of care that must be given or supervised by licensed nurses under the general direction of a doctor. Skilled nursing care might include intravenous injections or tube feeding.

Any service that could be safely performed by the average nonmedical person (such as bathing or dressing) without the direct supervision of a licensed nurse would not be considered skilled nursing care.

sleep problems See FATIGUE.

Social Security Disability Insurance (SSDI) A type of government insurance funded by the Social Security Act. To obtain disability insurance, a person's physical condition must be severe enough to prohibit working and must have lasted (or be expected to last) at least a year. The primary criteria for assessing impairment caused by multiple sclerosis include visual problems, mental problems, fatigue, and motor function.

In order to qualify for SSDI, an individual must have accumulated a certain amount of work cred-

its in a job covered by Social Security. Work credits are determined by earnings; the older a person is, the more credits he or she will need.

Social Security Income (SSI) Although SOCIAL SECURITY DISABILITY INSURANCE is based on work history, SSI is based on economic need. A person with multiple sclerosis under the age of 65 can qualify for SSI.

socioeconomic status and MS Statistics suggest that multiple sclerosis (MS) seems to occur more often among people in the middle-to-high socioeconomic ranges. MS also seems to occur more often in urban areas than in rural locations. Both of these associations are not a cause, however; researchers do not yet understand why the link exists.

Solu-Medrol treatment See METHYLPRED-NISOLONE.

spasticity Stiff, tight muscles and involuntary muscle contractions that are not coordinated with other muscles. Spasticity is one of the most common symptoms of multiple sclerosis (MS). Spasticity usually affects the larger, stronger muscles needed to keep the human body upright—the gastrocnemius muscles in the calf, the quadriceps at the front of the thigh, the adductor in the groin—as well as the biceps of the upper arm and the pronator in the forearm. However, spasticity can affect almost any muscle pair in the body. Repetitive muscle spasms (CLONUS) are often associated with spasticity.

Most muscles in the human body are paired and are designed to work in opposite ways so that when one is contracted, its twin is stretched. The regulation of the action of these paired muscles is complex. The brain sends messages are sent to the muscles, and receives sensory feedback from them. Spastic muscles, however, garble these messages to the brain so that both muscles in a pair contract at the same time.

People with MS who have spasticity problems experience the problem not only as a muscle contraction but as a stiffness. In mild cases, this may cause FOOT DROP, a knee that refuses to bend, an awkward arm posture, or a hunched posture. In extreme cases, the spastic limbs can force a person into the fetal position.

Symptoms and Diagnostic Path

Spasticity can be very painful. Depending on the affected muscles, it can result in an uncoordinated gait, stiff or deformed posture, and shortening of the range of limb movement. Spasticity may also produce feelings of pain or tightness in and around joints and can cause low back pain. It can cause permanent muscle shortening (contracture) and problems around the joints against which the two spastic muscles are supposed to move.

On the other hand, the increased muscle tone typical of spastic muscles often prevents the atrophy that can occur through lack of use. Some people who experience significant leg weakness find that spasticity makes the legs stiffer and helps them to stand or walk.

In MS, spasticity is usually caused by damage to the nerves that control muscles or those that receive sensory information. Reflexive spasms generated by the spinal cord are not inhibited by the brain, and increased muscle tone results. The lesions responsible for spasticity are usually located in the cerebellum or the white matter tracts that connect the cerebellum to the peripheral motor and sensory nerves.

There are two types of severe MS-related spasticity: flexor and extensor spasticity. Flexor spasticity involves the muscles on the back of the upper leg (hamstrings) so that the hips and knees are bent and difficult to straighten. Extensor spasticity involves the muscles on the front of the upper leg (quadriceps); the hips and knees remain straight with the legs very close together or crossed over at the ankles. Less often, spasticity may affect the arms.

Treatment Options and Outlook

Fortunately, several antispasticity medications are available that can relieve this crippling condition. Because spasticity varies so much from person to person, it must be treated on an individual basis in partnership with the physician, nurse, PHYSICAL THERAPIST, and OCCUPATIONAL THERAPIST.

Exercise/stretching Treatment begins with various self-help ways to ease symptoms, including EXERCISE and changes in daily activities. Relaxation techniques (breathing deeply while consciously relaxing a muscle) may help ease mild cases of spasticity.

PHYSICAL THERAPY focuses on strengthening and stretching exercises. Physical therapists stretch shortened muscles and increase movement in the joints, holding the stretch for one minute and then easing off. If these are effective or the spasticity is mild, drug treatments are often not necessary. Although research has not proven the helpfulness of stretching in easing spasticity, most doctors believe it can help at least temporarily.

On the person's first appointment, the physical therapist assesses the degree to which the muscle tone is affected, pulling and pushing the individual's arms and legs to gauge the level of resistance. In addition, the therapist evaluates the person's coordination, strength, and ability to perform ACTIVITIES OF DAILY LIVING. After pinpointing areas of significant spasticity, the therapist will work to extend contracted muscles, increase circulation, relax muscle fibers, stimulate sensory receptors in the muscles, and try to help the individual become more flexible.

To improve range of motion, the therapist rotates the hips, knees, or arms in the sockets, loosening the joints, restoring elasticity, and increasing circulation. To improve spastic ankles, the patient rises up and down on the toes, which exercises the Achilles tendon. Therapists also work directly on this area with a series of stretches, applying gentle but firm twisting and pulling motions to the affected ankles. To improve extension and flexion, the therapist extends and rotates weakened arms or legs, including the feet, ankles, calves, thighs, hamstrings, hips, lower back, arms, neck, and head. Patients are also encouraged to do these movements at home.

The therapist may also pull, rotate, stretch, or manipulate problem areas with the patient lying prone. Patients whose legs or spine are flexed may be placed in a standing frame to work on weight-bearing exercises to improve posture.

Other exercises may include lying on the back, hugging the knees, and rocking to stretch the spine. In addition, therapists may help muscles to relax by stroking and massaging spastic areas, with deep pressure to the stomach, groin, and lower back.

At home, patients should practice their exercises at least once a day. They may find they are particularly stiff in the morning and may benefit more from exercising once they have been moving around. Individuals should not exercise to the point of exhaustion or overheating. All exercises should be done very slowly.

Water exercise Exercising in a pool (WATER EXERCISE) can help ease spasticity because the water helps patients move their limbs more easily. The cool temperature of the water also helps to ease symptoms in many patients. Ideally, the pool water should not be warmer than 80–84 degrees F.

Medication In severe cases, drug treatments for spasticity may be needed. These may include two major antispasticity drugs with good safety records: BACLOFEN (Lioresal) and TIZANIDINE (Zanaflex). Although no drug can cure spasticity, certain drugs may be especially helpful for patients confined to a wheelchair who are having trouble with leg or arm stiffness or whose leg spasms are particularly painful.

Baclofen is a muscle relaxant, the most common drug used to treat spasticity. It works on the central nervous system and can dramatically decrease spasms while improving muscle tone and posture. This medication acts on the lower spinal cord and its descending motor pathways where MS lesions are often found. Researchers believe the drug affects the reflex involved in maintaining muscle tone, relaxing the main muscle groups in the arms, legs, and trunk. This has an overall inhibiting effect on spasms. Therefore, if the patient has a GAIT PROBLEM, walking will almost always get better after Baclofen is administered. Fluidity of movement, range of joint motion, and quickness of movement also improve. People with spasticity in the legs typically improve more than those with spasticity in the arms.

Unfortunately, strength and coordination are not improved with this drug. Moreover, the dosage must be carefully determined. Physicians typically start off with a low dose and slowly increase it until maximum benefit is reached. (Taking too high a dose at first can trigger fatigue and weakness.) The correct dose may vary considerably, from 5 mg to 80 mg daily. Patients often take this drug in the morning, when getting out of bed is usually difficult. Baclofen can be taken as needed, and patients usually can regulate the dosage themselves after an initial discussion with the doctor.

Baclofen is usually administered orally has few serious side effects other than fatigue or weakness, although it may interact dangerously with alcohol and other drugs. It can cause seizures and hallucinations if stopped suddenly. Baclofen should be used cautiously in women with MS who are pregnant, in alcoholics, in those with diabetes, and in those with kidney disease. Patients taking other medications such as central nervous system depressants, muscle relaxants, and the insomnia drug ethinamate should be particularly careful about using Baclofen. Some research also suggests that smoking may interfere with the absorption of Baclofen, especially if the patient smokes more than a pack a day.

Baclofen can also be given by an implanted pump (intrathecal baclofen), which is placed under the skin of the abdomen and connected directly to the lower half of the spinal cord. Because the implant is technically difficult to place and involves higher risks and costs, intrathecal baclofen is used only for severe spasticity that cannot be managed with oral medication. It can, however, produce dramatic improvement when the oral medication is ineffective.

Tizanidine also quickly relaxes muscles through its affects on the central nervous system, although it is less likely to cause muscle weakness than other spasticity treatments. Typically, this oral drug works after one week. In one study, 75 percent of subjects taking tizanidine reported improvement without the leg muscle weakness that is often experienced when using baclofen. Side effects include drowsiness and occasionally low blood pressure, dry mouth, dizziness, and hallucinations. It can cause liver damage in a minority of users.

GABAPENTIN (Neurontin) is an antiseizure medication that may help reduce spasticity without increasing fatigue or impairing concentration. It may also help reduce facial pain and improve vision.

Other drugs are used less often, including the benzodiazepines and DANTROLENE sodium (Dantrium). The benzodiazepines (diazepam

[Valium] and clonazepam [Klonopin and Rivotril]) work by relaxing the central nervous system, reducing muscle overactivity and painful spasms. They are particularly helpful for patients who also struggle with anxiety. However, these drugs are physically addictive, with a number of side effects including drowsiness and muscle weakness. They are not usually helpful on a day-to-day basis and should not be used by seriously depressed patients.

Dantrolene sodium (Dantrium) is usually prescribed only if Lioresal or Valium are not adequate. It works directly on chemicals in muscles, increasing passive movement, decreasing muscle tone, and reducing muscle spasms, tightness, and pain. Because dantrolene causes muscle weakness, it is best suited for either those who are wheelchair bound but still suffer from spasticity or those whose muscles are still strong so that the drug-induced weakness is not unduly debilitating. Unfortunately, this drug often produces a number of other side effects, including drowsiness, dizziness, fatigue, diarrhea, photosensitivity, and rarely, liver damage. The longer a patient takes this medication, the more likely it is that problems may develop.

Many people also report that CANNABIS works for both the muscle spasms and the pain involved with spasticity.

Tonic spasms—sudden cramps in an arm or leg that draws itself up into a stiff, flexed, or extended position—may respond to low doses of carbamazepine or phenytoin.

Patients who decide to stop taking any of these drugs listed above should consult with their physician first, because these drugs need to be tapered slowly rather than stopped abruptly. Withdrawing suddenly can lead to seizures.

Mechanical aids   Braces or splints may help prevent contracture (locked joints). For example, a brace may help keep a foot or hand in a neutral position, helping movement and preventing deformity. These mechanical devices are also called ORTHOTICS.

Injection therapy   If exercise, stretching, mechanical aids, and medication do not help spasticity, injections of chemicals to paralyze nerves may help.

This method, called chemodenervation, can be either temporary or permanent. It will affect the

nerves as a way of reducing spasms. The chemicals used include phenol and BOTULINUM TOXIN type A (Botox).

Botulinum is a toxin produced by the bacteria that causes the often-fatal food poisoning botulism. When a small amount of this substance is injected into a spastic muscle, it can temporarily paralyze the muscle, which eases the spasticity. This type of treatment is typically used to ease spasticity in the large muscle of the thigh, although it can also be used on the face.

Each Botox injection lasts for approximately three months. Although repeated injections can become expensive, doctors generally prefer Botox injections to the second alternative: phenol injections, which permanently destroy the nerve.

In very severe cases, administering phenol via spinal injections in the lower back may reduce pain and spasms for some patients, but most patients are not appropriate candidates for this approach. When phenol is injected, the muscle becomes limp, but this injection carries the risk of unwanted side effects. For example, phenol injections into the leg muscles may trigger a temporary loss of bladder and bowel control.

Surgery   For very severe spasticity that does not respond to medication or exercise, doctors may decide to destroy nerves or tendons surgically so that muscles cannot contract, destroying either the peripheral or the central nerves involved in the spasms. Although this severe treatment is rarely required, it can provide dramatic improvement in leg spasticity.

spastic small bladder   A type of bladder problem common in multiple sclerosis in which muscle contraction and SPASTICITY make the bladder "small," so that it fills more quickly with urine. When this happens, urination is no longer under conscious control but becomes a reflex reaction to the brain signal that the bladder is full. As a result, the bladder signals the need to empty when only a small amount of urine is present. Normally, the voiding signal is blocked by messages from the brain until the bladder has about a cup of urine. Sometimes referred to as a disinhibited bladder, spastic small bladder is caused by a loss of the protective MYELIN sheath along nerves between the brain and the voiding reflex center (a group of nerves at the base of the spinal cord that send emptying messages to the brain). It is the more common and less debilitating of the two common types of bladder problems (the other is FLACCID BIG BLADDER).

Symptoms and Diagnostic Path

A spastic small bladder may lead to urinary urgency, frequency, dribbling, or incontinence.

Bladder problems can be diagnosed with urodynamic testing, a simple examination combined with a cystoscopy, in which the UROLOGIST inserts a small telescope into the bladder. This can reveal whether the bladder is too small. In addition, the urologist will measure how much urine remains in the bladder after urination. Less than 100 cc of urine suggests either a normal or a small spastic bladder.

Treatment Options and Outlook

A spastic small bladder is usually treated with medications to slow down the bladder's response to the voiding reflex, which lessens the transmission of impulses from the voluntary reflex center. Medication can prolong the intervals between urination and decrease the sense of urgency, allowing patients more time to get to the bathroom and lessening the chance of incontinence. In some cases, taking the antispasticity drug Lioresal (BACLOFEN)—used by patients with spasticity problems—can relax the bladder enough so that the spastic bladder problem goes away.

More commonly, the drug oxybutynin (Ditropan) may be prescribed once or twice a day to stop leakage and frequency. It can be taken as needed, such as before leaving the house. However, this drug has a narrow therapeutic range before it becomes toxic, so dosage levels must be carefully monitored.

Another common drug is Pro-Banthine, an anticholinergic, antispasmodic muscle relaxant that is less effective—but less toxic—than oxybutynin. Pro-Banthine works by blocking nerve impulses in the parasympathetic nerve endings, blocking muscle contractions and bladder spasms. Although it has fewer side effects than oxybutynin, it may cause drowsiness, rapid heartbeat, and CONSTIPATION. This drug should not be taken with megadoses of vitamin C or antacids, which may make Pro-Banthine less effective.

The antidepressant imipramine (Tofranil) is occasionally prescribed to relax the mechanism that opens the bladder. This drug can also boost mood and combat depression.

If medication does not control the spastic bladder, the next step is catheterization. INTERMITTENT SELF-CATHETERIZATION, in which a catheter is placed by the patient, is safe and effective. For those who cannot manage this, however, an INDWELLING CATHETER may be used. This type of catheter is placed by a doctor and left in place.

See also BLADDER DYSFUNCTION; CATHETER; NEUROGENIC BLADDER; UNCOORDINATED BLADDER.

speech-language pathologist   A health care professional who specializes in the diagnosis and treatment of speech and SWALLOWING PROBLEMS. A person with multiple sclerosis (MS) may be referred to a speech-language pathologist for help with either or both of these problems.

Speech-language pathologists can evaluate and treat speech and communication problems, and they can recommend appropriate communication technologies that will aid in daily activities. Because of their expertise with speech and language difficulties, they may also provide cognitive remediation for individuals with COGNITIVE DYSFUNCTION.

Speech-language pathologists can also help people with MS maintain as many verbal communication skills as possible. They can teach techniques that conserve energy, including nonverbal communication.

See also DYSARTHRIA; SPEECH PROBLEMS AND MS; SPEECH THERAPY.

speech problems and MS   Speech problems in patients with multiple sclerosis (MS) may result from DEMYELINATION of certain areas of the brain, such as the CEREBELLUM. Tremor affecting the lips or tongue may also affect speech. The exact type of speech problem a patient may develop depends on what part of the brain is demyelinated and which parts of the tongue, lips, larynx, vocal cords, and throat are subsequently affected.

Typically, speech problems in people with MS include slurring, slowing, and lack of fluency. SPEECH THERAPY may be recommended, which may include techniques such as mouth and throat exercises, posture changes, and muscle-retraining techniques.

See also DYSARTHRIA.

speech therapy Special treatment designed to help improve communication skills in people who have difficulty speaking because of WEAKNESS or uncoordination of face and tongue muscles. Speech therapists often work with people who have multiple sclerosis, providing exercises and ASSISTIVE DEVICES. Speech therapists are also trained to evaluate SWALLOWING PROBLEMS (dysphagia).

See also DYSARTHRIA.

sphincterotomy A surgical enlargement of the urinary sphincter in a man whose SPASTICITY is so severe that he cannot empty his bladder. Once the surgery is performed, the man loses urinary control and must wear an external condom catheter to collect the urine. This procedure is seldom required in patients with multiple sclerosis.

spinal cord The very center of the nervous system, the spinal cord is a long bundle of nerves extending downward from the base of the brain along the inside of the spinal column. The spinal cord is the main link between the body and the brain. The lower end is about two-thirds of the way down the spine. Below this, the spinal cord splits to form several main nerves that continue within the spine, ending up at the legs and feet. Multiple sclerosis (MS) may cause scarring on the spinal cord that may be due to active or chronic inflammation.

Like the brain, the spinal cord contains both gray and white matter. The gray matter lies in the center of the cord and consists of thousands of the cell bodies of the motor neurons that pass signals to body muscles. A thick layer of WHITE MATTER surrounds the gray matter. White matter is made up of axons (long, thin, wiry extensions of the cells) and contains the nerve fibers that pass signals to and from the brain.

The spinal cord is almost totally enclosed by the spinal bones; 31 pairs of large nerves called spinal nerves branch off the spinal cord at regular intervals and pass through the narrow gaps between the spinal bones. Each spinal nerve contains both sensory and motor neurons. Spinal nerves in the neck handle signals to and from the head, arms, and hands. Nerves in the chest lead to the chest muscles, skin, and other organs such as lungs and heart. Nerves from the lower end of the cord branch out through the stomach, down into the legs and feet.

Some parts of the nerves carry information to the spinal cord, which relays the messages to the brain. These include nerve messages from the skin and messages from internal organs and muscles. Nerves that carry incoming messages are called sensory nerves.

Motor nerve carry outgoing information—signals from the brain traveling down the spinal cord that activate muscles and control body movements.

spinal lesions Scars on the spinal cord. These may be caused by multiple sclerosis due to active or chronic inflammation.

spinal multiple sclerosis Damage to the spinal cord caused by multiple sclerosis, resulting in slowed or blocked nerve signals.

spinal tap A procedure that tests fluid removed from the spinal canal to help diagnose disorders of the brain and spinal cord, including multiple sclerosis (MS). This cerebrospinal fluid (CSF) contains glucose, proteins, and other substances also found in the blood. Analysis of the fluid includes a count of the number and types of white blood cells, the amount of glucose, the types and levels of various proteins (especially immune system proteins called antibodies or immunoglobulins), and testing for bacteria, fungi, or other abnormal cells.

MS is suspected if the CSF reveals a large number of immunoglobulins (antibodies) as well as OLIGO-CLONAL BANDS (the pattern of immunoglobulins on a more specific test) or certain breakdown products of myelin. These findings indicate an abnormal autoimmune response within the brain and spinal cord, meaning that the body is attacking itself.

More than 90 percent of people with MS have oligoclonal bands in their CSF. Although increased immunoglobulins in the CSF and oligoclonal bands are seen in many other brain and spinal cord conditions, their presence is often useful in helping to establish an MS diagnosis. However, a negative spinal tap, one without abnormal findings, does not rule out MS. An abnormal autoimmune response in CSF is found in a number of other diseases, so the test is not specific for MS. Conversely, between 5 and 10 percent of people with MS never show these CSF abnormalities. This is why a spinal tap by itself cannot confirm or rule out a diagnosis of MS. It must be part of the total clinical picture that takes into account other diagnostic procedures such as EVOKED POTENTIALS and MAGNETIC RESONANCE IMAGING.

Procedure

To perform a spinal tap, the skin around the spine is cleansed and covered. A local anesthetic numbs the area so a long, thin, hollow needle can be inserted between two bones in the lower spine and into the spinal canal. One to two tablespoonfuls of fluid are withdrawn; the spinal cord itself is never touched. After the fluid is collected and the needle is removed, patients must lie flat for at least an hour to prevent a spinal headache. If a headache develops anyway, patients should lie down as much as possible and drink plenty of caffeine-containing beverages. All patients should drink 2½ quarts of liquid the day of the test and the day after. They should avoid strenuous or vigorous exercise for a day or so following the procedure.

Risks and Complications

Spinal taps are safe, although there are some risks. The procedure is not painful, but momentary twinges of pain may be felt if the needle brushes against nervous system tissue. About 10 percent of people develop a spinal headache (one that worsens when sitting or standing). Although the risk of infection is extremely low, it is still possible. Occasionally, a small blood vessel is pierced during the procedure, causing a bloody tap. No treatment is needed to repair the blood vessel; it heals on its own.

splint A type of brace that can be used for some patients with multiple sclerosis who have signifi-

cant GAIT PROBLEMS, especially foot dragging or weak or inturned ankles. In these cases, the patients strap on a splint instead of resorting to a WALKER or CANE.

Types of Splints

Several types of splints can be used by patients with multiple sclerosis. The ankle splint is a lightweight plastic ankle brace that fits over the foot, ankle, and lower leg, fastening with a Velcro strap. It is available in flexible, semirigid and rigid frames and can provide substantial walking support.

A dorsiflexion elastic assist is especially beneficial for patients with FOOT DROP. The shoe-clasp ankle-foot ORTHOTIC is a short leg brace that clips onto the back of a shoe, runs up the back of the leg, and fastens below the knee.

A double-strap ankle support is a slip-on ankle brace with an open heel that compresses both sides of the ankle. An athletic knee pad can give extra support to the knee and the leg, as can the overlock knee brace, which is a felt and elastic device that braces the entire leg. Likewise, the adjustable thigh support is a flannel-lined foam support that fastens around the thigh and strengthens the entire leg.

stance ataxia An inability to stand upright due to disturbed coordination of the involved muscles, which results in swaying and a tendency to fall in one or another direction.

statins Common cholesterol-lowering medications. Preliminary studies suggest statins may be also helpful in improving symptoms in patients with relapsing-remitting multiple sclerosis (MS). Statins help block production of immune factors involved in MS that lead to disability. Their ability to promote an anti-inflammatory response from the immune system suggests a potential treatment for MS.

Because standard MS drug treatments are expensive and only partly effective, scientists are always looking for newer, better medications. New research is needed to determine more precisely the clinical effects, best dose, therapeutic window, and potency of statins and also to evaluate whether using a combination of drugs might be more effective than using one drug alone. The most significant advantage of statins over existing MS therapies is that statins can be administered by mouth.

Atorvastatin (Lipitor) was the drug used in a 2002 animal study that suggested statins might improve symptoms. Other statin drugs include lovastatin (Mevacor), pravastatin (Pravachol), simvastatin (Zocor), and fluvastatin (Lescol).

statistics   An estimated 2,500,000 people in the world have multiple sclerosis (MS). Women outnumber men with the disease by 50 percent (that is, three women have the condition for every two men). About 33 percent of people with MS are not severely affected by MS and live normal and productive lives. On the other hand, in a significant group (33 percent), the disease becomes more progressive and disabling.

stem cell transplantation   See BONE MARROW TRANSPLANTATION.

steroids   See CORTICOSTEROIDS.

stress   Although stress does not cause multiple sclerosis (MS), it may temporarily worsen symptoms. Such symptoms may include poor concentration, MEMORY LOSS, ANXIETY, poor problem solving, or a host of physical problems. Some people with MS report having relapses after experiencing a severe emotional trauma such as the death of a close relative or the breakup of a relationship, but the relationship between stress and the onset or worsening of MS has not been confirmed in controlled research.

Extensive research suggests that although some types of physical stress (such as whiplash following a car accident) do not cause a relapse, physical stress such as HEAT does seem to worsen symptoms in many patients. However, there is no proof that heat can trigger a relapse.

Although exercise could be considered somewhat stressful, research suggests that moderate exercise boosts patients' feelings of well-being and modestly increases strength and conditioning.

Avoiding stress is a good idea for anyone, but it is not always possible. Learning how to handle stress

makes particular sense for patients with MS. In fact, one 2002 study reported fewer stress-related brain lesions in patients who reduced stress by learning how to cope using cognitive-behavioral methods.

Relaxation techniques (such as meditation, controlled breathing, and listening to soothing music) can be helpful. Other patients find a lukewarm bath or watching TV can ease stress. Hot baths should be avoided since they can temporarily worsen symptoms. If stress continues to be a problem, patients may want to consult a mental health expert.

superior colliculus   Nuclei within the thalamus (part of the brain) that are most critical in carrying out the function of vision. This structure got its name by the way it looked to early scientists. The colliculi are two pairs of "hills" on top of the midbrain (brain stem); the highest (or superior) two deal with vision.

supplementary motor area   A structure in the frontal lobe of the brain that receives input fibers from the basal ganglia and sends output back to the basal ganglia, the reticular formation, and the motor cortex. The supplementary motor area is involved in planning and initiating movement. A malfunction in this area can interfere with voluntary movement and speech.

surgery and MS   No evidence suggests that surgery triggers a worsening of symptoms in multiple sclerosis (MS). Most people with MS can tolerate standard anesthesia without extra risk. Most people with MS are young, otherwise healthy adults whose risks during elective surgical procedures are about the same as those of the general population. Having MS is not usually a reason to avoid having surgery.

Some people with MS who are severely disabled or have breathing problems may require special anesthesia considerations. In general people with MS who have surgery do not experience flares; however, infection or fever may aggravate MS symptoms. Moreover, patients with MS who have muscle WEAKNESS and who have been confined to bed may find recovering from surgery to be harder. PHYSICAL THERAPY is often useful in these instances and should be started as soon after surgery as possible.

swallowing problems   Having problems with swallowing food and beverages is a common symptom in patients with advanced multiple sclerosis (MS).

Symptoms and Diagnostic Path

A SPEECH-LANGUAGE PATHOLOGIST can best diagnose and treat swallowing problems in people with MS. To evaluate a swallowing problem, the speech-language pathologist first takes a careful history and neurologic examination of the tongue and swallowing muscles. The patient will probably be asked to swallow a barium liquid while X-rays of the mouth and throat are taken. This can identify the precise location and manner of a swallowing defect.

Treatment Options and Outlook

Swallowing problems can be treated with specific exercises to improve muscle strength or coordination. The therapist may recommend a change in the position of the head or certain head movements to improve swallowing and reduce coughing.

Risk Factors and Preventive Measures

Certain food safety rules may help those with swallowing problems avoid dehydration, poor nutrition, or the risk of ASPIRATION PNEUMONIA. Patients should:

- sit upright or lean slightly forward when eating or drinking
- keep the chin parallel with the table or slightly tucked down
- begin a meal with something cold, such as a sherbet shake or a fruit or vegetable smoothie
- take one small bite or sip at a time
- never try swallowing twice in a row
- never wash down food with a liquid
- eat soft, moist foods and drink thick, cold liquids first since these are easiest to swallow; dry solids and thin liquids are more difficult to swallow
- avoid drinking thin liquids when tired; thin beverages are best drunk in the morning and thick beverages in the evening
- drink something cold if swallowing becomes more difficult
- try to be calm and quiet during a meal
- swallow solids at least two times per mouthful (the first time to get the food down, followed by a dry swallow to catch any leftover bits)
- when drinking hot, thin liquids, swallow, clear the throat, and then swallow again before taking another sip

Swank low-fat diet   A DIET developed for people with multiple sclerosis (MS) that is low in saturated fat and relatively rich in polyunsaturated oils (supplemented with fish oil). The meal plan, developed by Roy L. Swank, M.D., Ph.D., also advocates getting plenty of rest, relieving stress, and maintaining a positive mental attitude. The diet has been used by patients with MS for more than 35 years. Dr. Swank developed the unsaturated-fatty-acid hypothesis, showing that a reciprocal relationship of fat and oil consumption existed in his MS patients on the low-fat diet. Dr. Swank found that although the diet was not a cure, his subjects did best when the fat intake was very low and oil intake was relatively high. His patients fared less well with high fat intake.

To obtain maximum benefit from treatment, Dr. Swank advocates that patients go on the diet as early as possible, while their symptoms are transient and before a major disabling MS attack occurs.

Symadine   See AMANTADINE.

Symmetrel   See AMANTADINE.

symptoms of MS   See CLINICAL SIGNS AND SYMPTOMS.

synapse   The point at which a nerve impulse passes from the AXON of one NEURON to a DENDRITE of another. To send a signal, one neuron transmits an electrical signal to another by firing across the synapse gap between adjacent dendrites, which triggers the release of chemical messengers that diffuse across the spaces between cells, attaching themselves to receptors on the neighboring nerve cell. The receiving dendrite has receptors that recognize the chemical transmitter and speeds the signal through the neuron. The human brain contains about 10 billion neurons joined together by about 60 trillion synapses.

tactile vibration test A sensory challenge test, often used as part of a NEUROLOGICAL EXAMINATION in the assessment of multiple sclerosis, that measures a patient's ability to perceive tactile vibrations. In this assessment, a doctor taps a tuning fork and touches the fork to a part of the person's body (such as a toe bone). If the person's ability to perceive vibrations is not dysfunctional, he or she will be able to identify the moment when the vibration stops. Those who cannot identify the ceasing of the vibration may have neurological problems.

tandem gait A test of balance and coordination that involves alternately placing the heel of one foot directly against the toes of the other foot.

Taxol See PACLITAXEL.

T cell A white blood cell that develops in the bone marrow, matures in the thymus, and works as part of the immune system to increase the production of antibodies by B-cells. These suppressor T cells suppress B-cell activity; their levels fall during a flare-up of multiple sclerosis activity.

Most experts believe that the destruction of MYELIN (DEMYELINATION) seen in multiple sclerosis (MS) is caused by an abnormal autoimmune process—by activation of T cells against some component of central nervous system myelin. Myelin is the fatty substance that covers and protects nerves. Demyelination slows or stops nerve impulses and produces the symptoms of MS.

Types of T Cells

There are three broad types of T cells—helper T cells, suppressor T cells, and killer T cells. Helper T cells boost the immune response by recognizing the presence of a foreign antigen and then triggering antibody production, producing cytokines that activate other T cells. Suppressor T cells function in the opposite way, turning off the immune response. Killer T cells (also called cytotoxic T cells) directly attack and destroy antigenic material.

Individual T cells are able to recognize only certain antigens. Their ability to discriminate among antigens is conferred by protein molecules on each T cell's surface called receptors. A receptor and an antigen fit together only when their shapes match perfectly. The number and specificity of T cell receptors appear to be determined by the cell's genes.

Scientists have learned a great deal about the specific roles of T cells in MS. For example, researchers have discovered that suppressor T cell function drops in the peripheral blood of MS patients during an acute flare. They also have discovered higher numbers of helper T cells in the spinal fluid and higher numbers of helper T cells passing into the brain from peripheral blood, which then attract other immune cells into the brain. Moreover, there are T cells in MS lesions and an increased frequency of activated T cells against the myelin seen in MS patients as compared with healthy controls.

The abnormal autoimmune process that causes the destruction of the myelin typical in MS seems to involve selective activation of helper T cells and killer T cells, with a corresponding decrease in suppressor T cells. These findings suggest ways to treat MS, such as by using therapies that target only specific T cells or T cell receptors that are sensitized to myelin. Some of these approaches, such as the use of MONOCLONAL ANTIBODIES against certain T cells, have been successful in treating animals with EXPERIMENTAL AUTOIMMUNE ENCEPHALOMYELITIS, an animal model of MS.

In the future, treatments may involve antibodies directed against the cytokines that turn on the T cells or therapy designed to desensitize or inhibit T cell activity. Scientists have concluded that T cells and their cytokines are the keys to the autoimmune process of MS. Continuing research may provide new, specific immunotherapies that will stop the progression of MS without harming any immune cells that are not involved in myelin destruction.

Tegretol   See CARBAMAZEPINE.

tenotomy   An irreversible surgical procedure that cuts severely contracted tendons attached to muscles that do not respond to any other type of SPASTICITY control and are causing intractable pain and skin complications related to lack of physical movement.

thalamotomy   A type of surgery, in which the part of the THALAMUS generating a tremor is destroyed by freezing or cutting. This rare surgery is sometimes recommended for people with MS with extreme chronic cerebellar tremor that has not responded to other types of treatment.

thalamus   The first part of the brain to receive messages from the body about heat and cold, pain, and pressure. As the part of the brain that automatically responds to extremes in temperature and pain, the thalamus is critical to states of awareness and all sensor-motor function. Named for the Greek word for "chamber," the thalamus serves as the entrance chamber to the perceptual cortex and is also important in the factual memory circuit.

The thalamus is a bit smaller than the cerebellum. It is found deep inside the hemispheres of the cerebrum, above the hypothalamus.

tic doloreux   See TRIGEMINAL NEURALGIA.

tickle sensation test   A type of sensory test used as part of a NEUROLOGICAL EXAMINATION, in which a doctor uses a feather or bit of tissue paper to stroke the patient's cheek. Healthy patients should be able to feel the same sensation on both sides of the face; people with a neurological problem may not.

timed 25 foot walk (T25-FW)   A mobility and leg function performance test based on a timed 25-foot walk. Gait speed in general has been demonstrated to be a useful and reliable functional measure of walking ability. It is one component of the Multiple Sclerosis Functional Composite test.

For this test, the person is directed to one end of a clearly marked 25-foot course and instructed to walk as safely and quickly as possible. The time begins with the instruction to start, and ends when the person has reached the 25-foot mark. The task is immediately administered again by having the person walk back the same distance. During the test, patients may use assistive devices, such as canes or crutches.

The test should take between one to five minutes; the score is calculated by averaging two completed trials.

Tinetti Assessment Tool   This easily administered test measures gait and balance, and is scored on a three-point scale to assess a person's ability to perform specific tasks. Scores are combined to form three measures: an overall gait assessment, an overall balance assessment, and a gait and balance score. The scores can be interpreted with regard to risk for falls.

tissue donor programs   A type of research program that provides BRAIN tissue for researchers studying the pathology of multiple sclerosis (MS)—its nature, cause, and effects on the brain. When a patient with MS dies, the brain can be donated to an MS tissue bank—an area in a laboratory or medical center where tissue specimens are stored for later use by researchers studying MS. The MS tissue banks store brain and spinal cord tissues, spinal fluid, and other specimens from persons who had the disease during their lifetimes. These samples must be frozen or otherwise preserved immediately after the death of the donor and carefully cataloged with information about each donor's medical history.

For those considering donating tissue, planning ahead is essential. Brain tissue must be prepared within hours after death to be of use in research. For contact information for tissue banks, see Appendix I.

titubation   A form of tremor, typically appearing primarily in the head and neck, caused by DEMYELINATION in the cerebellum.

tizanidine (Zanaflex)   A short-acting drug used in multiple sclerosis (MS) to treat the increased muscle tone associated with SPASTICITY. Although tizanidine does not provide a cure for the problem, it is designed to provide short-term relief from the spasms, cramping, and tightness of muscles. In order to minimize unwanted side effects with this medication, the physician typically starts the patient on a low dose and gradually increases it until a well-tolerated and effective level is reached.

Because peak effectiveness occurs one to two hours after dosing and ends between three to six hours after dosing, a physician will prescribe a dosing schedule that provides the most relief during activities and periods of time when it is most important that the patient have symptom relief.

Side Effects

Common side effects that should be reported to the doctor as soon as possible include burning, prickling, or tingling sensations; diarrhea; fainting; fever; loss of appetite; nausea; nervousness; pain or burning during urination; skin sores; stomach pain or vomiting; yellow eyes or skin; and blurred vision. Since telling the difference between common symptoms of MS and some side effects of tizanidine may be difficult, patients should consult a doctor if a symptom suddenly appears while on this drug.

This medication will also increase the effects of alcohol and other central nervous system depressants (such as antihistamines, sedatives, tranquilizers, prescription pain medications, seizure medications, and other muscle relaxants), possibly causing drowsiness.

Common side effects include: dryness of mouth; sleepiness or sedation; weakness, fatigue, and or tiredness; dizziness or light-headedness, especially when getting up from a sitting or lying position;

increase in muscle spasms, cramps, or tightness; and back pain. These side effects may go away as the body adjusts to the medication and do not require medical attention unless they continue for more than two weeks or are bothersome.

Because birth control pills may slow the release of tizanidine, women using this type of contraception should tell their doctor so that the dose level of tizanidine can be reduced.

Studies of tizanidine have not been conducted in pregnant women. Animal studies, using significantly higher doses than those prescribed for humans, have resulted in damage to the offspring. If a patient is pregnant or planning to become pregnant, she should discuss this with her physician before starting this medication. It is not known whether tizanidine is passed into breast milk, so women should not take tizanidine while nursing unless told to do so by a physician.

Tofranil   See IMIPRAMINE.

toileting aids   See BATHROOM AIDS.

tolterodine tartrate (Detrol)   An antispasmodic medication used to treat overactive bladder with symptoms of urinary incontinence, urgency, and frequency. This medication is used to relax the bladder muscle and is designed to cause some urine retention and slow the frequency of urination.

T1 (enhancing) lesions   Lesions that indicate current inflammatory disease activity. To detect these enhancing lesions, a T1 MAGNETIC RESONANCE IMAGING (MRI) scan is prescribed. During the test, GADOLINIUM is injected to highlight the areas with active lesions on the MRI scan.

tonic seizure   An intense spasm that lasts for a few minutes and affects one or both limbs on one side of the body. Like other types of PAROXYSMAL SYMPTOMS in multiple sclerosis, these spasms occur abruptly and fairly frequently in those individuals who have them and are similar from one brief episode to the next. The attacks may be triggered by movement or occur spontaneously.

transcutaneous electric nerve stimulation (TENS)
A nonaddictive and noninvasive method of pain control that applies electric impulses to nerve endings via electrodes attached to a stimulator placed onto the skin. The electric impulses block the transmission of pain signals to the brain.

transverse myelitis   An acute attack of inflammatory DEMYELINATION that involves both sides of the spinal cord so that nerve impulses can no longer be transmitted up and down. Paralysis, weakness and numbness are experienced in the legs and trunk below the level of the inflammation. Symptoms develop rapidly and may also include back pain, bowel dysfunction, and bladder dysfunction. There is no cure, but medications may be used to treat symptoms.

trauma (injury) and MS   Although a link between traumatic injury and multiple sclerosis (MS) has been debated for years, most recent research has concluded that physical trauma does not exacerbate or trigger the onset of symptoms of MS.

In one prospective study conducted by researchers at the University of Arizona, 170 patients with MS and 134 controls were followed for eight years. The results of this study, published in 1991 in the journal *Neurology, Neurosurgery, and Psychiatry,* concluded that except for electrical injuries, there was no evidence of a direct relationship between traumatic injury and an MS flare. A second study at the Mayo Clinic supported the Arizona findings. The Mayo study also indicated there is no relationship between traumatic injury and MS onset. This study, published in 1993, was based on the detailed clinical records of 164 long-term patients with definite MS who were actively followed at the Mayo Clinic.

Both studies also showed that people with MS experienced more traumatic events than did the healthy control group, probably because many traumas were caused by MS symptoms such as UNCOORDINATION, BALANCE PROBLEMS, GAIT PROBLEMS, or VISUAL PROBLEMS. However, researchers emphasized that these events did not trigger the onset or worsening of the disease.

treatment of MS   See MULTIPLE SCLEROSIS.

tremor   See MULTIPLE SCLEROSIS.

trigeminal neuralgia   A problem with the fifth cranial nerve (trigeminal nerve) that causes brief episodes of stabbing PAIN in the face, involving the cheek, lips, chin, or gums on one side. Typically, it is one of the first signs of multiple sclerosis (MS) and usually begins in one particular trigger point. It is often brought on by touching the face, talking, chewing, or swallowing. Its nickname, tic douloureux (painful twitch), refers to the fact that the intense pain often causes wincing.

Attacks recur in clusters of brief episodes that may last for weeks; the recurrences tend to occur closer and closer together with time. The problem often waxes and wanes, and successive recurrences may be incapacitating. Due to the intensity of the pain, even the fear of an impending attack may interfere with activities of daily living.

Treatment Options and Outlook
If nonprescription painkillers fail to alleviate facial pain, it can be treated with the anticonvulsive medication CARBAMAZEPINE (Tegretol), which may suppress the pain in most people. (Carbamazepine is also effective on other types of MS pain and spasm-related symptoms, including itching and aching.) However, others develop a resistance to the drug.

Another antiseizure drug, GABAPENTIN (Neurontin), however, may be particularly effective for MS. This medication also appears to improve blurred vision associated with MS and may help spasticity in general.

Phenytoin (Dilantin), BACLOFEN, clonazepam, diazepam (Valium), pimozide (Orap), the antidepressant amitriptyline (Elavil), or valproic acid may also be effective. They may be used in combination to achieve pain relief.

If severe pain persists and interferes with function, some patients choose to have a section of a nerve surgically removed or blocked, stopping the pain but causing NUMBNESS. Before patients commit to such a procedure, experts suggest they ask the doctor to block the nerve temporarily with an anesthetic in order to experience the effect of numbness before undergoing irreversible surgery.

See also TRIGEMINAL NEURALGIA ASSOCIATION.

types of MS   There are several types of multiple sclerosis (MS), each of which might be mild, moderate, or severe. Although every individual will experience a different combination of MS symptoms, there are a number of distinct patterns relating to the course of the disease.

Relapsing-Remitting MS

This type of MS is the most common, and is characterized by clearly defined flare-ups (also called relapses, flares, attacks, or exacerbations). These are episodes of acute worsening of neurologic function, followed by partial or complete recovery periods (remissions) free of disease progression.

Primary-Progressive

People with this type of MS experience a slow but nearly continuous worsening of their disease from the onset, with no distinct relapses or remissions. However, there are variations in rates of progression over time, occasional plateaus, and temporary minor improvements. This form of MS is relatively rare, affecting about 10 percent of patients.

Secondary Progressive MS

People with this type of MS experience an initial period of relapsing-remitting disease followed by a steadily worsening disease course, with or without occasional flares, minor remissions, or plateaus. Before introduction of the DISEASE-MODIFYING AGENTS, about half of those with relapsing-remitting MS developed this form of the disease within 10 years of their initial diagnosis. Long-term data are not yet available to demonstrate if this development is significantly delayed by treatment.

Progressive-Relapsing MS

This form of the disease that steadily worsens from the beginning with obvious, acute attacks along the way, with or without recovery. In contrast to relapsing-remitting MS, the periods between relapses are characterized by continuing disease progression. This type of MS is relatively rare and occurs in about 5 percent of people with MS.

Tysabri   See DISEASE-MODIFYING AGENTS.

U

Uhthoff's sign A symptom of multiple sclerosis in which a person's vision becomes blurred when the body gets overheated.

umbilical cord blood donation The blood in umbilical cords is being studied for potential use in a wide variety of life-threatening diseases because it is a rich source of blood stem cells. There is no solid evidence, however, that umbilical cord blood stem cells can be transformed into other types of cells such as replacement nerve tissue or MYELIN-producing cells in multiple sclerosis (MS).

Although transplantation of blood stem cells from umbilical cords has been used successfully to treat several pediatric blood diseases, including sickle cell anemia, leukemia, and lymphoma, the procedure is still considered experimental. Currently, research is being conducted using umbilical cord blood cells to analyze immune response and other factors that may eventually shed light on the causes and treatment of MS.

In addition, researchers are studying BONE MARROW TRANSPLANTATION (also called hemopoietic stem cell transplantation) for the treatment of severe forms of MS. However, the long-term benefits of this experimental procedure have not yet been established. In this procedure, the individual receives grafts, often of his or her own blood stem cells.

The American Academy of Pediatrics and the National Marrow Donor Program both strongly encourage umbilical cord donations for general research purposes. Potential donors should contact a cord blood bank by the 35th week of pregnancy. To obtain the cord blood, the umbilical cord is clamped after the baby has been delivered. The small amount of blood remaining in the umbilical cord is drained and taken to a cord blood bank. It is free to donate for public storage, but donation sites are not available in all communities at this time. Pregnant women interested in donating their baby's cord blood may contact the National Marrow Donor Program at www.marrow.org for a list of sites.

Some relatives of MS patients wonder whether it is possible to store their newborn's cord blood for the child's or a family member's future use. The American Academy of Pediatrics and the National Marrow Donor Program have issued a joint policy calling private cord blood banking for future transplantation "unwise." This is particularly pertinent to individuals with MS, for whom no research is available on the benefits of umbilical stem cell transplantation.

uncoordination One of the primary symptoms of multiple sclerosis (MS) involves loss of coordination, most typically affecting balance, so that walking becomes quite difficult. People with MS find climbing up and down stairs or riding a bike to be difficult. Fine-motor coordination also may be affected, so writing neatly or putting a key into a lock becomes difficult for the person.

See also BALANCE PROBLEMS; GAIT PROBLEMS.

urinary tract infection (UTI) Infection in the urinary tract (including the bladder) is a common symptom of people with multiple sclerosis (MS). Infections should be treated promptly, and their cause identified. Because infections can increase body temperature, patients may notice MS symptoms worsen in the presence of infection.

A urine culture can confirm the diagnosis of a UTI. Oral antibiotics are required for patients who have urinary frequency or urgency, fever, burning, or discomfort while urinating; blood or mucus in their urine; or foul-smelling urine. Intravenous antibiotics are required only for severe infections.

urologist A physician who specializes in the anatomy, physiology, disorders, and care of the male and female urinary tracts as well as the male genital tract.

vaccines and MS   Most vaccines are safe for people with multiple sclerosis (MS) and are not associated with an increased risk for the development of MS or OPTIC NEURITIS. Vaccines found to be safe for people with MS in a recent study published in the *Archives of Neurology* in 2003 include influenza (flu—shot only), hepatitis B, tetanus, measles, and rubella (German measles). The study evaluated data on vaccinations and other risk factors from medical records and telephone interviews with 440 people with MS or optic neuritis and 950 control subjects without neurologic disease.

In addition, a report released by the National Academy of Sciences' Institute of Medicine (IOM) says that no evidence indicates that hepatitis B vaccination causes MS or triggers MS attacks. Hepatitis B is a serious disease, complications of which can be fatal, and it is usually prevented by vaccination. This independent study by the IOM confirms previous findings of no link between vaccinations against hepatitis B and the onset or worsening of MS.

Immunizations and Multiple Sclerosis, a clinical practice guideline published by the Multiple Sclerosis Council for Clinical Practice Guidelines in 2001, concluded that people with MS should not be denied access to potentially life-saving vaccines because of their MS. The expert panel used the recommendations of the Centers for Disease Control and Prevention (CDC) as a foundation for the development of its guideline and recommended that people with MS should follow the CDC guidelines for any given vaccine.

For example, an annual flu shot is recommended for:

- adults 50 years of age and older
- residents of long-term care facilities
- individuals with chronic heart or lung conditions or other chronic diseases such as diabetes or renal dysfunction
- women who will be in their second or third trimester of pregnancy during influenza season
- groups, including household members and caregivers, who can infect high-risk persons
- any person who wants to reduce his or her chances of catching influenza

Other Vaccines

Although other vaccinations such as pneumococcus and hepatitis A do not have published studies addressing their safety in patients with MS, clinical practice guidelines recommend that people with MS who meet the CDC criteria for these vaccinations should be given them.

People with MS do have specific considerations about having a vaccine, however. For example, patients who are experiencing a serious RELAPSE that affects their ability to carry out ACTIVITIES OF DAILY LIVING should wait to be vaccinated until four to six weeks after the onset of the relapse.

People who have received immune globulin preparation in the past three months should not receive live, attenuated virus vaccinations, such as varicella or MMR (measles, mumps, rubella). Live, attenuated vaccines are those whose biological activity has been reduced so that their ability to cause disease has been weakened but not totally inactivated.

People taking IMMUNOSUPPRESSANTS such as MITOXANTRONE, AZATHIOPRINE, METHOTREXATE, CYCLOPHOSPHAMIDE, or CORTICOSTEROIDS should not receive live, attenuated vaccines. A person with a suppressed immune system would be at greater risk for developing the disease against which the vaccine is supposed to protect. (INTERFERON medications and glatiramer acetate are not immunosuppressants; people who are taking any of these medications can be given all of the vaccines mentioned above.)

Smallpox Vaccine

The smallpox vaccine has never been studied in people with MS. This vaccine, however, is used to prevent a serious, generally fatal illness and should be made available to any person with MS who is exposed to smallpox, because the risks associated with not getting vaccinated would be too great.

However, because of the serious adverse events that can occur with this vaccine, the NATIONAL MULTIPLE SCLEROSIS SOCIETY recommends that no person with MS be given it unless he or she has been directly exposed to smallpox.

Valium See DIAZEPAM.

vertigo A dizzying sensation that one is spinning or that the environment is spinning, often accompanied by nausea and vomiting. It is a fairly common symptom of multiple sclerosis (MS). Vertigo in patients with MS is due to lesions in the complex pathways that coordinate visual and spatial information sent to the brain and needed to produce and maintain equilibrium. It is often accompanied by a feeling of unsteadiness.

Treatment Options and Outlook

Usually the symptoms respond to antimotion sickness drugs such as meclizine (Antivert or Bonine), dimenhydrinate, prochlorperazine, or ondansetron. Some of these drugs may cause sedation, but they can be quite helpful in treating vertigo. In very severe cases of vertigo, a short course of corticosteroids may be needed.

In addition, PHYSICAL THERAPISTS can teach exercises to help control vertigo caused by head position changes. After determining which positions worsen vertigo, the therapist holds the patient's head in that position for a period of time. Eventually, this can produce tolerance.

vestibular nerve Part of the vestibulocochlear nerve, this nerve carries sensory impulses from the semicircular canals in the inner ear to the CEREBEL-LUM. When combined with information from the eyes and joints, this nerve helps control balance.

vestibular system The system found in the inner ear that helps a person maintain balance and allows someone to judge his or her position in space, even with the eyes shut. The three looped semicircular ducts of the system communicate with saclike structures known as the saccule and the utricle. Hair cells on each structure are linked to nerve fibers. When a person moves his or her head, fluid flows through the ducts and sacs, moving hair cells that trigger signals from nerve fibers to the brain via the eighth cranial nerve. Since different movements of the head can activate different sets of fibers, the semicircular ducts can register nodding, turning, or tilting of the head. The saccule and utricle relay to the brain the position of the head in relation to gravity. This is how a person can stand or walk in the dark.

vestibulocochlear nerve Another name for the eighth cranial nerve, this nerve is concerned with balance and hearing. It carries sensory impulses from the inner ear to the brain. The nerve enters the brain between the pons and the medulla oblongata (parts of the brain stem).

The vestibulocochlear nerve is actually made up of two parts: the vestibular nerve and the acoustic nerve (also called the cochlear or auditory nerve).

vestibulo-ocular reflex This visual reflex located in the brain stem permits continued fixation of the eyes on an object while the head is in motion. With this sophisticated reflex, the neurons of the retina, the oculomotor system, and the vestibular system combine. It can best be understood by a simple test: a person who stares at an index finger while turning the head rapidly from side to side can easily retain focus on the finger. Focusing on the finger when the head is still and the finger is moved rapidly back and forth is far more difficult.

Viagra See SILDENAFIL.

vibration sense The ability to feel vibrations against various parts of the body. Vibration sense is tested with a tuning fork as part of the sensory portion of a NEUROLOGICAL EXAMINATION.

videofluoroscopy　A radiographic study of a person's swallowing mechanism that is recorded on videotape and used to help diagnose SWALLOWING PROBLEMS in people with multiple sclerosis. Videofluoroscopy shows the physiology of the pharynx and the location of the swallowing difficulty. It also confirms whether or not food particles or fluids are being aspirated into the airway.

viruses　One of the contenders for a cause of multiple sclerosis (MS) is some type of slow virus—one that is acquired early in life but that begins its destructive effects much later. Slow viruses are known to cause other diseases, including AIDS and other autoimmune diseases.

Many claims have been made for the role of viruses as a trigger for MS; two of these include EPSTEIN-BARR VIRUS and the HERPESVIRUS 6. How a virus could trigger an autoimmune reaction is unclear.

Some experts believe that MS occurs when the immune system actually attacks a virus (one too well hidden for detection in the laboratory), and MYELIN damage is an unintentional consequence of fighting the infection. Others suggest that the immune system mistakes myelin for a viral protein, one it encountered during a prior infection. When primed for the attack, it destroys myelin because the myelin resembles the previously recognized viral invader.

Either of these models allows a role for genetic factors since certain genes can increase the likelihood of autoimmunity. Environmental factors may also change the sensitivity of the immune system or interact with myelin to provide the trigger for the secondary immune response. Possible environmental triggers that have been invoked in MS include viral infection, trauma, electrical injury, and chemical exposure.

visual evoked potentials　A test in which the brain's electrical activity in response to visual stimuli (such as a flashing light) is recorded by an electroencephalograph and analyzed by computer. DEMYELINATION (loss of the protective coating of the nerves) results in a slowing of response time. Because this test is able to confirm the presence of a suspected area of demyelination in the brain as well as identify the presence of an unsuspected lesion that has produced no symptoms, it is extremely useful in diagnosing multiple sclerosis (MS). Visual EVOKED POTENTIALS are abnormal in about 90 percent of people with MS.

visual occipital cortex　The area at the back of each cerebral hemisphere, this is the part of the brain where humans "see"—that is, where a person registers electrochemical impulses that arrive from the eyes. In the primary visual cortex, different columns of brain cells register signals from different parts of the retina. From here, the signals are passed on to nearby visual areas for more refinement. In each visual area in the visual cortex, special cells react only to signals produced by particular visual stimuli such as movements in certain directions. By working together, these visual areas of the brain help understand the size, shape, and position of objects a person sees.

visual problems　Visual symptoms are very common in people with multiple sclerosis (MS), but these conditions rarely result in total blindness. Typical visual problems common in MS include OPTIC NEURITIS, uncontrolled eye movements (NYSTAGMUS), or DOUBLE VISION.

The visual problems typically found in MS can be caused by damage to the optic nerve or by uncoordinated eye muscles, neither of which can be corrected with glasses.

Damage to the optic nerve can also cause blurred vision, which may or may not improve completely. This blurring cannot be corrected with glasses, because it is the result of nerve damage—not changes in eye shape typical of normal short- or farsightedness.

A person's ability to perceive color is especially vulnerable to damage as a result of demyelination since accurate color vision involves accurate sensory transmission along many nerve fibers from the eye to the brain.

Optic Neuritis

Messages from the eye to the brain travel along the optic nerve, which can be affected by the inflammation or demyelination so common in MS. Lesions along the nerve pathways that control eye movements and visual coordination can also cause visual problems. When these things happen, the patient may experience optic neuritis, causing a pain or a temporary loss or problem with vision. Typically, some or all of the patient's vision returns to normal within a few weeks of the attack. Although a person with MS rarely becomes totally blind, it is not unusual for a person to experience recurrent episodes of optic neuritis, usually in one eye at a time.

Optic neuritis may cause blurring or graying of vision, or blindness in one eye. It may also lead to a dark spot (SCOTOMA) in the center of the visual field that is experienced as a visual image with a dark, blank area in the middle. This is not correctable with either eyeglasses or medication, although steroids may be helpful in the early, acute phase.

Optic neuritis almost always improves by itself, and patients generally make a good recovery. If visual loss is relatively mild and manageable, experts usually recommend that the patient simply wait for the episode to end on its own.

Although episodes of optic neuritis typically improve spontaneously, in the past, acute loss of vision used to be treated fairly routinely with low doses of oral cortisone in order to end the episode more quickly. Recent research has demonstrated that high-dose corticosteroids such as methylprednisolone (Solu-Medrol) or dexamethasone (Decadron) are more effective in the treatment of optic neuritis. Today, a course of high-dose corticosteroids may be prescribed if everyday functioning becomes too impaired.

Uncontrolled Eye Movements

Uncontrolled, rhythmic horizontal or vertical eye movements (nystagmus), is another common symptom of MS. Nystagmus can range from a mild irritation (occurring only when looking to the side) so slight that the person does not perceive a problem to a severe problem that can impair vision. If nystagmus becomes troublesome, clonazepam (Klonopin) can be effective in reducing this annoy-ing but painless problem. Special prisms have also been successful in treating the visual deficits caused by nystagmus and its close cousin, jumping vision (opsoclonus).

Double Vision (Diplopia)

When the pair of muscles that control eye movement is not perfectly coordinated because of weak eye muscles, images that are not properly fused create the illusion of a double image. Diplopia usually improves without treatment, but sometimes a brief course of corticosteroids may help. During a diplopia episode, patching one eye can make driving or other short tasks easier. However, permanent patching is not recommended because it interferes with the brain's unusual ability to accommodate to the problem and produce a single image in spite of the weakened muscles. Special lenses are rarely recommended because the symptom tends to improve on its own, although some doctors prescribe glasses with special prisms to help minimize the double vision.

vitamin D and MS   A high intake of vitamin D has been linked to a lower risk of multiple sclerosis (MS), according to studies linking low vitamin D intake to a higher risk of MS and two studies linking low sunlight exposure to MS.

In the first prospective study to assess the relationship between vitamins and MS, researchers at the Harvard School of Public Health found that women with the highest intake of vitamin D supplements had a 40 percent lower risk of developing MS as compared with women who did not use supplements.

More than 185,000 healthy women from the Brigham and Women's-based Nurses' Health Study and Nurses' Health Study II filled out dietary questionnaires every four years between 1980 and 1999 that assessed their vitamin D intake along with other dietary information. During the span of the study, 173 women developed MS. When compared with women who did not use vitamin supplements, those taking the highest levels of vitamin D supplements (400 IU a day or more) had a reduced risk of 40 percent of developing MS. No reduction in risk was associated with vitamin D intake through food alone. (Foods such as milk and fish are good sources of vitamin D; the vitamin is also manufactured by the body via exposure to the Sun.)

Experts suspected that vitamin D may play a role in reducing the risk of developing MS. Since the main source of vitamin D intake among women in the study was multivitamins, isolating the effects of vitamin D use from those of other vitamins is difficult. However, none of the other vitamins was itself significantly associated a with risk of MS after adjusting for total vitamin D intake or vitamin D from supplements.

Meanwhile, two other studies pointed to the benefit of exposure to sunlight by linking a lack of exposure to vitamin D—created naturally by sunshine or artificial ultraviolet light—to a significantly increased risk for developing MS.

According to the findings of an Oxford University study, the exact causes of MS remain unknown. However, the disease becomes more common the farther away people live from the equator. Records spanning more than 35 years—from 1963 up to 1999—of people with MS and other autoimmune or neurological diseases were included in the study.

According to the study authors, a minimum level of UV exposure throughout the year might be important in conferring protection by beneficially influencing the immune system response. This may possibly occur through changes to the production of vitamin D and melanin, the substance involved in acquiring a tan.

A major problem with generating sufficient vitamin D is that so many humans live in high latitudes where, for climatic and other reasons, they are not exposed to sufficient natural sunlight.

Vitamin D is produced naturally by the body when exposed to UVB sunlight. Appropriate exposure to either natural or artificial sources of this ultraviolet light, such as tanning beds, can produce the same levels of vitamin D in the human body.

This research adds to the growing body of knowledge that points to the benefits of moderate and responsible exposure to naturally or artificially produced UVB sunlight and of the risks that come from insufficient exposure to this critical element of sunlight. Other studies in 2002 and 2003 have linked

insufficient UVB exposure to a host of other serious health problems, including rickets and diabetes.

Earlier research also points to the role of vitamin D in MS. Since levels of vitamin D in the body can predict periods of low or high MS disease activity, the higher the vitamin D, the lower the disease activity.

Although the Harvard and Oxford studies are among the first to address vitamin D deficiency and the onset of MS specifically, animal research has shown that appropriate levels of vitamin D in mice can stop or slow the progress of autoimmune diseases such as MS.

vitamins While vitamins are necessary for general good health, a well-balanced diet can usually supply all requirements. There is little evidence that multiple sclerosis (MS) is caused by a vitamin deficiency and, therefore, most experts do not suggest adding vitamins to the diet or take vitamin injections as a treatment for MS.

There have been few controlled studies to support claims that vitamins have improved MS symptoms. Most MS specialists note that people who believe vitamins are making them feel better are most probably experiencing a "placebo response." This occurs when a person who is ill perceives or actually experiences an improvement because of the psychological effect of receiving treatment, rather than from any medical or therapeutic value of the treatment.

Many experts do not recommend vitamin therapy as a treatment for MS and large doses of certain vitamins are harmful. Too much vitamin A may cause increased pressure within the skull. Too much B_6 is known to cause nerve damage and may produce symptoms similar to those seen in MS, such as numbness or tingling. Too much VITAMIN D may cause liver damage.

People with MS who believe that they are not getting sufficient nutrients in their diet should ask their health-care provider for referral to a registered dietitian.

vocational rehabilitation A program of services designed to enable people with disabilities to become or remain employed. Originally mandated by the Rehabilitation Act of 1973, vocational rehabilitation programs are carried out by individually created state agencies. These programs typically involve evaluation of the disability and need for adaptive equipment or mobility aids, vocational guidance, training, job placement, and follow-up.

See also VOCATIONAL REHABILITATION SPECIALISTS.

vocational rehabilitation specialists   Health care experts who help people with multiple sclerosis recognize their skills and abilities, explore new careers, find a job, and prepare for interviews. They also help develop safe work sites and help clients cope with work-related issues.

walkers　A metal device with four legs that can be used by a person with gait difficulties to maintain balance. Walkers may be more appropriate when there is significant leg weakness or balance problems that make walking with canes difficult.

Several different types of walkers are available, including rigid, folding, and wheeled versions. The standard walker is a rigid device usually made of aluminum whose frame can be readjusted if needed. A folding walker can be collapsed and stored when not needed. However, these walkers tend to be heavier than standard models with a more complex frame. Wheels may be added to two of the four wheels on a walker if necessary; this device is then called a ROLLATOR. Although many patients find this type of walker handy, a wheeled walker may be too unstable for some people.

Additional add-on items may include a wire basket or a utility pouch that fits across the handles to hold small items, a platform attachment for supporting arms and wrists, and a sling seat to transform a walker into a chair. In a two-story house, individuals may find that keeping two walkers, one on each floor, is more convenient.

See also ASSISTIVE DEVICES; CANES; CRUTCHES; QUAD CANE; WHEELCHAIRS.

walking　Problems in walking are some of the most common problems for patients with multiple sclerosis (MS). These problems are often related to muscle weakness, which can lead to problems such as toe drag, FOOT DROP, and other gait abnormalities. Weakness in both legs is known as PARAPARESIS; weakness in only one leg is called monoparesis. Weakness can often be compensated for with appropriate exercises and the use of assistive devices, including braces, canes, or walkers. Still, approximately 65 percent of people with MS are

able to walk 25 years after diagnosis, depending on how well they manage symptoms of weakness, tremor, balance, and coordination, and training in the use of physical aids. Exercises that help maintain range of motion and limiting stiffness play an important part in keeping a person walking in a safe and less tiring manner.

SPASTICITY or tight muscles can also cause walking problems; these can be treated with antispasticity medications such as BACLOFEN or TIZANIDINE. Stretching exercises may also help.

BALANCE PROBLEMS among people with MS typically result in a swaying gait called ATAXIA. People with severe ataxia usually require an ASSISTIVE DEVICE, such as a CANE or WALKER, in order to walk. Other patients with sensory ataxia have such severe NUMBNESS in their feet that they cannot feel the floor or know where their feet are. As FATIGUE worsens, many patients experience more problems walking.

Most gait problems can be helped to some extent by PHYSICAL THERAPY (including exercises and gait training), by the use of appropriate assistive devices, and in some cases, by medications. Each person's walking problem needs to be evaluated by a trained health care professional to determine an appropriate therapy program for that particular individual.

See also SPLINT.

water exercise　Aquatic exercise can help people with multiple sclerosis (MS) maintain muscle strength, balance, and coordination. Swimming has been called the "perfect exercise." For these patients, the cool water is an ideal place to work out, since one of the classic symptoms of MS is sensitivity to heat. The natural resistance of the water provides a source of resistance to every part of the body.

Exercise has the same benefits for people with MS that it has for everyone. However, people with poor balance, impaired coordination, and difficulty WALKING need to exercise with care, because they are at higher risk of self-injury. The risk diminishes in a swimming pool, because swimmers cannot fall and break a bone if they lose their balance. MS patients also benefit from the water's buoyancy, allowing swimmers to work with less than 20 percent of their full body weight. This is why many patients who cannot lift a foot or leg on dry land can do so in a cool pool.

The cooling effect of water at 85 degrees Fahrenheit—the temperature of a typical swimming pool—is more than 10 degrees cooler than human body temperature, which allows someone to be active without overheating. The water continuously lowers the body heat generated by the exercise.

Some MS patients do walking exercises in the pool (forward, backward, and sideways to ensure that they use as many different muscles as possible). Others do leg and arm lifts, using the resistance of the water to press against their muscles. Some use lightweight dumbbells. For people who sit most of the day, walking or even just floating in the water helps the circulation in the lower part of their bodies. The benefits include improved endurance and flexibility plus the self-esteem and sense of accomplishment of a good physical workout.

Cautions

Swimmers with MS should not swim in a pool warmer than 80–84 degrees Fahrenheit. Doing so may temporarily worsen symptoms just as would a hot shower or sauna. People with MS should also be wary of potential muscle spasms and should stay out of deep water unless another swimmer is nearby and if there is a lifeguard on duty.

Those with more severe MS who have trouble moving their arms and legs can wear inflatable floatation cuffs around their arms to maintain buoyancy.

weakness   One of the most disabling symptoms of multiple sclerosis (MS) is a feeling of weakness in the arms, legs, or face, either on one entire side of the body or in only one leg or one arm. The amount of weakness varies and may range from a slight loss of strength to total paralysis. It may appear gradually over a number of years, or it may appear quite suddenly over a period of hours.

The most common symptom of weakness is heaviness affecting one leg, making it difficult to lift, especially at the end of the day. Anyone with MS could have both legs affected. Such weakness may be particularly evident when stepping up onto a stair or curb.

Some people may experience similar sensations of heaviness or clumsiness in one or both of their arms and hands. This may affect their ability to grip, push, or lift.

Weakness caused by disuse can improve through EXERCISE to strengthen the muscle. Weakness caused by fatigue can often be treated by getting more rest. However, if the weakness is caused by poor nerve communication due to the lesions of MS, exercise or rest will not help.

No medications can improve the nerve signaling that would help strengthen weak muscles, but potassium channel blockers are being studied as a possible treatment. Early research suggests that these drugs may help, although they also cause dizziness and seizures.

weighting for tremor   Adding a weight to a part of the body may help provide increased control over movements. Weights fastened to the wrists or ankles with Velcro strips can stabilize an affected limb. Weighted boots are also used. Putting weights on canes or walkers, or using weighted spoons or forks can make these tools easier to use when tremor is active. The use of weighted devices has to be balanced against the added fatigue they might cause. Therapists commonly offer samples for a try-out.

The West Wing   A television show about a president of the United States, who has multiple sclerosis (MS). In the show, President Josiah "Jed" Bartlet, played by actor Martin Sheen, has RELAPSING-REMITTING MS. However, he did not tell either voters or his staff that fact when he ran for and won his first term as president. The character finally discloses his condition to the public when he decides to run for reelection. The show has been praised for accurately depicting the physical and emotional problems common to patients with MS.

wheelchairs Wheelchairs or three-wheeled scooters may provide more independence for people with multiple sclerosis (MS) who have little ability to walk. They make a good choice for those who experience FATIGUE, unsteadiness, or occasional falls. Eventually, about 25 percent of people with MS will need a wheelchair.

See also ASSISTIVE DEVICES; CANES; CRUTCHES; ROLLATOR; WALKERS.

white matter Another term for white nerve fibers (as opposed to cell bodies, which appear as gray). The white appearance comes from MYELIN, a fatty substance that surrounds axons, acting as an insulator to enhance electrical signals moving along the nerves. Multiple sclerosis typically affects white matter.

Williams, Montel (1956–) TV personality who was diagnosed with multiple sclerosis (MS) in 1999. Born in Baltimore, Maryland, Williams joined the U.S. Marine Corps in 1974. The next year, he became the first African-American marine selected to the Naval Academy Prep School who then went on to graduate from the Naval Academy. Upon graduation, he received a presidential appointment to the U.S. Naval Academy in Annapolis, Maryland. While at Annapolis, Williams studied Mandarin Chinese and graduated with a degree in general engineering and a minor in International Security Affairs.

He began hosting and producing his Emmy award–winning talk show, *The Montel Williams Show,* in 1990. When Williams was diagnosed with MS, he pledged to use his celebrity to help find a cure. He formed the Montel Williams MS Foundation, an organization that raises awareness of MS, educate the public about the disease, and provides financial assistance to organizations conducting MS research. Every penny of all donations goes toward the research that will lead to a cure. By 2003, the foundation granted $470,000 to MS research.

Williams wrote a book about his experience with MS, *Climbing Higher,* to share his story and encourage others with MS.

See also FAMOUS PEOPLE WITH MS.

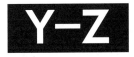

yoga and MS   Yoga—an Eastern discipline featuring controlled exercises and body positions—may be just as good as more conventional forms of EXERCISE in reducing FATIGUE caused by multiple sclerosis (MS), according to a 2004 study. Researchers at the Oregon Health Sciences University found six months of weekly yoga classes together with home practice significantly reduced general fatigue while improving vitality in people with MS. Fatigue is one of the most common and potentially disabling symptoms of the disease. The cause of MS-related fatigue is unknown, and there are no approved treatments for the problem.

Researchers say this is the first randomized, controlled trial of yoga in people with MS and shows that the mind-body exercise is as effective as traditional aerobic exercise in improving MS-related fatigue. The study involved 69 people with MS who were divided into three groups: one taking weekly Iyengar yoga classes along with home practice, another taking a weekly aerobics class using a stationary bicycle and home exercise, and a third group who did no exercise. Of the active (or hatha) yoga techniques, researchers say Iyengar yoga is the most common type of yoga practiced in the United States. The technique uses a series of stationary positions that use isometric contraction and relaxation of different muscle groups. Participants also perform breathing exercises to promote concentration and relaxation.

The study showed that MS patients in both exercise groups experienced significant improvements in two different measures of fatigue (vitality and general fatigue) compared with the control group who did no exercise. Neither exercise group reported improvements in attention or alertness.

Researchers say the study shows that regardless of the workout method, exercise seems to help MS patients reduce fatigue symptoms. This is true whether the regular exercise is yoga, swimming, using a stationary bicycle, or any other physical activity. Everyone with MS who exercises regularly reports benefit.

Zanaflex   See TIZANIDINE.

Zenapax   See DACLIZUMAB.

Zocor   See SIMVASTATIN.

APPENDIXES

APPENDIX I
ORGANIZATIONS

ADVOCACY

CLAMS: Computer Literate Advocates for Multiple Sclerosis

http://www.clams.org

This Internet support network tries to reach those who are not involved in those telephone and in-person support networks already available. CLAMS promotes activities that improve worldwide knowledge and research about MS and its etiology, diagnosis, treatments, prevention, and cure. CLAMS supports activities worldwide that make it easier for physicians, families, and caretakers to get the most recent, reliable local and international information. It maintains an up-to-date national list of GOOD-DOCS (a list prepared by people with MS featuring the names of physicians or other health-care professionals from whom they feel they have received extraordinary care).

ASSISTED LIVING

Assisted Living Federation of America (ALFA)

11200 Waples Mill Rd
Suite 150
Fairfax VA 22030
(703) 691-8100
http://www.alfa.org

An association that represents more than 7,000 for-profit and nonprofit providers of assisted living, continuing-care retirement communities, independent living, and other forms of housing and services. Founded in 1990 to support the assisted-living industry and enhance the quality of life for the consumers it serves, ALFA broadened its membership in 1999 to embrace the full range of housing and care providers who share a consumer-focused philosophy of care.

ASSISTIVE TECHNOLOGY

ABLEDATA

8630 Fenton Street
Suite 930
Silver Spring, MD 20910
(800) 227-0216 (Voice)
(301) 608-8912 (TTY)
http://www.abledata.com
E-mail: abledata@macroint.com

Sponsored by the National Institute on Disability and Rehabilitation Research, U.S. Department of Education, ABLEDATA is a source for information on assistive technology.

Center for Assistive Technology

University of Buffalo
322 Stockton Kimball Tower
Buffalo NY 14214
(800) 628-2281
http://cat.buffalo.edu

The center at the University of Buffalo that operates a free information service called Link to Assistive Products (LINK) to help people learn about assistive products and where to get them. Users will be asked to answer a few question by mail or over the telephone; the center then mails catalogs and brochures on the products that meet individual needs.

LINK is a nonprofit service to inform consumers about available products. Interested persons are under no obligation to buy anything, and no sales person has access to the names of LINK users. All personal information is held in strictest confidentiality. The project is supported by the National Institute on Disability and Rehabilitation Research.

ATAXIA

National Ataxia Foundation

2600 Fernbrook Lane

Suite 119
Minneapolis, MN 55477
(763) 553-0020
http://www.ataxia.org
E-mail: naf@ataxia.org

Nonprofit organization with 45 chapters that supports research and offers information and educational programs.

AUTOIMMUNE DISEASES

American Autoimmune Related Diseases Association
22100 Gratiot Avenue
East Detroit, MI 48201-2227
(586) 776-3900
http://www.aarda.org
E-mail: aarda@aol.com

BREAST-FEEDING AND MULTIPLE SCLEROSIS

La Leche League
1400 North Meacham Road
Schaumburg, IL 60173
(847) 519-7730
http://www.lalecheleague.org

La Leche League was founded to give information and encouragement, mainly through personal help, to all mothers who want to breast-feed their babies. While complementing the care of the physician and other health care professionals, it recognizes the unique importance of one mother helping another to perceive the needs of her child and to learn the best means of fulfilling those needs.

CAREGIVERS

Family Care America
http://www.familycareamerica.com

Family Caregiver Alliance
180 Montgomery Street
Suite 1100
San Francisco, CA 94104
(415) 434-3388
(800) 445-8106
http://www.caregiver.org

The first community-based nonprofit organization in the country to address the needs of families and friends providing long-term care at home.

During the 1980s, a small task force of families and community leaders in San Francisco created support services for those struggling to care for a loved one who did not fit into traditional health systems. This included patients with a wide variety of conditions. Although the diagnoses were different, the families shared common challenges: isolation, lack of information, few community resources, and drastic changes in family roles. FCA is now a nationally recognized information center on long-term care and the lead agency in California's system of Caregiver Resource Centers. FCA serves as a public voice for caregivers, illuminating the daily challenges they face, offering them the assistance they so desperately need and deserve, and championing their cause through education, services, research, and advocacy.

National Adult Day Services Association
2519 Connecticut Avenue NW
Washington DC 20008
(800) 558-5301
http://www.nadsa.org

The only organization that provides a focal point for adult day services at the national level. The association, formerly known as the National Institute on Adult Daycare, tries to promote the concept of adult day services as a workable community-based option for disabled older persons.

The group provides information on all aspects of adult day services; provides help to adult day service programs; works closely with national, state, and local organizations and governmental agencies; and supports research projects. The group is also interested in stimulating action on legislative, public policy, and service delivery issues.

National Association for Home Care (NAHC)
228 Seventh Street SE
Washington DC 20003
(202) 547-7424
http://www.nahc.org

The nation's largest trade association representing the interests and concerns of home care agencies, hospices, home care aide organizations, and medical equipment suppliers. NAHC members are primarily corporations or other organizations providing care directly in the home in addition to state home care associations, medical equipment suppliers, and schools. NAHC also offers individual memberships.

The association believes that Americans should receive health care and social services in their own homes as often as possible and that institutionalization should be a last resort. The association was founded in Washington, DC, in 1982 through a merger of the National Association for Home Health Agencies and the Council of Home Health Agencies/Community Health Services. In 1986, NAHC merged with the National Homecaring Council, which became part of NAHC's related Foundation for Hospice and Home Care.

National Center for Assisted Living
1201 L Street, NW
Washington, DC 20005
(202) 842-4444
http://www.ncal.org

A nonprofit organization specializing in information about assisted living as part of the American Health Care Association, the nation's largest organization representing long-term care. The diversification of long-term care has brought rapid growth to the assisted living profession, and NCAL is an essential resource for professionals in the field. The organization offers consumer education, publications, an Internet site, educational programs, and public policy advocacy. NCAL supports lobbying efforts at both the state and federal level on assisted living issues.

National Family Caregivers Association (NFCA)
10400 Connecticut Avenue
Suite 500
Kensington, MD 20895-3944
(800) 896-3650
http://www.thefamilycaregiver.org
E-mail: info@thefamilycaregiver.org

A grassroots organization created to educate, support, and empower Americans who care for chronically ill or disabled loved ones. NFCA is the only constituency organization that reaches across the boundaries of different diagnoses, different relationships, and different life stages to address the common needs and concerns of all family caregivers. Through its services in the areas of information, education, support, validation, public awareness, and advocacy, NFCA strives to minimize the disparity between a caregiver's quality of life and that of mainstream Americans.

Well Spouse Foundation
63 West Main Street
Suite H
Freehold, NJ 07728
(800) 838-0879
http://www.wellspouse.org

A national, nonprofit membership organization providing information and support to wives, husbands, and partners of patients with multiple sclerosis, among other conditions. Well Spouse support groups meet monthly to share thoughts and feelings openly, with others facing similar circumstances, in a supportive, nonjudgmental environment. Well Spouse also publishes a bimonthly newsletter, *Mainstay,* and helps set up letter writing round-robins to contact more-isolated members. Well Spouse also works to make health care professionals and the general public aware of the difficulties caregivers face.

CHILDREN AND MULTIPLE SCLEROSIS

American Academy of Child and Adolescent Psychiatry (AACAP)
3615 Wisconsin Avenue, NW
Washington, DC 20016-3007
(202) 966-7300
http://www.aacap.org

The leading national nonprofit professional medical association dedicated to treating and improving the quality of life for children, adolescents, and families affected by mental disorders. Established in 1953, its members actively research, evaluate, diagnose, and treat psychiatric disorders. The AACAP widely distributes information on mental illnesses, advances efforts in the prevention of mental illnesses, and assures proper treatment and access to services for children and adolescents.

Association on Higher Education and Disability (AHEAD)
P.O. Box 540666
Waltham, MA 02454
(781) 788-0003
http://www.ahead.org

International, multicultural organization of professionals committed to full participation in higher education for persons with disabilities.

Children's Defense Fund
25 E Street, NW
Washington, DC 20001
(202) 628-8787
http://www.childrensdefense.org
E-mail: cdinfo@childrensdefense.org

A nonprofit research and advocacy organization that provides a strong voice for children who cannot speak for themselves, including children with disabilities. The organization has regional offices throughout the country.

Disability Rights Education and Defense Fund
2212 Sixth Street
Berkeley, CA 94710
(510) 644-2555
http://www.dredf.org

A national law and policy center dedicated to protecting and helping people with disabilities through legislation, litigation, advocacy, technical help, and education.

Family Center on Technology and Disability
Academy for Educational Development (AED)
1825 Connecticut Avenue, NW
7th Floor
Washington, DC 20009-5721
(202) 884-8068
http://www.fctd.info

A resource designed to support organizations and programs that work with families of children and youth with disabilities, offering a range of information and services on the subject of assistive technologies.

Family Resource Center on Disabilities
20 East Jackson Boulevard
Room 300
Chicago, IL 60604
(800) 952-4199
(312) 939-3513
http://www.frcd.org

Coalition of parents, professionals, and volunteers dedicated to improving services for all children with disabilities.

Federation of Families for Children's Mental Health
1101 King Street
Suite 420
Alexandria, VA 22314
(703) 684-7710
http://www.ffcmh.org

A nonprofit group working for mental health rights of children.

National Clearinghouse on Women and Girls with Disabilities
114 East 32nd Street
Suite 701
New York, NY 10016
(212) 725-1803

Clearinghouse that publishes manuals, directories, and videos, many of which deal with sexual issues faced by women and girls with disabilities.

National Dissemination Center for Children with Disabilities
P.O. Box 1492
Washington, DC 20013
(800) 695-0285 (Voice/TTY)
http://www.nichcy.org

The national information center that provides information on disabilities and disability-related issues. With a special focus on children and youth, the Web site provides information about specific disabilities, special education and related services for children in school, individualized education programs, parent materials, disability organizations, professional associations, education rights, and transition to adult life.

National Parent Network on Disabilities
1130 17th Street, NW
Suite 400
Washington, DC 20036
(202) 434-8686
http://www.npnd.org

Membership advocacy organization open to all agencies, organizations, parent centers, parent groups, professionals, and individuals concerned with the quality of life for people with disabilities. Provides weekly e-mail newsletter with legislative news and more.

National Pediatric MS Center at Stony Brook University Hospital
Department of Neurology
HSC-T12-020
Stony Brook University
Stony Brook, NY 11794-8121
(631) 444-7802
http://www.pediatricmscenter.org
E-mail: info@pediatricmscenter.org

The only medical center in the United States with research and clinical programs focused on the special problems of multiple sclerosis (MS) in people younger than 17. The center offers evaluations by a treatment team that includes a pediatric neurologist, an MS specialist, a pediatric nurse practitioner, and a pediatric neuropsychologist. Children and their parents are also evaluated for counseling needs as part of good symptom management.

The center, which is affiliated with Stony Brook University, is committed to the care of children and adolescents with MS as well as those for whom the diagnosis of MS is being considered. The center's goal is to improve the diagnosis and treatment of MS in the pediatric age group and better define the emotional, clinical, and neurological complications of the disorder. The center provides clinical services, research, community, and educational outreach for all children and adolescents with MS, regardless of a family's ability to pay. The center also spearheads a nationwide research program whose ultimate goal is to find a cure for MS.

North American Children with MS Family Support Network
National MS Society
733 3rd Avenue
6th Floor
New York, NY 10017
(866) KIDS-W-MS

A collaborative program of the U.S. and Canadian MS Societies that provides multiple options for families living with a child who has been diagnosed with multiple sclerosis (MS). The network targets both children with MS under age 18 who live with their parents or guardian and the parents of a child with MS. The group provides parent teleconferences, parent support groups, short-term counseling, bulletin boards, information, referrals, and a pen pal program.

Pediatric Physical Therapy
Therapy Market Incorporated
219 Appoquin Drive
Middletown, DE 19709
http://www.pediatricphysicaltherapy.com

This site is designed for pediatric physical therapists but has helpful resources and information about current research in the field.

Sibling Support Project
Children's Hospital and Medical Center
P.O. Box 5371 CL-09
Seattle, WA 98105
(206) 368-0371
http://www.thearc.org/siblingsupport/

National program dedicated to the interests of brothers and sisters of those with special health and developmental needs.

STARBRIGHT Foundation
1850 Sawtelle Boulevard
Suite 450
Los Angeles, CA 90025
(310) 479-1212
http://www.starbright.org

Foundation dedicated to projects that empower seriously ill children to combat medical and emotional challenges. STARBRIGHT projects address the pain, fear, loneliness, and depression that can be as damaging as the sickness itself. Through the efforts of STARBRIGHT Chairmen Steven Spielberg and General H. Norman Schwarzkopf, a computer network is available where hospitalized children and teens can interact with a community of peers and help each other cope with the day-to-day realities of living with illness.

Young People with MS Connect
http://www.ms-forums.org/cgi-bin/ubbcgi/
    ultimatebb.cgi?ubb=forum;f=18

Bulletin board for young people with MS to allow communication via e-mail.

COMPLEMENTARY AND ALTERNATIVE MEDICINE
MS-CAM
http://www.ms-cam.org/
E-mail: contactus@mscenter.org

Internet Web Site sponsored by the Rocky Mountain MS Center, a nonprofit Colorado corporation. The Web Site is designed to create a worldwide community of people interested in complementary and alternative medicine (CAM) and multiple sclerosis (MS); to provide accurate, unbiased, and up-to-date information about CAM and MS; and to share the experiences of patients with particular CAM therapies.

DEPRESSION
(See also MENTAL HEALTH)

Anxiety Disorders Association of America (ADAA)
8730 Georgia Avenue
Suite 600

Silver Spring, MD 20910
(240) 485-1001
http://www.adaa.org

The ADAA promotes the prevention and cure of anxiety disorders and works to improve the lives of all people who suffer from them.

Depression and Bipolar Support Alliance (DBSA)
730 North Franklin Street
Suite 501
Chicago, IL 60610
(800) 826-3632
(312) 642-0049
http://www.dbsalliance.org

The nation's largest patient-directed, illness-specific organization, incorporated in 1986 and based in Chicago. It represents the voices of the more than 23 million Americans living with depression and another 2.5 million living with bipolar disorder (manic depression.) DBSA was formerly the National Depressive and Manic-Depressive Association.

DISABILITY

American Association of People with Disabilities
1629 K Street, NW
Suite 503
Washington, DC 20006
(800) 840-8844
http://aapd-dc.org

Organization offering emotional support, information, and support for full implementation and enforcement of disability nondiscrimination laws.

Association on Higher Education and Disability (AHEAD)
P.O. Box 540666
Waltham, MA 02454
(781) 788-0003
http://www.ahead.org

International, multicultural organization of professionals committed to full participation in higher education for persons with disabilities.

Clearinghouse on Disability Information
U.S. Department of Education
400 Maryland Avenue, SW
Washington, DC 20202
(202) 205-5465
http://www.ed.gov/about/offices/list/osers

Provides support in three key areas: special education, vocational rehabilitation, and research. Works with states, school districts, and individuals and funds programs for infants, toddlers, children, and adults with disabilities, with the goal of improving opportunities for people with disabilities of all kinds.

Commission on Mental and Physical Disability Law
American Bar Association (ABA)
740 15th Street, NW
Washington, DC 20005
(202) 662-000
http://www.abanet.org/disability/home.html

This ABA-affiliated group is committed to justice for those with physical disabilities and maintains resources and references for helping the disability community.

Disability Rights Education and Defense Fund
2212 Sixth Street
Berkeley, CA 94710
(510) 644-2555
http://www.dredf.org

A national law and policy center dedicated to protecting and helping people with disabilities through legislation, litigation, advocacy, technical help, and education.

National Association of Protection and Advocacy Systems
900 Second Street NE
Suite 211
Washington, DC 20002
(202) 408-9514
http://www.napas.org

A national membership organization for the federally mandated nationwide network of disability rights agencies, protection and advocacy systems, and client assistance programs.

National Clearinghouse on Women and Girls with Disabilities
114 East 32nd Street
Suite 701
New York, NY 10016
(212) 725-1803
E-mail: 75507.1306@compuserve.com

Clearinghouse that publishes manuals, directories, and videos, many of which deal with sexual issues faced by women and girls with disabilities.

National Institute for People with Disabilities
460 West 34th Street
New York, NY 10001
(212) 563-7474
http://www.yai.org

Nonprofit agency serving children and adults with developmental disabilities in New York, including information and referrals.

National Institute on Disability and Rehabilitative Research (NIDRR)
Office of Special Education and Rehabilitative
  Services
U.S. Department of Education
400 Maryland Avenue, SW
Washington, DC 20202
(202) 245-7468
http://www.ed.gov/offices/OSERS/NIDRR/nidrr/
  index.html

The NIDRR conducts research and administers Americans with Disabilities Act technical assistance centers.

National Organization on Disability
910 16th Street, NW
Suite 600
Washington, DC 20006
(202) 293-5960
http://www.nod.org

National disability network group concerned with all disabilities in people of all ages.

Protection and Advocacy
100 Howe Avenue
Suite 185-N
Sacramento, CA 95825
(800) 776-5746
http://www.pai-ca.org

Nonprofit agency that provides legal assistance to those with physical, developmental, and psychiatric disabilities. Services include information and referral to other help, peer, and self-advocacy training; representation in administrative and judicial proceedings; investigation of abuse and neglect; and legislative advocacy.

World Institute on Disability
510 16th Street
Suite 100
Oakland, CA 94612
(510) 763-4100
http://www.wid.org

Nonprofit public policy center dedicated to the independence and inclusion of people with disabilities.

FINANCIAL HELP

Cost Containment Research Institute
4200 Wisconsin Avenue, NW
Suite 106-222
Washington, DC 20016
(202) 318-0770
http://www.institute-dc.org

For patients concerned about the cost of getting treatment for multiple sclerosis, this organization publishes the pamphlet *Free and Low Cost Drugs* (item PD-370), available in a printed version for $5, an electronic version online for $4, or both for $7. Payment can be made online via credit card.

Needy Meds
P.O. Box 63716
Philadelphia, PA 19147
http://www.needymeds.com

For information on drug company programs that can help people obtain health supplies and equipment.

The Medicine Program
P.O. Box 515
Doniphan, MO 63935
(573) 996-7300
http://themedicineprogram.com

Provides a list of company programs that contribute drugs to physicians treating patients who could not otherwise afford medication.

GOVERNMENT AGENCIES

Food and Drug Administration (FDA)
5600 Fishers Lane
Rockville, MD 20857
(888) 463-6332
http://www.fda.gov

The FDA regulates drugs and medical devices to ensure that they are safe and effective. This government agency publishes a number of publications for consumers.

National Dissemination Center for Children with Disabilities
P.O. Box 1492
Washington, DC 20013

(800) 695-0285 (Voice/TTY)
http://www.nichcy.org/

The national information center that provides information on disabilities and disability-related issues. With a special focus on children and youth (birth to age 22), the Web site can provide information about specific disabilities; special education and related services for children in school; individualized education programs; parent materials; disability organizations; professional associations; education rights; early intervention services for infants and toddlers; and transition to adult life.

National Center for Complementary and Alternative Medicine (NCCAM)
NCCAM Clearinghouse
P.O. Box 7923
Gaithersburg, MD 20898
(888) 644-6226 (Toll-free)
(866) 464-3615 (TTY)
http://www.nccam.nih.gov

One of the 27 institutes and centers that make up the National Institutes of Health, the mission of this center is to support rigorous research on complementary and alternative medicine (CAM), to train researchers in CAM, and to provide information about which CAM modalities work, which do not, and why. Information specialists at the NCCAM Clearinghouse can answer questions about the center and CAM.

National Institute of Child Health and Human Development
P.O. Box 3006
Rockville, MD 20847
(800) 370-2943
http://www.nichd.nih.gov

Institute that supports research into the health of children and offers information on a wide variety of topics relevant to children and maternal health.

National Institute of Mental Health (NIMH)
Office of Communications
6001 Executive Boulevard
Room 8184, MSC 9663
Bethesda, MD 20892-9663
(301) 443-4513
http://www.nimh.nih.gov

The foremost mental health research organization in the world.

National Institute of Neurological Disorders and Stroke
NIH Neurological Institute
P.O. Box 5801
Bethesda, MD 20824
(800) 352-9424
(301) 496-5751
http://www.ninds.nih.gov

This federal institute conducts and supports research on many serious diseases affecting the brain.

Rehabilitation Services Administration (RSA)
400 Maryland Avenue SW
Washington, DC 20202-7100
(202) 245-7488
http://www.ed.gov/offices/OSERS/RSA/rsa.html

The RSA guides programs that help those with physical or mental disabilities get hired by providing counseling, health services, job training, and other support.

Veterans Affairs MS Centers of Excellence
http://www.va.gov/ms/

The Veterans Affairs MS Centers of Excellence states their mission as being "to provide the best possible care for veterans with MS and provide a valuable resource for MS health care providers."

HEALTH SERVICES

HRSA Information Center
Parklawn Building
5600 Fishers Lane
Rockville, MD 20857
(888) 275-4772
http://www.ask.hrsa.gov

A federal agency that can provide publications and resources on health care services for low-income, uninsured individuals and those with special health care needs. Publications are available in Spanish; Spanish speakers on staff.

National Health Information Center (NHIC)
P.O. Box 1133
Washington, DC 20013-1133
(800) 336-4797
(301) 565-4167
http://www.health.gov/nhic/

A federal health information referral service that puts health professionals and consumers who have health questions in touch with those organizations that are best able to provide answers. NHIC was established in 1979 by the Office of Disease Prevention and Health Promotion, Office of Public Health and Science, Office of the Secretary, U.S. Department of Health and Human Services.

INTERNATIONAL

European Charcot Foundation
Heiweg 97, 6533 PA Nijmegen
The Netherlands
31-24-3561954
http://www.charcot-ms.org
E-mail: info@charcot-ms.org

A nonprofit, independent organization dedicated to the advancement of multiple sclerosis (MS) research in Europe, sponsored by private organizations, MS societies, and industry. The organization was established in the Netherlands in 1990 and organized a European database for clinical description of MS (EDMUS). Its working base in Europe now consists of more than 500 institutions and 950 investigators that organize meetings and workshops, exchange MS researchers among various groups, provide information, recruit young researchers, and organize treatment trials.

International MS Support Foundation (IMSSF)
9136 East Valencia
Suite 110–PMB–83
Tucson, AZ 85747
http://www.imssf.org/ms/

A nonprofit organization devoted to multiple sclerosis (MS) education and founded in Tucson, Arizona, in 1996 by Jean Sumption, a nurse with MS. The IMSSF is independent of all other MS organizations and is staffed entirely by volunteers who have been diagnosed with MS. The foundation provides information, education, workshops, and a support network for people with MS, their families, their friends, and physicians.

Multiple Sclerosis International Foundation
3rd floor Skyline House
200 Union St.
London
SE1 OLX
+44(0) 20 7620 1911
http://www.msif.org

An international group established in 1967 to link national multiple sclerosis (MS) societies around the world. The federation's goals are to eliminate MS, support those affected by MS, and support global research and the exchange of information.

International Neural Network Society
2810 Crossroads Drive
Madison, WI 53718
(608) 443-2461
http://www.inns.org

A professional group for those interested in a theoretical and computational understanding of the brain. The group promotes research into behavioral processes and models of the brain, and it encourages development of computing applications that use neural modeling concepts. Founded in 1978, the group sponsors an annual world congress.

World Institute on Disability
510 16th Street, Suite 100
Oakland, CA 94612
(510) 763-4100
http://www.wid.org

A nonprofit public policy center dedicated to the independence and inclusion of people with disabilities.

MEDICAL MAIL-ORDER PRODUCTS

UroMed
1095 Windward Ridge Parkway
Suite 170 Alpharetta, GA 30005
(800) 403-9189
http://www.uromed.com/MS_Home.asp

Aids for daily living, incontinence supplies, and wheelchair accessories.

Walking Equipment
5539 Park Street N
St. Petersburg, FL 33709
(877) 890-7677
http://www.walkingequipment.com/lofstrand.htm

A retail outlet for walking aids of all kinds from canes to crutches.

The Wright Stuff
75 Esaias Road
Grenada, MS 38901
(662) 294-1444; (877) 750-0376 (toll-free)
http://www.thewright-stuff.com
E-mail: info@thewright-stuff.com

Products include kitchen accessories, walkers, canes, walker accessories, wheelchair accessories, magnets, exercise videos, gel cushions, gel mattresses, bathing and dressing aids, joint supports, splints, wraps, adapted utensils, reachers, bathroom safety equipment, skin creams, and more.

MENTAL HEALTH

American Psychiatric Association
1000 Wilson Boulevard
Arlington, VA 22209-3901 Suite 1825
(703) 907-7300
http://www.psych.org

A medical specialty society that works to ensure humane care and effective treatment for everyone with mental disorders, mental retardation, or substance-related disorders.

American Psychological Association
750 First Street, NE
Washington, DC 20002-4242
(800) 374-2721 (202) 336-5510
http://www.apa.org

A scientific and professional organization that represents psychology in the United States and has more than 155,000 members—the largest association of psychologists worldwide.

Center for Mental Health Services
P.O. Box 42557
Washington, DC 20015
http://www.mentalhealth.org

Federal agency that provides information and resources on mental health, including a database of community resources, an extensive catalog, events, and more. The goal of this agency is to provide the treatment and support services needed by adults with mental disorders and children with serious emotional problems.

National Institute of Mental Health (NIMH)
Office of Communications
6001 Executive Boulevard
Room 8184, MSC 9663
Bethesda, MD 20892-9663
(301) 443-4513
http://www.nimh.nih.gov

The foremost mental health research organization in the world.

MULTIPLE SCLEROSIS

Heuga Center
27 Main Street
Suite 303
Edwards, CO 81632
(800) 367-3101
http://www.heuga.org

A nonprofit organization dedicated to improving the lives of people with multiple sclerosis (MS) through educational and wellness programs. The Heuga Center was founded by former Olympic ski racer Jimmy Heuga, who was diagnosed with MS in 1970 at the height of his racing career.

The Heuga Center's programs are based on the philosophy that patients can have a chronic condition but still be healthy. By drawing on a wide range of medical professionals and focusing on many aspects of health—including exercise, nutrition, social support, and disease management—The Heuga Center helps people with MS learn how to live healthier, happier, more active lives. Programs include education, nutrition, mental well-being, and exercise as well as teaching specific, individualized life management skills and ways to integrate wellness activities into everyday life.

The center's CAN DO Program is an intensive five-day event offering comprehensive education about MS, including effects, treatment options, and lifestyle adaptations. During this program, participants develop a lifestyle prescription designed just for them. In addition, sessions for support partners provide education for parents and friends. The CAN DO Program has a two-to-one staff-to-participant ratio and provides 45 hours of group and individual service in five days.

CAN DO2 is a follow-up program for CAN DO graduates, offering a two-day educational/wellness program designed to refresh and remotivate past participants. Each CAN DO Program is limited to 15 participants and their support partners.

The Jumpstart Program introduces The Heuga Center education/wellness model and philosophy. Jumpstart Programs are held throughout the country, often in collaboration with other MS organizations or care providers.

The center is a member of the Consortium of Multiple Sclerosis Centers and works closely with the National Multiple Sclerosis Society and the American Academy of Neurology.

Multiple Sclerosis Association of America

706 Haddonfield Road
Cherry Hill, NJ 08002
(856) 488-4500
http://www.msaa.com

A national nonprofit organization established in 1970 dedicated to enhancing the quality of life for those affected by multiple sclerosis (MS) and providing support and direct services to individuals with MS. In addition to a variety of programs and services, including consultations, support groups, equipment distribution, home modifications, magnetic resonance imaging, diagnostic funding, and public awareness campaigns, the association also provides valuable information through its quarterly magazine and other literature.

Multiple Sclerosis Foundation

6350 North Andrews Avenue
Fort Lauderdale, FL 33309
(800) 225-6495
(888) MSFocus (673-6287)
htpp://www.msfocus.org
E-mail: support@msfocus.org

A national support group that provides funding for research into the cause, prevention, treatment, and cure of multiple sclerosis. The foundation also provides information, referrals, and support services. Founded in 1986, the foundation publishes a number of brochures and a quarterly newsletter.

National Institute of Neurological Disorders and Stroke

NIH Neurological Institute
P.O. Box 5801
Bethesda, MD 20824
(800) 352-9424
http://www.ninds.nih.gov

This federal institute conducts and supports research on many serious diseases affecting the brain.

National Multiple Sclerosis Society

733 3rd Avenue
6th Floor
New York, NY 10017
(212) 986-3240
(800) 344-4867
http://www.nmss.org

Through the society's 50-state network of chapters, assistance is provided to more than 1 million people each year, including people with MS, their families, employers, and caregivers. In 2003, the society had an estimated 497,000 general members; 342,000 of them indicate that they have MS.

Programs for everyone affected by MS are available at every chapter, including an equipment loan closet, a library, and an information service. Information about MS and referrals to area health care professionals and resources, and to chapter-affiliated self-help groups, are free. Free and nominal-fee programs may include education, counseling, and recreational events.

Each chapter organizes a variety of special events to raise funds and awareness. The top nationwide events are the MS 150 Bike Tours and the MS Walk, which includes more than 250,000 people each year. Many participants join teams formed at their workplace or by family and friends of people with MS.

The National Multiple Sclerosis Society spends more money on MS research than any other voluntary agency in the world. By the end of 2004, the society had invested $420 million in research since it was founded in 1946. This support has resulted in improved diagnosis, important new treatments, and better rehabilitation and symptom treatments for all forms of MS. The society supports more than 300 research projects in the U.S. and abroad every year.

The society also advocates on public policies that affect all people with MS on the local, state, and national levels. It works to improve medical care for people with MS by improving professional understanding of clinical issues. The society sponsors professional meetings, teleconferences, and accredited continuing medical education courses in collaboration with major medical centers. In addition, the Professional Resource Center provides educational materials and programs, consultation, and library search services.

Linking all these efforts is a wide-ranging communications program including the locally edited chapter newsletters, *MSConnection;* an award-winning national magazine, *InsideMS;* a Web site including individual chapter sites; professional bulletins, white papers, and other publications for the health care community; publications for people with MS (including many in Spanish); and *Keep S'myelin,* a quarterly newsletter for children.

Veterans Affairs MS Centers of Excellence

http://www.va.gov/ms/

The Veterans Affairs MS Centers of Excellence states their mission as "to provide the best possible care for veterans with MS and provide a valuable resource for MS health care providers."

MULTIPLE SCLEROSIS CLUSTERS

U.S. Centers for Disease Control Agency for Toxic Substances and Disease Registry

(888) 422-8737

http://www.atsdr.cdc.gov

E-mail:ATSDRIC@cdc.gov

Anyone can report a suspected multiple sclerosis cluster to this agency.

OCCUPATIONAL THERAPY

American Occupational Therapy Association (AOTA)

4720 Montgomery Lane

P.O. Box 31220

Bethesda, MD 20824-1220

(301) 652-2682

(800) 377-8555 (TDD)

http://www.aota.org

The AOTA Web site provides national and regional news and information about occupational therapy and related issues.

PAIN

American Chronic Pain Association (ACPA)

P.O. Box 850

Rocklin, CA 95677-0850

(916) 632-0922

(800) 533-3231

http://www.theacpa.org

Founded in 1980, the American Chronic Pain Association maintains a network of support groups to raise awareness of chronic pain and help chronic pain sufferers live a normal life.

National Chronic Pain Outreach Association (NCPOA)

P.O. Box 274

Millboro, VA 24460

(540) 862-9437

http://www.chronicpain.org

E-mail: ncpoa@cfw.com

NCPOA disseminates literature about chronic pain, including the quarterly newsletter Lifeline. The group also keeps a list of support groups and can provide aid in establishing new support groups.

National Foundation for the Treatment of Pain

P.O. Box 70045

Houston, TX 77270-0045

(713) 862-9332

http://www.paincare.org

NFTP strives to educate the public, health-care workers, insurance providers, lawyers, and others about pain and pain medication with the goal of achieving adequate pain care for all patients.

PARALYSIS

American Pain Foundation

201 North Charles Street

Suite 710

Baltimore, MD 21201

(888) 615-PAIN (7246)

(410) 783-7292

http://www.painfoundation.org

E-mail: info@painfoundation.org

Created in 1997 to increase awareness of pain management as a national health-care issue and work toward the elimination of under treatment of pain.

PEDIATRIC MS

See CHILDREN AND MULTIPLE SCLEROSIS

PHYSICAL THERAPY

American Physical Therapy Association

1111 North Fairfax Street

Alexandria, VA 22314

(800) 999-2782

(703) 684-2782 (Voice)

(703) 683-6748 (TTY)

http://www.apta.org

This site provides information on almost every aspects of physical therapy, from therapists in each state to current research.

Pediatric Physical Therapy

Therapy Mamet Incorporated

219 Appoquin Drive

Middletown, DE 19709

http://www.pediatricphysicaltherapy.com

This site is designed for pediatric physical therapists but has helpful resources and information about current research in the field.

PROFESSIONAL

American Academy of Neurological and Orthopaedic Surgeons
10 Cascade Creek Lane
Las Vegas NV 89113
(702) 388-7390
http://www.aanos.org

A professional organization of neurological and orthopedic surgeons, neurologists, and professionals in allied medical or surgical specialties. The group provides information about neurological and orthopedic medicine and surgery and seeks to improve patient care. It maintains the American Board of Neurological and Orthopedic Medicine and Surgery and the American Board of Medical-Legal Analysis in Medicine and Surgery and the American Board of Medical-Legal Analysis in Medicine and Surgery.

The group publishes the quarterly *Journal of Neurological and Orthopedic Surgery* and holds an annual scientific meeting in Las Vegas.

American Academy of Neurology
1080 Montreal Avenue
Saint Paul, MN 55116
(800) 879-1960
(651) 695-2717
http://www.aan.com

An international professional association of neurologists and neuroscience professionals specializing in nervous system diseases, dedicated to providing the best possible care for patients with neurological disorders. The academy is a medical specialty society established to advance the art and science of neurology and thereby promote the best possible care for patients with neurological disorders.

American Neurological Association
5841 Cedar Lake Road
Suite 204
Minneapolis, MN 55416
(952) 545-6284
http://www.aneuroa.org

A professional society of academic neurologists and neuroscientists devoted to advancing the goals of academic neurology; to training and educating neurologists and other physicians in the neurologic sciences; and to expanding both physicians' understanding of diseases of the nervous system and their ability to treat them. Founded in 1875, the group promotes research, bestows awards, sponsors an annual convention, and publishes the monthly *Annals of Neurology.*

International Organization of Multiple Sclerosis Nurses (IOMSN)
P.O. Box 450
Teaneck, NJ 07666
(201) 837-9241
http://www.iomsn.org

The first and only international organization focused solely on the need and goals of professional nurses throughout the world who care for people with multiple sclerosis (MS). The mission of the organization is to establish and perpetuate a specialized branch of nursing in MS, to establish standards of nursing care in MS, to support MS nursing research, and to educate the health care community. Ultimately, the IOMSN tries to improve the lives of all those persons affected by MS through the provision of appropriate health care services.

REHABILITATION

National Rehabilitation Information Center (NARIC)
4200 Forbes Boulevard
Suite 202
Lanham, MD 20706-4829
(301) 459-5900
(301) 459-5984
(800) 346-2742 (TTY)
http://www.naric.com
E-mail: naricinfo@heitechservices.com

Rehabilitation Services Administration (RSA)
400 Maryland Avenue, SW
Washington, DC 20202-7100
(202) 245-7488
http://www.ed.gov/about/offices/OSERS/RSA/rsa.html

The RSA guides programs that help those with physical or mental disabilities get hired by providing counseling, health services, job training, and other support.

RESEARCH

Boston Cure Project for MS
300 Fifth Avenue
Waltham, MA 02451

(781) 487-0008
http://www.bostoncure.org
E-mail: info@bostoncure.org

A national nonprofit organization dedicated to curing multiple sclerosis (MS) by determining its cause. The project was begun by Art Mellor, a patient with MS, and Dr. Timothy Vartanian at Beth Israel Deaconess Medical Center in Boston. The project's mission is to cure MS as quickly as possible by concentrating on the causes of the disease and by improving the way research is orchestrated, conducted, and funded.

Dana Alliance for Brain Initiatives

745 Fifth Avenue
Suite 900
New York, NY 10151
http://www.dana.org
E-mail: dabiinfo@dana.org

The Dana Alliance, a nonprofit organization of 150 neuroscientists, was formed to help provide information about the personal and public benefits of brain research.

Montel Williams MS Foundation

331 West 57th Street
PMB 420
New York, NY 10019
http://www.montelms.org
E-mail: msfoundation@montelshow.com

Nonprofit foundation founded by TV host Montel Williams, dedicated to funding research into a cure for multiple sclerosis.

Myelin Project

2136 Gallows Road
Suite E
Dunn Loring, VA 22027
(703) 560-5400
(800) 869-3546
http://www.myelin.org
E-mail: mp@myelin.org

An international grassroots organization whose mission is to accelerate medical research on myelin repair, with scientists located in the United States, Britain, France, Germany, Italy, Switzerland, and Dubai. The Myelin Project has set up a work group from among the top international laboratories specializing in myelin repair. Researchers come from Yale University and the University of Wisconsin at Madi-

son in the U.S., the Istituto Superiore di Sanità and San Raffaele Scientific Institute in Italy, the Hôpital de la Salpêtrière and the Institut Pasteur in France, the Queen's University at Kingston in Canada, the University of Cambridge in the United Kingdom, and the Max-Planck-Institut in Germany. Project funds are targeted toward clinically oriented experiments on the cutting edge of remyelination research. As of March 2004, the Myelin Project has financed 36 experiments.

National Institute of Neurological Disorders and Stroke

NIH Neurological Institute
P.O. Box 5801
Bethesda, MD 20824
(800) 352-9424
(301) 496-5751
http://www.ninds.nih.gov

This federal institute conducts and supports research on many serious diseases affecting the brain, including multiple sclerosis.

Society for Neuroscience

11 Dupont Circle, NW
Suite 500
Washington, DC 20036
(202) 462-6688
http://apu.sfn.org/
E-mail: info@sfn.org

A nonprofit professional organization of scientists and physicians who study the brain and the nervous system. Founded in 1970, the society is one of the largest organizations of scientists devoted to the study of the brain. The society's primary goal is to promote the exchange of information among researchers. The group publishes *The Journal of Neuroscience* and holds an annual convention each fall.

SERVICE DOGS

Delta Society's National Service Dog Center

875 124th Avenue, NE
Suite 101
Bellevue, WA 98005
(425) 226-7357
http://www.deltasociety.org
E-mail: info@deltasociety.org

Delta Society is a leading international resource for promoting and implementing the improvement of human health through the use of service and therapy animals.

Canine Partners for Life
P.O. Box 170
Cochranville, PA 19330
(610) 869-4902
http://www.k94life.org
E-mail: info@k94life.org

A nonprofit organization that trains and places assistance dogs with individuals who have mobility impairments to help increase independence and quality of life. Each dog is trained to meet the specific needs of the individual recipient. The organization's efforts are focused on (but not limited to) an area within a 250-mile radius of Cochranville, Pennsylvania.

Typically the waiting period for an assistance dog is six to 18 months to allow the staff to get to know applicants and their needs. The group asks for a $900 donation to be made to CPL at time of placement.

Guide Dog Foundation for the Blind, Inc.
371 East Jericho Turnpike
Smithtown, NY 11787
(631) 930-9091
http://www.guidedog.org

Through the foundation, guide dogs are available free of charge to blind or visually impaired people who seek enhanced mobility and independence.

International Association of Assistance Dog Partners (IAADP)
38691 Filly Drive
Sterling Heights, MI 48310
(586) 826-3938
http://www.iaadp.org

This nonprofit, cross-disability organization represents people partnered with guide, hearing, and service dogs.

National Education for Assistance Dog Services (NEADS)
P.O. Box 213
West Boylston, MA 01583
(978) 422-9064 (voice; TTY)
http://www.neads.org

A national, nonprofit organization established to train and provide rescued dogs and donated puppies to help people who are deaf or physically disabled in leading more independent lives at work, at home, and at school. These service dogs bring security, freedom, independence, and relief from social isolation to their human partners.

Founded in 1976, NEADS is the oldest continuing hearing dog program in the country as well as one of the largest. NEADS has trained well over 850 assistance dog teams. Among the types of dogs trained are hearing, service, social, specialty, classroom SERVICE DOGS, ministry, therapy, laptop (small lapdogs), and walker dogs. NEADS trains all breeds and mixed breeds of dogs to help people who are physically disabled, such as people with multiple sclerosis.

Most service dogs are donated as puppies by breeders throughout the country. Although most are golden or labrador retrievers, many other breeds are also suitable.

People who get dogs stay at the NEADS residence for two weeks. With careful supervision from the trainers, clients learn to handle their dogs and develop strong working relationships with them. Although the new owners pay for their dog and equipment, NEADS raises sponsorships for each person to cover the balance of the costs.

NEADS relies solely on the support of individuals, foundations, corporations, service organizations, bequests, and workplace campaigns. It receives no government funding.

SPASTICITY

Worldwide Education & Awareness for Movement Disorders (WE MOVE)
204 West 84th Street
New York, NY 10024
(800) 437-MOV2 (6682)
(212) 875-8312
http://www.wemove.org
E-mail: wemove@wemove.org

A nonprofit organization that promotes public education of movement problems, such as spasticity, plus research, rehabilitation, and support services.

SPEECH PROBLEMS

National Aphasia Association
29 John Street
Suite 1103
New York, NY 10038
(800) 922-4622
http://www.aphasia.org

A nonprofit organization that promotes public education, research, rehabilitation, and support services to assist people with aphasia and their families.

SPORTS

National Sports Center for the Disabled
Winter Park Office:
P.O. Box 1290
Winter Park, Colorado 80482
(970) 726-1540
(303) 316-1540
http://www.nscd.org

Denver Office:
633 17th Street
#24
Denver, CO 80202
(303) 293-5711
E-mail: info@nscd.org

The National Sports Center for the Disabled has specialty trained instructors and its own adaptive equipment to accommodate children and adults with almost any physical or developmental disability.

SUICIDE

American Association of Suicidology
4201 Connecticut Avenue, NW
Suite 408
Washington, DC 20008
(202) 237-2280
http://www.suicidology.org

This organization provides information on current research, prevention, ways to help a suicidal person, and surviving suicide. A list of crisis centers is available.

American Foundation for Suicide Prevention
120 Wall Street
22nd Floor
New York, NY 10005
(888) 333-AFSP
(212) 363-3500
http://www.afsp.org
E-mail: inquiry@afsp.org

This organization provides research, education, and current statistics regarding suicide. Links to other suicide and mental health sites are offered.

TISSUE DONATION

MS Human Neurospecimen Bank
Veteran Administration Medical Center
11301 Wilshire Boulevard
Los Angeles, CA 90073
(310) 268-3536
(310) 478-3711 (after hours and weekends; ask for the Brain Bank)
http://www.loni.ucla.edu/~nnrsb/NNRSB/

Individuals interested in the possibility of tissue donation can contact this tissue bank.

Rocky Mountain MS Center/Research Division
701 East Hampden
Suite 420/530
Englewood, CO 80110
(303) 788-4806
http://www.mscenter.org/pages/index2.html

Individuals interested in the possibility of tissue donation can contact this tissue bank.

TREMOR

International Essential Tremor Foundation
P.O. Box 14005
Lenexa, KS 66285-4005
(913) 341-3880
(888) 387-3667
http://www.essentialtremor.org
E-mail: staff@essentialtremor.org

Provides information, services, and support to individuals and families affected by essential tremor.

International Tremor Foundation
P.O. Box 14005
Lenexa KS 66285
(913) 341-3880
http://www.essentialtremor.org

A national support group for those suffering from tremor, their families, and their friends. Tremor is a common symptom of multiple sclerosis. The foundation promotes research and development of clinical care programs and provides patient information and referrals. The group also publishes a quarterly newsletter and sponsors educational meetings.

Tremor Action Network
P.O. Box 5013
Pleasanton, CA 94566-0513
(510) 559-4669
http://www.tremoraction.org
E-mail: Tremor@TremorAction.org

This organization works to spread awareness of essential tremor by advocating for a cure through research.

TRIGEMINAL NEURALGIA

Trigeminal Neuralgia Association
2810 SW Archer Road
Gainesville, FL 32608
(352) 376-9955
(800) 923-3608
http://www.TNA-support.org

A support group for those with trigeminal neuralgia, a neurological disorder that often accompanies multiple sclerosis and is characterized by sudden attacks of pain along the trigeminal nerve in the face and head. The group works to increase public and professional awareness, and coordinates the exchange of information.

VISUAL PROBLEMS

American Council of the Blind
1155 15th Street, NW
Suite 1004
Washington, DC 20005
(800) 424-8666
(202) 467-5081
http://www.acb.org

The nation's leading membership organization of blind and visually impaired people, founded in 1961. The council strives to improve the well-being of all blind and visually impaired people by serving as a representative national organization of blind people; elevating the social, economic, and cultural levels of blind people; improving educational and rehabilitation facilities and opportunities; cooperating with the public and private institutions and organizations concerned with services for the blind; and encouraging and assisting all blind persons to develop their abilities and conducting a public education program to promote greater understanding of blindness and the capabilities of blind people.

American Foundation for the Blind (AFB)
11 Penn Plaza
Suite 300
New York, NY 10001
(800) AFB-LINE
(212) 502-7600
http://www.afb.org

Since 1921, the AFB—to which Helen Keller devoted her life—has been eliminating barriers that prevent the 10 million Americans who are blind or visually impaired from reaching their potential. The AFB is dedicated to addressing the most critical issues facing this growing population: independent living, literacy, employment, and technology.

American Nystagmus Network
303-D Beltline Place
#321
Decatur, AL 35603
http://www.nystagmus.org

A nonprofit organization established in February 1999, to serve the needs and interests of those affected by nystagmus.

Association for Education and Rehabilitation of the Blind and Visually Impaired
1703 North Beauregard Street
Suite 440
Alexandria, VA 22311
(877) 492-2708
http://www.aerbvi.org

The only international membership organization dedicated to helping professionals in all phases of education and rehabilitation of blind and visually impaired children and adults. It was formed in 1984 as the result of a consolidation between the American Association of Workers for the Blind and the Association for Education of the Visually Handicapped.

Helen Keller National Center for Deaf/Blind Youth and Adults (HKSB)
111 Middle Neck Road
Sands Point, NY 11050
(516) 944-8900
http://www.helenkeller.org

A nonprofit agency with a spectrum of special services that guide legally blind New Yorkers toward a life of independence and success. With its diverse services, the HKSB often works one-on-one to teach, educate, and rehabilitate thousands of clients according to their individual needs. Its facilities throughout metropolitan New York serve residents of Brooklyn, Queens, Staten Island, and Nassau and Suffolk Counties. The HKSB, founded in 1893 as the Industrial Home For The Blind, is one of the oldest continuously operated rehabilitation agencies in the United States. In 1986, the agency was renamed after Helen Keller.

National Association for the Visually Handicapped

22 West 21st Street
6th Floor
New York, NY 10010
(212) 889-3141

3201 Balboa Street
San Francisco, CA 94121
(415) 221-3201
http://www.navh.org

This nonprofit association works with millions of people worldwide coping with difficulties of vision impairment.

National Federation of the Blind (NFB)

1800 Johnson Street
Baltimore, MD 21230
(410) 659-9314
http://www.nfb.org

Founded in 1940, the NFB is a consumer and advocacy organization and the nation's largest membership organization of blind persons.

National Library Service for the Blind and Physically Handicapped (NLS)

Library of Congress
1291 Taylor Street, NW
Washington, DC 20011
(202) 707-5100 (Voice)
(202) 707-0744 (TTY)
http://www.loc.gov/nls

Through a national network of cooperating libraries, the NLS administers a free library program of braille and audio materials circulated to eligible borrowers in the United States by postage-free mail.

APPENDIX II
NATIONAL MS SOCIETY–
AFFILIATED CLINICAL FACILITIES

ALABAMA

Joanne P. LaGanke MS Center
North Central Neurology
1890 Alabama Highway 157
Suite 420
Cullman, AL 35058
(256) 739-1210

Neurology Department, University of Alabama at Birmingham, School of Medicine
Health Services Foundation, PC
Kirklin Clinic
2000 6th Avenue South
5th Floor
Birmingham, AL 35233
(205) 934-1885

Tanner Center for Multiple Sclerosis
HealthSouth Medical Center
1201 11th Avenue South
Birmingham, AL 35205
(205) 930-6767

ARIZONA

Barrow Neurology Clinic
MS and Related Diseases Clinic
500 W. Thomas Road
Suite 300
Phoenix, AZ 85013
(602) 406-6209

Mayo Clinic, Scottsdale
13400 East Shea Boulevard
Scottsdale, AZ 85259
(480) 301-8111

CALIFORNIA

Cedars Sinai Medical Center MS Treatment Center
8631 West 3rd Street

Suite 215 East Tower
Los Angeles, CA 90048
(310) 423-2474

East Bay Neurology
3000 Colby Street
#101
Berkeley, CA 94705
(510) 849-0499

Fountain Valley MS Clinic
11190 Warner Avenue
Fountain Valley, CA 92708
(714) 545-8016

HealthSouth Tustin Rehabilitation
Outpatient Clinic
621 West 1st Street
Tustin, CA 92780
(714) 838-7705

Kaiser-Permanente Medical Center
900 Kiely Boulevard
Santa Clara, CA 95051
(408) 236-4999

MS Clinic
Department of Rehabilitation
Santa Clara Valley Medical Center
751 South Bascom Avenue
San Jose, CA 95128
(408) 885-2000

MS Clinic
Loma Linda University Neurology Associates
Medical Group
11370 Anderson Street
Suite 2400

Loma Linda, CA 92354
(909) 558-2120

**MS Comprehensive Care Center at USC
University Hospital**
1510 San Pablo Street
Suite HCC 637
Los Angeles, CA 90033-4606
(323) 442-6870

MS Service
1844 San Miguel Drive
#316
Walnut Creek, CA 94596
(925) 938-5252

**Multiple Sclerosis Clinic at Harbor-UCLA
Medical Center**
1000 West Carson Street
Torrance, CA 90505
(310) 222-3897

Neurology Group of Diablo Valley
130 La Casa Via
#206
Walnut Creek, CA 94520
(925) 939-9400

Northridge MS Center
18433 Roscoe Blvd.
Suite 206
Northridge, CA 91325
(818) 349-2503

**Rancho Los Amigos Medical Center Multiple
Sclerosis Clinic**
Division of Neurosciences
7601 East Imperial Way
Building 100
Downey, CA 90242
(562) 401-7115
(562) 401-7093

Reed Neurological Research Center, UCLA
P.O. Box 951769
Los Angeles, CA 90095-1769
(310) 825-7313

St. Mary's Hospital, MS Clinic
2250 Hayes Street
Level C
San Francisco, CA 94117
(415) 750-5762

**Transitions Rehabilitation Multiple Sclerosis
Clinic**
7101 Monterey Street
Suite A
Gilroy, CA 95020
(408) 842-6868

**UCLA Medical Center, Multiple Sclerosis
Center**
300 Medical Plaza
Suite B200
Los Angeles, CA 90024-6975
(310) 794-1195

UCSD MS Center
200 West Arbor Drive
Neurology, 3rd Floor
San Diego, CA 92103
(858) 642-1279

UCSF Multiple Sclerosis Center
350 Parnassus Avenue
Suite 908
San Francisco, CA 94117
(415) 514-1684

University of California
100 Irvine Hall
Irvine, CA 92717
(714) 824-5692

West Los Angeles VAMC
11301 Wilshire Boulevard
Los Angeles, CA 90073
(310) 268-3891
(310) 268-3013

COLORADO

MS Center of Southern Colorado
HealthSouth Rehabilitation Hospital
325 Parkside Drive
Colorado Springs, CO 80910
(719) 630-2338

MS Clinic at Denver Health Medical Center
700 Delaware Street
Denver, CO 80204
(303) 436-6065

Western Slope Multiple Sclerosis Clinic
St. Mary's Hospital
Grand Junction, CO 81506
(970) 241-9329

CONNECTICUT

Gaylord Hospital Multiple Sclerosis Clinic
P.O. Box 400
Wallingford, CT 06492
(203) 284-2888

West Haven VAMC
Multiple Sclerosis Program
950 Campbell Avenue
West Haven, CT 06516
(203) 937-4735

Yale University School of Medicine MS Clinic
40 Temple Street
Suite 7-I
New Haven, CT 06510-8018
(203) 764-4280

FLORIDA

Halifax Multiple Sclerosis Center
303 North Clyde Morris Boulevard
201 Building
Daytona Beach, FL 32114
(386) 226-4506

HealthSouth Doctors' Hospital
5000 University Drive
Miami, FL 33146
(305) 666-2111

HealthSouth Sea Pine Rehabilitation Hospital
101 East Florida Avenue
Melbourne, FL 32901
(321) 984-4600

MS Clinic at North Ridge Neuroscience Center
5757 North Dixie Highway
Ft. Lauderdale, FL 33334
(954) 928-0611

MS Clinic HealthSouth Rehabilitation
3251 Proctor Road
Sarasota, FL 34231
(941) 921-8600

**North Florida Multiple Sclerosis
  Comprehensive Care Center**
St. Luke's Hospital
4203 Belfort Road
Rodger Main Building
Suite 115
Jacksonville, FL 32216
(904) 296-5731

South Tampa Multiple Sclerosis Center
2829 West Deleon Street
Tampa, FL 33609
(813) 872-1548

USF Physicians Group Neurological Center
12901 Bruce B. Downs Boulevard
Tampa, FL 33612
(813) 974-2722

GEORGIA

Augusta Multiple Sclerosis Center
Department of Neurology
1120 15th Street
Augusta, GA 30912
(706) 721-4581

MS Center at Shepherd Center
2020 Peachtree Road NW
Atlanta, GA 30309
(404) 350-7392

Multiple Sclerosis Center of Atlanta
3200 Downwood Circle
Suite 550
Atlanta, GA 30327
(404) 351-0205

ILLINOIS

Central Illinois MS Center
Koke Mill Medical Center
3132 Old Jacksonville Road
Springfield, IL 62704
(217) 862-0422

Consultants in Neurology MS Center
1535 Lake Cook Road
Suite 601
Northbrook, IL 60062
(847) 509-0270

3545 Lake Avenue
Wilmette, IL 60091
(847) 251-1800

Loyola University Medical Center MS Clinic
1S260 Summit Ave.
Oakbrook Terrace, IL 60187
(630) 953-6600

Loyola University Medical Center MS Clinic
Mulcahy Outpatient Center

2160 South First Avenue
Room 2300
Maywood, IL 60153
(708) 216-4702

Northwestern University Medical Faculty
Galter Outpatient Facility
675 North Saint Clair Street
Ste. 20-100
Chicago, IL 60611
(312) 695-7950

Rush Presbyterian–St. Luke's MS Center
1725 West Harrison Street
Professional Building
Suite 309
Chicago, IL 60612
(312) 942-8011

University of Chicago MS Center
Center of Advanced Medicine
5758 Maryland Avenue
Room 4D
Chicago, IL 60637
(773) 702-6222

INDIANA

Fort Wayne Neurological Center
2622 Lake Avenue
Fort Wayne, IN 46805
(260) 460-3100

**Indiana Center for MS and
    Neuroimmunopathologic Disorders**
8424 Naab Road
#1A
Indianapolis, IN 46260
(317) 614-3100

**Indiana University Multiple
    Sclerosis Center**
541 Clinical Drive
Room 365
Indianapolis, IN 46202-5111
(317) 278-2771

Physiotherapy Associates
10601 North Meridian Street
Suite 110
Indianapolis, IN 46290
(317) 575-2100

IOWA

Physicians Clinic of Iowa
Neurology Department
600 7th Street, SE
Cedar Rapids, IA 52401
(319) 398-1721

Ruan Neurological Center
1111 6th Avenue
Suite 400
Des Moines, IA 50314
(515) 643-4500

University of Iowa Hospitals and Clinics
Department of Neurology
200 Hawkins Drive
Iowa City, IA 52242
(319) 356-7680

KANSAS

MS Clinic
University of Kansas Medical Center
Department of Neurology
3901 Rainbow Boulevard
Kansas City, KS 66160
(913) 588-6970

KENTUCKY

Baptist Hospital East MS Center
4002 Kresge Way
Louisville, KY 40207
(502) 895-7456

LOUISIANA

MS Clinic
Louisiana State University
2020 Gravier Street
7th Floor
New Orleans, LA 70112
(504) 568-4082

MS Clinic, Neurology Clinic
Tulane Medical Center
1415 Tulane Avenue
New Orleans, LA 70112
(504) 588-5231

Our Lady of Lourdes MS Center
406 Dunreath Street
Lafayette, LA 70506
(337) 289-4978

MAINE

MS Center of Maine
Maine Neurology, PA
49 Spring Street
Scarborough, ME 04074
(207) 883-1414

MARYLAND

Johns Hopkins Hospital
Multiple Sclerosis Center
John Hopkins Outpatient Center
601 North Caroline Street
Baltimore, MD 21287-7613
(410) 955-9441

Maryland Center for MS
University of Maryland Medical Center
16 South Eutaw Street
Third Floor
Frenkil Building
Baltimore, MD 21201
(410) 328-5858

MASSACHUSETTS

Metro West Medical Center
115 Lincoln Street
Framingham, MA 01702
(508) 383-8765

MS Center at Sturdy Memorial Hospital
211 Park Street
Attleboro, MA 02703
(508) 236-7170

Multiple Sclerosis Care Center
Mount Auburn Hospital
300 Mount Auburn Street
Suite 316
Cambridge, MA 02138
(617) 499-5014

Partners Multiple Sclerosis Center
333 Longwood Avenue
Boston, MA 02115
(617) 713-2030

UMass Memorial Medical Center
MS Clinical Center Neurology Department
55 Lake Avenue North
Worcester, MA 01655
(508) 856-2527

MICHIGAN

Department of Neurology
Henry Ford Hospital
2799 West Grand Boulevard
Detroit, MI 48202
(313) 876-7207

Michigan State University
138 Service Road
A-217 Clinical Center
East Lansing, MI 48824
(517) 353-8122

Mid-Michigan Regional Medical Center
4011 Orchard Drive
Suite 4010
Midland, MI 48640
(517) 835-8744

University of Michigan MS Center
Department of Neurology, Taubman Center
    1324/0322
1500 East Medical Center Drive
Ann Arbor, MI 48109
(734) 615-7920

Wayne State University
School of Medicine
Department of Neurology
University Health Center,
8D4201 Saint Antoine
Detroit, MI 48201
(313) 577-1249

West Michigan MS Clinic
Michigan Medical PC
3322 Beltline Court NE
Grand Rapids, MI 49525
(616) 456-9104

MINNESOTA

Fairview MS Center
Riverside Park Plaza
701 25th Avenue South
#200
Minneapolis, MN 55454
(612) 672-6100

The Minneapolis Clinic of Neurology
Golden Valley Office
4225 Golden Valley Road
Golden Valley, MN 55422
(763) 588-0661

Noran Neurological Clinic
910 East 26th Street
Suite 210
Minneapolis, MN 55404
(612) 879-1000

SMDC Comprehensive MS Program
400 East 3rd Street
Duluth, MN 55805
(218) 786-3925

MISSOURI

MS Clinic
Washington University School of Medicine
Department of Neurology
Box 8111
660 South Euclid
St. Louis, MO 63110
(314) 362-3293

West County MS Center
Saint John's Mercy Medical Center
621 South New Ballas Road
Tower B
Suite 5018
St. Louis, MO 63141
(314) 569-6507

NEBRASKA

University of Medical Associates at the University of Nebraska
Medical Clinic
South Tower Doctors Building
Suite 222
Omaha, NE 68198
(402) 559-7857

NEVADA

MS Service
50 Kirman Avenue
#201
Reno, NV 89502
(775) 324-2234

NEW HAMPSHIRE

Upper Valley Neurology Neurosurgery
106 Hanover Street
Lebanon, NH 03766
(603) 448-0447

NEW JERSEY

Gimbel MS Care Center
718 Teaneck Road
Teaneck, NJ 07666
(201) 837-0727

Kennedy Hospital at Statford
Voorhees Professional Building
102 White Horse Pike
Suite 101
Voorhees, NJ 08043
(856) 784-6800

MS Center
Saint Barnabas Hospital
101 Old Short Hills Road
West Orange, NJ 07052
(973) 322-6600

MS Research and Treatment Center of UMDNJ
185 South Orange Avenue
H506
Newark, NJ 07103
(973) 972-2550

NEW MEXICO

University of New Mexico
Department of Neurology
1201 Yale Boulevard NE
Albuquerque, NM 87131
(505) 272-3342

NEW YORK

Bronx-Lebanon Hospital
1770 Grand Concourse
Bronx, NY 10457
(718) 960-1335

Center for the Disabled
314 South Manning Boulevard
Albany, NY 12208
(518) 437-5623

Corrine Goldsmith Dickinson Center for Multiple Sclerosis at Mount Sinai Medical Center
Mount Sinai School of Medicine
5 East 98th Street
First Floor
New York, NY 10029
(212) 241-7317

Helen Hayes Hospital MS Clinic
Route 9W
West Haverstraw, NY 10993
(845) 947-3000

**Jacobs Neurological Institute and
William C. Baird MS Research Center**
Buffalo General Hospital
100 High Street
Buffalo, NY 14203
(716) 859-7592

Maimonides Medical Center
Multiple Sclerosis Care Center
4802 10th Avenue
Brooklyn, NY 11219
(718) 283-7470

Multiple Sclerosis Treatment Center
200 Old Country Road
Suite 125
Mineola, NY
(516) 663-4525

National Pediatric MS Center
HSC-T12-020
Stony Brook University Medical Center
Stony Brook, NY 11794-8121
(631) 444-7802

New York Medical Center of Queens
Multiple Sclerosis Care Center
56-45 Main Street
Flushing, NY 11355
(718) 460-6765
(718) 460-2903

New York Presbyterian Hospital
Cornell Medical Center
Multiple Sclerosis Care Center
525 East 68th Street
New York, NY 10021
(212) 746-4504

**New York University Hospital for Joint
Diseases**
Multiple Sclerosis Comprehensive Care Center
301 East 17th Street
New York, NY 10003
(212) 598-6305

North Shore MS Care Center at East Meadow
801 Merrick Avenue
East Meadow, NY 11554
(516) 496-6502

**Saint Luke's–Roosevelt MS Research and
Treatment Center**
425 West 59th Street
Suite 7C
New York, NY 10019
(212) 523-8070

South Shore Neurologic Associates, PC
877 East Main Street
Riverhead, NY 11901
(516) 727-0660

Staten Island University Hospital
Irving R. Boody Jr. Medical Arts Pavilion
475 Seaview Avenue
Staten Island, NY 10305
(718) 667-3800

Strong Memorial Hospital
University of Rochester
601 Elmwood Avenue
Rochester, NY 14642-8873
(716) 275-7854

SUNY at Stony Brook
Department of Neurology
Health Science Center, T-12
Room 020
Stony Brook, NY 11794-8121
(631) 444-1450

SUNY Upstate Medical University MS Clinic
Department of Neurology
University Health Care Center
90 Presidential Plaza
Syracuse, NY 13210
(877) 464-5540

NORTH CAROLINA

Duke Multiple Sclerosis Center
Duke University Hospital
3184 Duke South
Room 03102
Durham, NC 27710
(919) 684-4126

MS Center
Carolinas Medical Center
P.O. Box 32861
Charlotte, NC 28232-2861
(704) 446-1900

Triangle MS Center
3901 North Roxboro Road
Durham, NC 27704
(919) 479-4140 ext. 114

Raleigh Neurology Associates
1540 Sunday Drive
Raleigh, NC 27607
(919) 782-3456

Wake Forest University Health Sciences
Medical Center Boulevard
Winston-Salem, NC 27157
(336) 716-4101

OHIO

Medical College of Ohio MS Clinic
Multidisciplinary MS Clinic
3120 Glendale Avenue
RHC 1400, Neurology Clinic
Toledo, OH 43614
(419) 383-3760

Mellen Center
U-10, Cleveland Clinic Foundation
9500 Euclid Avenue
Cleveland, OH 44195
(216) 445-6800

Ohio State University Medical Center
Department of Neurology
466 West 10th Avenue
Columbus, OH 43210-1228
(614) 293-4964

OREGON

MS Center of Oregon
Department of Neurology, L226
Oregon Health Science University
3181 South West Sam Jackson Park Road
Portland, OR 97201
(503) 494-5759

PENNSYLVANIA

Allegheny MS Treatment Center
420 East North Avenue
Suite 206
Pittsburgh, PA 15212
(412) 359-8850

Geisinger Medical Center
100 North Academy Avenue
Danville, PA 17822-1405
(800) 275-6401

HealthSouth Rehab of Reading
1623 Morgantown Road
Reading, PA 19607-9455
(610) 796-6328

Hospital of the University of Pennsylvania
3 West Gates Building
3400 Spruce Street
Philadelphia, PA 19104-4283
(215) 662-6565

Knobler Institute of Neurologic Disease
467 Pennsylvania Avenue
Suite 108
Fort Washington, PA 19034
(215) 643-9045

Lehigh Valley Hospital
Neuroscience Research
1210 South Cedar Crest Boulevard
Suite 1800
Allentown, PA 18103
(610) 402-8420

Multiple Sclerosis Institute
1740 South Street
Suite 401
Philadelphia, PA 19146-1514
(215) 985-2245

Penn State Hershey Medical Center
500 University Drive
Hershey, PA 17033
(717) 531-8692

Temple University
Department of Neurology
Broad and Ontario Street
Philadelphia, PA 19140
(215) 707-7847

Thomas Jefferson University
Neurology Department
1025 Walnut Street
Suite 310
Philadelphia, PA 19107
(215) 955-2468

University of Pittsburgh
811 Lillian Kaufman Building
3471 Fifth Avenue
Pittsburgh, PA 15213
(412) 692-4920

RHODE ISLAND

MS Center of Care New England
Kent Hospital Outpatient Rehabilitation
Building 2
Suite 200
1351 South County Trail
East Greenwich, RI 02818
(401) 886-0629

SOUTH CAROLINA

Medical University of South Carolina
171 Ashley Avenue
Charleston, SC 29425
(843) 792-3223

TENNESSEE

Saint Thomas Neurosciences Institute
4230 Harding Road
Suite 809
Nashville, TN 37205
(615) 467-6256

Vanderbilt University Medical Center
Vanderbilt Stallworth Rehabilitation Hospital
2201 Capers Avenue
Nashville, TN 37212
(615) 320-7600

TEXAS

Ben Taub Neurology Clinic
1504 Taub Loop
Houston, TX 77030
(713) 793-3100

Maxine Mesinger Multiple Sclerosis Clinic
Baylor College of Medicine and the Methodist
   Hospital
One Baylor Plaza NB 302
Houston, TX 77030
(713) 798-7707

Saint David's Rehabilitation Center
1005 East 32nd Street
Austin, TX 78705
(512) 338-5042

Texoma Area MS Clinic
2201 S. Austin
Denison, TX 75020
(903) 463-4752

**University of Texas Southwestern Medical
   Center**
5323 Harry Hines Boulevard
J3134
Dallas, TX 75390-9036
(214) 648-9030

UTAH

School of Medicine
University of Utah
50 North Medical Drive
Salt Lake City, UT 84132
(801) 585-6032
(801) 581-4283

VERMONT

MS Center of Northern New England
FAHC-UHC Campus
1 South Prospect Street
Burlington, VT 05401
(802) 847-4589

VIRGINIA

Bon Secours DePaul Medical Center
Multiple Sclerosis Clinic
150 Kingsley Lane
Norfolk, VA 23505
(757) 889-5201

WASHINGTON

Holy Family Multiple Sclerosis Center
5901 North Lidgerwood
Suite 25B
Spokane, WA 99208
(509) 489-5019

Multiple Sclerosis Clinic
Overlake Hospital
1035 116th Avenue NE
Bellevue, WA 98004
(425) 688-5900

Swedish Medical MS Center
801 Broadway
Suite 830
Seattle, WA 98122
(206) 386-2700

VA MS Center
Rehabilitation Care Services
Veterans Affairs
Puget Sound Health Care System
1660 South Columbian Way
117-RCS
Seattle, WA 98108-1597
(206) 768-5462

Virginia Mason MS Center
Mailstop: X7-NEU
1100 Ninth Avenue
P.O. Box 900
Seattle, WA 98111
(206) 341-0420

Western MS Center
University of Washington Medical Center
    Rehabilitation Unit
1959 NE Pacific Street
P.O. 356157
Seattle, WA 98195
(206) 598-3344

WEST VIRGINIA

Charleston Area Medical Center
501 Morris Street
Charleston, WV 25301
(304) 388-6304

WISCONSIN

Marshfield Clinic MS Center
1000 North Oak Avenue
Marshfield, WI 54449
(715) 387-5350

Medical College of Wisconsin MS Clinic
MCW Clinic at Froedtert
9200 West Wisconsin Avenue
Milwaukee, WI 53226
(414) 454-5200

Saint Luke's Medical Center
2801 W. Kinnickinnic River Parkway
Suite 630
Milwaukee, WI 53215
(414) 385-1801

**University of Wisconsin Hospitals and Clinics
    MS Clinic**
600 Highland Avenue
Madison, WI 53792
(608) 262-0546

APPENDIX III
CLINICAL TRIALS IN MULTIPLE SCLEROSIS

Clinical trials change constantly. To obtain up-to-date information concerning clinical trials access the National MS Society website at http//:www.nationalmssociety.org

Clinical trials in multiple sclerosis (MS) are studies to see if a promising new drug or other medical therapy is actually safe and effective in the treatment of this disease. The studies must be carefully controlled to make sure that the results are valid and not due to factors other than the drug or therapy being tested. This means that clinical trials must have strict criteria for participation. Not everyone who wants to participate in a particular study may be eligible.

Most well-controlled clinical trials involve two groups: one who receives the experimental treatment and the other who receives either a placebo (inactive substance) or a previously approved treatment. Patients in these studies must understand that there is a 50/50 chance that they will not receive the experimental treatment. Other trial designs involve a crossover of treatment. This usually means that the type of treatment given to each group is switched during the course of the trial. In these types of trials, all groups eventually receive the active treatment under study.

The actual design and circumstances of the trial are explained by the investigators before a patient is asked to consent to participate.

The patient must often meet requirements to participate in a clinical trial. They include the following:

- The patient should live near the research facility, usually within 150 miles.

- The patient must usually have a specific type of MS. (Trials will often specify which clinical type of MS is being studied—relapsing-remitting, secondary progressive, primary progressive, or progressive-relapsing).

- The patient must fall within the guidelines of age, sex, level of disability, and duration of disease.

- Previous or current treatment with certain drugs (such as drugs that suppress the immune system) may exclude a patient from a study.

Patients who are eligible and who choose to enter clinical trials should be fully aware of the potential risks and benefits of the study. All aspects of a clinical trial should be discussed with the patient's neurologist. Physicians may also be able to help patients locate appropriate clinical research programs. Before participating in a clinical trial, patients must sign consent forms stating they know the purpose of the trial and how it will be conducted. Patients can leave a clinical trial at any time for any reason.

ALABAMA

Tanner Center for MS, Birmingham
Information: (205) 930-7151

This randomized, double-blind, placebo-controlled study of patients with relapsing-remitting MS is testing the safety and effectiveness of Avonex in combination with oral methotrexate, intravenous methylprednisolone, or both.

ARIZONA

Barrow Neurological Institute, Phoenix
Information: (800) 669-0281
http://www.pseudobulbar.com

This double-blind, placebo-controlled study of patients with relapsing-remitting MS is designed to determine the safety and effectiveness of AVP-923 (an orally administered combination of dextromethorphan and quinidine sulfate). This drug is designed to improve the symptom of emotional lability (uncontrollable laughing or crying).

Barrow Neurological Institute, Phoenix
Information: (800) 972-2505

This randomized, double-blind, placebo-controlled study of patients with relapsing-remitting and secondary progressive MS is designed to evaluate the safety, tolerability, and effectiveness of NBI-5788 (an altered peptide ligand; a modified portion of a myelin protein that induces an immune response).

Mayo Clinic, Scottsdale
Information: (480) 301-8260

This randomized, double-blind, placebo-controlled study of patients with relapsing-remitting MS is testing the safety and effectiveness of Avonex in combination with oral methotrexate, intravenous methylprednisolone, or both.

Mayo Clinic, Scottsdale
Information: (480) 301-8788

This open-label study of patients with relapsing-remitting MS is designed to compare low-dose Campath versus high-dose Campath versus high-dose Rebif.

Phoenix Neurological Associates, Ltd.
Information: (602) 259-3354

This randomized, double-blind, placebo-controlled study of patients with relapsing-remitting MS is testing the safety and effectiveness of Avonex in combination with oral methotrexate, intravenous methylprednisolone, or both.

Phoenix Neurological Associates, Ltd.
Information: (602) 259-3354

This open-label study of patients with relapsing-remitting MS is designed to compare low-dose Campath versus high-dose Campath versus high-dose Rebif.

ARKANSAS

Clinical Trials, Inc., Little Rock
Information: (501) 227-6179 ext. 115

An open-label study of patients with relapsing-remitting MS designed to compare low-dose Campath versus high-dose Campath versus high-dose Rebif.

CALIFORNIA

East Bay Region Associates in Neurology, Berkeley
Information: (510) 849-0499

This open-label study of patients with relapsing-remitting MS is designed to compare low-dose Campath versus high-dose Campath versus high-dose Rebif.

Multiple Sclerosis Service, Walnut Creek
Information: (925) 938-5252

This open-label study of patients with relapsing-remitting MS is designed to compare low-dose Campath versus high-dose Campath versus high-dose Rebif.

NervePro Research, Irvine
Information: (949) 753-1570

This open-label study of patients with relapsing-remitting MS is designed to compare low-dose Campath versus high-dose Campath versus high-dose Rebif.

Neurology Center, Oceanside
Information: (760) 732-0557 ext. 143

This open-label study of patients with relapsing-remitting MS is designed to compare low-dose Campath versus high-dose Campath versus high-dose Rebif.

Neuro-Therapeutics, Inc., Pasadena
Information: (626) 356-0800

This open-label study of patients with relapsing-remitting MS is designed to compare low-dose Campath versus high-dose Campath versus high-dose Rebif.

UC Davis, Sacramento
Information: (916) 734-6276

This randomized, double-blind, placebo-controlled study of patients with relapsing-remitting MS is designed to test the safety and effectiveness of Avonex in combination with oral methotrexate, intravenous methylprednisolone, or both.

UC Davis Medical Center
Information: (800) 972-2505

This randomized, double-blind, placebo-controlled study of patients with relapsing-remitting and secondary progressive MS is designed to evaluate the safety, tolerability, and effectiveness of NBI-5788 (an altered peptide ligand; a modified portion of a myelin protein that induces an immune response).

University of California, Irvine
Information: (800) 972-2505

This randomized, double-blind, placebo-controlled study of patients with relapsing-remitting and secondary progressive MS is designed to evaluate the safety, tolerability, and effectiveness of NBI-5788 (an altered peptide ligand; a modified portion of a myelin protein that induces an immune response).

University of California, Irvine
Information: (949) 824-7524

This randomized, double-blind study of patients with relapsing-remitting MS is designed to compare the safety and effectiveness of Betaseron and Avonex.

University of California, Irvine
Information: (949) 824-7524

This randomized, double-blind, placebo-controlled study of patients with relapsing-remitting MS is designed to test the safety and effectiveness of Avonex in combination with oral methotrexate, intravenous methylprednisolone, or both.

University of Southern California, Los Angeles
Information: (323) 224-5333

This randomized, double-blind, placebo-controlled study of patients with relapsing-remitting MS is designed to test the safety and effectiveness of Avonex in combination with oral methotrexate, intravenous methylprednisolone, or both.

CONNECTICUT

Associated Neurologists of Southern Connecticut, Fairfield
Information: (203) 333-1151

This randomized, double-blind, placebo-controlled study of patients with relapsing-remitting MS is testing the safety and effectiveness of Avonex in combination with oral methotrexate, intravenous methylprednisolone, or both.

MS Treatment Center at Griffin, Derby
Information: (203) 732-1290

This randomized, double-blind, placebo-controlled study of patients with relapsing-remitting MS is testing the safety and effectiveness of Avonex in combination with oral methotrexate, intravenous methylprednisolone, or both.

Yale Center for MS Treatment and Research, New Haven
Information: (203) 764-4280 (option #2)

This randomized, double-blind, placebo-controlled study of patients with relapsing-remitting MS is testing the safety and effectiveness of Avonex in combination with oral methotrexate, intravenous methylprednisolone, or both.

Yale Center for MS Treatment and Research, New Haven
Information: (800) 972-2505

This randomized, double-blind, placebo-controlled study of patients with relapsing-remitting and secondary progressive MS is designed to evaluate the safety, tolerability, and effectiveness of NBI-5788 (an altered peptide ligand; a modified portion of a myelin protein that induces an immune response).

DISTRICT OF COLUMBIA

Georgetown University Medical Center
Information: (202) 444-2658

This randomized, double-blind, placebo-controlled study of patients with relapsing-remitting MS is testing the safety and effectiveness of Avonex in combination with oral methotrexate, intravenous methylprednisolone, or both.

George Washington University Medical Faculty Associates
Information: (800) 669-0281
http://www.pseudobulbar.com

This double-blind, placebo-controlled study will determine the safety and effectiveness of AVP-923 (an orally administered combination of dextromethorphan and quinidine sulfate). This drug is designed to improve the symptom of emotional lability (uncontrollable laughing or crying).

FLORIDA

Cancer Research Network
Information: (954) 475-8171

This open-label study of patients with relapsing-remitting MS is designed to compare low-dose Campath versus high-dose Campath versus high-dose Rebif.

MS Center, University of Miami
Information: (305) 243-1088

This randomized, double-blind, placebo-controlled study of patients with relapsing-remitting MS is testing the safety and effectiveness of Avonex in combination with oral methotrexate, intravenous methylprednisolone, or both.

MS Center of Brevard, Melbourne
Information: (321) 253-0880

This randomized, double-blind, placebo-controlled study of patients with relapsing-remitting MS is testing the safety and effectiveness of Avonex in combination with oral methotrexate, intravenous methylprednisolone, or both.

MS Center of Sarasota
Information: (941) 917-6222

This randomized, double-blind, placebo-controlled study of patients with relapsing-remitting MS is testing the safety and effectiveness of Avonex in combination with oral methotrexate, intravenous methylprednisolone, or both.

MS Center of Vero Beach
Information: (772) 299-4304

This randomized, double-blind, placebo-controlled study of patients with relapsing-remitting MS is testing the safety and effectiveness of Avonex in combination with oral methotrexate, intravenous methylprednisolone, or both.

Neurological Associates, Ft. Lauderdale
Information: (800) 669-0281
http://www.pseudobulbar.com

This double-blind, placebo-controlled study of patients with relapsing-remitting or progressive MS will determine the safety and effectiveness of AVP-923 (an orally administered combination of dextromethorphan and quinidine sulfate). This drug is designed to improve the symptom of emotional lability (uncontrollable laughing or crying).

Neurological Associates, Ft. Lauderdale
Information: (954) 202-2246

This open-label study of patients with relapsing-remitting MS is designed to compare low-dose Campath versus high-dose Campath versus high-dose Rebif.

Neurological Services of Orlando
Information: (407) 540-1097 ext. 25

This open-label study of patients with relapsing-remitting MS is designed to compare low-dose Campath versus high-dose Campath versus high-dose Rebif.

Neurology Associates, PA, Maitland
Information: (407) 647-5996 ext. 204

This randomized, double-blind, placebo-controlled study of patients with relapsing-remitting MS is testing the safety and effectiveness of Avonex in combination with oral methotrexate, intravenous methylprednisolone, or both.

Tampa Neurology Associates
Information: (813) 353-9613

This open-label study of patients with relapsing-remitting MS is designed to compare low-dose Campath versus high-dose Campath versus high-dose Rebif.

University of Florida Health Science Center, Jacksonville
Information: (904) 244-9814

This randomized, double-blind, placebo-controlled study of patients with relapsing-remitting MS is testing the safety and effectiveness of Avonex in combination with oral methotrexate, intravenous methylprednisolone, or both.

GEORGIA
MS Center of Atlanta
Information: (404) 351-0205 ext. 104

This randomized, double-blind, placebo-controlled study of patients with relapsing-remitting MS is testing the safety and effectiveness of Avonex in combination with oral methotrexate, intravenous methylprednisolone, or both.

Neurology and Headache Specialist of Atlanta, LLC, Decatur
Information: (800) 669-0281
http://www.pseudobulbar.com

This double-blind, placebo-controlled study will determine safety and effectiveness of AVP-923 (an orally administered combination of dextromethorphan and quinidine sulfate). This drug is designed to improve the symptom of emotional lability (uncontrollable laughing or crying).

Neurotrials Research, Atlanta
Information: (404) 851-9934

This open-label study of patients with relapsing-remitting MS is designed to compare low-dose Campath versus high-dose Campath versus high-dose Rebif.

Shepherd Center, Atlanta
Information: (800) 972-2505

This randomized, double-blind, placebo-controlled study of patients with relapsing-remitting and secondary progressive MS is designed to evaluate the safety, tolerability, and effectiveness of NBI-5788 (an altered peptide ligand; a modified portion of a myelin protein that induces an immune response).

Sleep Medicine and Neurology
Information: (706) 653-8455

This open-label study of patients with relapsing-remitting MS is designed to compare low-dose Campath versus high-dose Campath versus high-dose Rebif.

ILLINOIS

Consultants in Neurology, Ltd., Northbrook
Information: (800) 669-0281
http://www.pseudobulbar.com

This double-blind, placebo-controlled study will determine safety and effectiveness of AVP-923 (an orally administered combination of dextromethorphan and quinidine sulfate). This drug is designed to improve the symptom of emotional lability (uncontrollable laughing or crying).

Consultants in Neurology, Ltd., Northbrook
Information: (847) 509-0270

This open-label study of patients with relapsing-remitting MS is designed to compare low-dose Campath versus high-dose Campath versus high-dose Rebif.

Radiant Research Alexian Brothers' Center for Clinical Research, Elk Grove Village
Information: (800) 669-0281
http://www.pseudobulbar.com

This double-blind, placebo-controlled study will determine safety and effectiveness of AVP-923 (an orally administered combination of dextromethorphan and quinidine sulfate). This drug is designed to improve the symptom of emotional lability (uncontrollable laughing or crying).

INDIANA

Fort Wayne Neurological Center
Information: (260) 460-3118

This open-label study of patients with relapsing-remitting MS is designed to compare low-dose Campath versus high-dose Campath versus high-dose Rebif.

Indiana University, Indianapolis
Information: (800) 972-2505

This randomized, double-blind, placebo-controlled study of patients with relapsing-remitting and secondary progressive MS is designed to evaluate the safety, tolerability, and effectiveness of NBI-5788 (an altered peptide ligand; a modified portion of a myelin protein that induces an immune response).

KENTUCKY

Associates in Neurology, PSC, Lexington
Information: (859) 296-1922 ext. 149

This open-label study of patients with relapsing-remitting MS is designed to compare low-dose Campath versus high-dose Campath versus high-dose Rebif.

Louisville Neurology Associates
Information: (502) 589-6177

This randomized, double-blind, placebo-controlled study of patients with relapsing-remitting MS is testing the safety and effectiveness of Avonex in combination with oral methotrexate, intravenous methylprednisolone, or both.

Riverhills Health Care, Crestview
Information: (859) 426-3547

This randomized, double-blind, placebo-controlled study of patients with relapsing-remitting MS is testing the safety and effectiveness of Avonex in combination with oral methotrexate, intravenous methylprednisolone, or both.

University of Kentucky, Lexington
Information: (859) 323-6702 ext. 252

This randomized, double-blind, placebo-controlled study of patients with relapsing-remitting MS is testing the safety and effectiveness of Avonex in combination with oral methotrexate, intravenous methylprednisolone, or both.

LOUISIANA

Our Lady of Lourdes Research and Grants, Lafayette
Information: (337) 289-4855

This randomized, double-blind, placebo-controlled study of patients with relapsing-remitting MS is testing the safety and effectiveness of Avonex in combination with oral methotrexate, intravenous methylprednisolone, or both.

MARYLAND

Johns Hopkins University, Baltimore
Information: (410) 614-4823

This randomized, double-blind, placebo-controlled study of patients with relapsing-remitting MS is testing the safety and effectiveness of Avonex in combination with oral methotrexate, intravenous methylprednisolone, or both.

Johns Hopkins University, Baltimore
Information: (410) 502-0514

Pilot study in aggressive MS for patients with aggressive relapsing-remitting disease, assessing treatment with high-dose cyclophosphamide.

National Institutes of Health, Bethesda
Information: (301) 496-0064

An open-label, crossover study of patients with relapsing-remitting and secondary progressive MS to determine the safety and effectiveness of Zenapax (daclizumab), a molecule that regulates the immune response.

University of Maryland, Maryland Center for MS, Baltimore
Information: (410) 328-7601

This open-label study of patients with relapsing-remitting MS is designed to compare low-dose Campath versus high-dose Campath versus high-dose Rebif.

University of Maryland, Maryland Center for MS, Baltimore
Information: (410) 328-7603

An open-label comparison between Avonex and Betaseron for relapsing-remitting MS patients.

MASSACHUSETTS

Beth Israel Deaconess Medical Center, Boston
Information: (617) 667-3744

This randomized, double-blind, placebo-controlled study of patients with relapsing-remitting MS is testing the safety and effectiveness of Avonex in combination with oral methotrexate, intravenous methylprednisolone, or both.

Brigham and Women's Hospital MS Center, Boston
Information: (617) 713-2006

A double-blind, placebo-controlled study to determine the safety and effectiveness of Copaxone and Proventil (albuterol).

Lahey Clinic, Burlington
Information: (781) 744-2950

This randomized, double-blind, placebo-controlled study of patients with relapsing-remitting MS is testing the safety and effectiveness of Avonex in combination with oral methotrexate, intravenous methylprednisolone, or both.

Newton Wellesley Hospital, Newton
Information: (617) 243-6517

This randomized, double-blind, placebo-controlled study of patients with relapsing-remitting MS is testing the safety and effectiveness of Avonex in combination with oral methotrexate, intravenous methylprednisolone, or both.

University of Massachusetts–Memorial Health Care, Worcester
Information: (508) 856-8568

This randomized, double-blind, placebo-controlled study of patients with relapsing-remitting MS is testing the safety and effectiveness of Avonex in combination with oral methotrexate, intravenous methylprednisolone, or both.

MICHIGAN

Michigan Medical PC West Michigan MS Clinic, Grand Rapids
Information: (616) 974-4722

This open-label study of patients with relapsing-remitting MS is designed to compare low-dose Campath versus high-dose Campath versus high-dose Rebif.

Michigan Neurological Associates, St. Claire
Information: (586) 552-1502

This randomized, double-blind, placebo-controlled study of patients with relapsing-remitting MS is testing the safety and effectiveness of Avonex in combination with oral methotrexate, intravenous methylprednisolone, or both.

Michigan State University, East Lansing
Information: (517) 353-8122 ext. 106

This randomized, double-blind, placebo-controlled study of patients with relapsing-remitting MS is testing the safety and effectiveness of Avonex in combination with oral methotrexate, intravenous methylprednisolone, or both.

University of Michigan, Ann Arbor
Information: dmiko@umich.edu

This open label, randomized, placebo-controlled study is addressing the effectiveness of the combined therapy in MS patients of Betaseron (interferon beta-1b) and CellCept (mycophenolate mofetil, an oral immune suppressant currently used to prevent rejection of organ transplants).

Wayne State University School of Medicine, Detroit
Information: (313) 966-5068

This open-label study of patients with relapsing-remitting MS is designed to compare low-dose Campath versus high-dose Campath versus high-dose Rebif.

MINNESOTA

MS Treatment and Research Center, Minneapolis Clinic of Neurology
Information: (763) 302-4072 (phone)
(763) 302-4068 (fax)

A randomized, double-blind, placebo-controlled study of relapsing-remitting MS patients to test the safety and effectiveness of a combination of Lipitor (atorvastatin, a cholesterol-lowering drug) and Rebif (interferon beta-1a).

Cleveland Clinic Foundation, Cleveland, and the Mayo Clinic, Rochester
Information: faticap@ccf.org

This open study of gender differences in the immune response in MS involves two blood draws to analyze the gene for the immune messenger protein interferon gamma, which has been linked to the immune attack in MS. The study is open to patients with all types of MS diagnosed within the past three years who are not on immunosuppressive therapy.

MISSOURI

Washington University, St. Louis
Information: (314) 362-3371

An open-label comparison between Avonex and Betaseron for relapsing-remitting MS patients.

Washington University, St. Louis
Information: (314) 362-3371

A double-blind, placebo-controlled study to compare the number of MS relapses in people who receive a bladder infection suppressant (trimethoprim antibiotic therapy and vitamin C) versus those who receive placebo and routine bladder care. This study is for those with relapsing-remitting and secondary progressive MS.

Washington University, St. Louis
Information: (314) 362-3371

This is an open-label study of Rituxan (rituximab, a molecule that regulates immune response) for the treatment of relapsing-remitting MS.

Washington University School of Medicine
Information: (800) 972-2505

This randomized, double-blind, placebo-controlled study of patients with relapsing-remitting and secondary progressive MS is designed to evaluate the safety, tolerability, and effectiveness of NBI-5788 (an altered peptide ligand; a modified portion of a myelin protein that induces an immune response).

MONTANA

Advanced Neurology Specialists, Great Falls
Information: (800) 669-0281
http://www.pseudobulbar.com

This double-blind, placebo-controlled study will determine the safety and effectiveness of AVP-923 (an orally administered combination of dextromethorphan and quinidine sulfate). This drug is designed to improve the symptom of emotional lability (uncontrollable laughing or crying).

NEBRASKA

Creighton University Medical Center, Omaha
Information: (402) 280-3550

This randomized, double-blind, placebo-controlled study of patients with relapsing-remitting MS is testing the safety and effectiveness of Avonex in combination with oral methotrexate, intravenous methylprednisolone, or both.

University of Nebraska Medical Center, Omaha
Information: pleusche@unmc.edu

An open-label, randomized study of the use of over-the-counter pain medications (Tylenol [acetaminophen], Advil [ibuprofen], or Aleve [naproxen]) to minimize side effects in two groups: those initiating Avonex therapy and those who continue to exhibit side effects after six months on Avonex. This study is for patients with relapsing-remitting MS.

NEVADA

Nevada Neurological Consultants, Henderson
Information: (702) 836-1241

This open-label study of patients with relapsing-remitting MS is designed to compare low-dose Campath versus high-dose Campath versus high-dose Rebif.

Washoe Comprehensive MS Center, Reno
Information: (775) 982-4602

This randomized, double-blind, placebo-controlled study of patients with relapsing-remitting MS is testing the safety and effectiveness of Avonex in combination with oral methotrexate, intravenous methylprednisolone, or both.

NEW JERSEY

Bernard W. Gimbel MS Center, Teaneck
Information: (201) 837-0727, ext. 128

This randomized, double-blind, placebo-controlled study of patients with relapsing-remitting MS is testing the safety and effectiveness of Avonex in combination with oral methotrexate, intravenous methylprednisolone, or both.

Bernard W. Gimbel MS Center, Teaneck
Information: UMDNJ—(973) 972-7395
Gimbel Center—(201) 837-0727

This is a phase IV, rater-blinded, randomized study comparing the effects of 250 mcg of Betaseron with 20 mg of Copaxone in patients with relapsing-remitting MS or clinically isolated syndrome—a single, isolated neurologic event suggesting loss of nerve-insulating myelin—using 3 tesla magnetic resonance imaging.

Kessler Medical Rehabilitation Research and Education Corporation, West Orange
Information: (973) 324-3533

A study examining three types of MS-related impairments and their impact on driving ability, including cognitive abilities, physical abilities, and visual abilities.

NEW MEXICO

University of New Mexico, Mind Imaging Center, Albuquerque
Information: (800) 972-2505

This randomized, double-blind, placebo-controlled study of patients with relapsing-remitting and secondary progressive MS is designed to evaluate the safety, tolerability, and effectiveness of NBI-5788 (an altered peptide ligand; a modified portion of a myelin protein that induces an immune response).

NEW YORK

Beth Israel Medical Center, New York
Information: (212) 844-1491

This randomized, double-blind, placebo-controlled, crossover pilot trial of oral lamotrigine (Lamictal) is open to patients with all types of MS.

Jacobs Neurological Institute, Buffalo
Information: (716) 859-7510

This randomized, double-blind, placebo-controlled study of patients with relapsing-remitting MS is testing the safety and effectiveness of Avonex in combination with oral methotrexate, intravenous methylprednisolone, or both.

Mount Sinai School of Medicine, Corinne Goldsmith Dickinson Center for MS, New York

Information: (212) 241-4264

multiple.scleroisis@mssm.edu

This research study will evaluate the safety and tolerability of two treatment groups. One group will be given glatiramer acetate (Copaxone), and the second group will receive mitoxantrone (Novantrone) for three consecutive months followed by starting glatiramer acetate.

MS Comprehensive Care Center, White Plains

Information: (914) 328-6410 ext. 223

This open-label study of patients with relapsing-remitting MS is designed to compare low-dose Campath versus high-dose Campath versus high-dose Rebif.

MS Research and Treatment Center, New York

Information: (212) 523-8070

This randomized, double-blind, placebo-controlled study of patients with relapsing-remitting MS is testing the safety and effectiveness of Avonex in combination with oral methotrexate, intravenous methylprednisolone, or both.

New York University Hospital for Joint Diseases, New York

Information: (212) 598-6305

This randomized, double-blind, placebo-controlled study of patients with relapsing-remitting MS is testing the safety and effectiveness of Avonex in combination with oral methotrexate, intravenous methylprednisolone, or both.

Stony Brook University Hospital, Stony Brook

Information: (800) 972-2505

This randomized, double-blind, placebo-controlled study of patients with relapsing-remitting and secondary progressive MS is designed to evaluate the safety, tolerability, and effectiveness of NBI-5788 (an altered peptide ligand; a modified portion of a myelin protein that induces an immune response).

SUNY Stony Brook

Information: pmelvill@neuro.som.sunysb.edu

This is an observational study of mild cognitive impairment in people with relapsing-remitting and secondary progressive MS.

SUNY Stony Brook

Information: (631) 444-8164

This randomized, double-blind, placebo-controlled study of patients with relapsing-remitting MS is testing the safety and effectiveness of Avonex in combination with oral methotrexate, intravenous methylprednisolone, or both.

University Hospital Stony Brook

Information: (631) 444-3448

This open-label study of patients with relapsing-remitting MS is designed to compare low-dose Campath versus high-dose Campath versus high-dose Rebif.

University of Rochester

Information: (585) 275-6120

This randomized, double-blind, placebo-controlled study of patients with relapsing-remitting MS is testing the safety and effectiveness of Avonex in combination with oral methotrexate, intravenous methylprednisolone, or both.

University of Rochester

Information: (585) 275-7854

This open-label study of patients with relapsing-remitting MS is designed to compare low-dose Campath versus high-dose Campath versus high-dose Rebif.

Upstate Clinical Research, LLC, Albany

Information: (518) 533-1500 ext. 546

This double-blind study will compare the safety and effectiveness of Avonex and Prozac (fluoxetine) versus Avonex and placebo in relapsing-remitting MS patients.

Upstate Medical University, Syracuse

Information: (315) 464-3935

This randomized, double-blind, placebo-controlled study of patients with relapsing-remitting MS is testing the safety and effectiveness of Avonex in combination with oral methotrexate, intravenous methylprednisolone, or both.

NORTH CAROLINA

MS Center, Carolinas Healthcare System, Charlotte

Information: (704) 446-1910

This randomized, double-blind, placebo-controlled study of patients with relapsing-remitting MS is testing the safety and effectiveness of Avonex in combination with oral methotrexate, intravenous methylprednisolone, or both.

Raleigh Neurology Associates
Information: (919) 420-1657

This randomized, double-blind, placebo-controlled study of patients with relapsing-remitting MS is testing the safety and effectiveness of Avonex in combination with oral methotrexate, intravenous methylprednisolone, or both.

Raleigh Neurology Associates, PA, Raleigh
Information: (800) 669-0281
http://www.pseudobulbar.com

This double-blind, placebo-controlled study will determine safety and effectiveness of AVP-923 (an orally administered combination of dextromethorphan and quinidine sulfate). This drug is designed to improve the symptom of emotional lability (uncontrollable laughing or crying).

Triad Neurology Services, Winston-Salem
Information: (336) 768-6347 ext. 228

This open-label study of patients with relapsing-remitting MS is designed to compare low-dose Campath versus high-dose Campath versus high-dose Rebif.

Triad Neurology Services, Winston-Salem
Information: (336) 659-1500 ext. 106

This open-label study of patients with relapsing-remitting MS is designed to compare low-dose Campath versus high-dose Campath versus high-dose Rebif.

Wake Forest University, Winston-Salem
Information: (800) 972-2505

This randomized, double-blind, placebo-controlled study of patients with relapsing-remitting and secondary progressive MS is designed to evaluate the safety, tolerability, and effectiveness of NBI-5788 (an altered peptide ligand; a modified portion of a myelin protein that induces an immune response).

OHIO

Cleveland Clinic Foundation
Information: (216) 444-4817

This randomized, double-blind, placebo-controlled study of patients with relapsing-remitting MS is testing

the safety and effectiveness of Avonex in combination with oral methotrexate, intravenous methylprednisolone, or both.

NeuroCare Center, Inc., Canton
Information: (800) 669-0281
http://www.pseudobulbar.com

This double-blind, placebo-controlled study will determine the safety and effectiveness of AVP-923 (an orally administered combination of dextromethorphan and quinidine sulfate). This drug is designed to improve the symptom of emotional lability (uncontrollable laughing or crying).

Neurological Associates, Inc., Columbus
Information: (614) 457-4880

This randomized, double-blind, placebo-controlled study of patients with relapsing-remitting MS is testing the safety and effectiveness of Avonex in combination with oral methotrexate, intravenous methylprednisolone, or both.

Ohio State University, Columbus
Information: (800) 972-2505

This randomized, double-blind, placebo-controlled study of patients with relapsing-remitting and secondary progressive MS is designed to evaluate the safety, tolerability, and effectiveness of NBI-5788 (an altered peptide ligand; a modified portion of a myelin protein that induces an immune response).

Ohio State University, Columbus
Information: (614) 293-7877

This randomized, double-blind, placebo-controlled study of patients with relapsing-remitting MS is testing the safety and effectiveness of Avonex in combination with oral methotrexate, intravenous methylprednisolone, or both.

Research Resources, Inc., West Chester
Information: (513) 233-2241

This open-label study of patients with relapsing-remitting MS is designed to compare low-dose Campath versus high-dose Campath versus high-dose Rebif.

OKLAHOMA

Medical Neurologists, Inc., Oklahoma City
Information: (405) 936-5822

This randomized, double-blind, placebo-controlled study of patients with relapsing-remitting MS is testing the safety and effectiveness of Avonex in combination with oral methotrexate, intravenous methylprednisolone, or both.

Neurological Associates of Tulsa, Inc.
Information: (918) 481-7711

This open-label study of patients with relapsing-remitting MS is designed to compare low-dose Campath versus high-dose Campath versus high-dose Rebif.

OREGON
MS Center of Oregon, Oregon Health and Science University, Portland
Information: (503) 494-7241

This double-blind, placebo-controlled study is designed to determine the effects of ginkgo biloba treatment on the cognitive function in people with relapsing-remitting, secondary progressive, and primary progressive MS.

Oregon Health and Science University, Portland
Information: (503) 494-5759

This randomized, double-blind, placebo-controlled study of patients with relapsing-remitting MS is testing the safety and effectiveness of Avonex in combination with oral methotrexate, intravenous methylprednisolone, or both.

Providence St. Vincents Medical Center, Portland
Information: (503) 296-4827

This randomized, double-blind, placebo-controlled study of patients with relapsing-remitting MS is testing the safety and effectiveness of Avonex in combination with oral methotrexate, intravenous methylprednisolone, or both.

PENNSYLVANIA
Allegheny Senger Research, Pittsburgh
Information: (412) 359-4782

This randomized, double-blind, placebo-controlled study of patients with relapsing-remitting MS is testing the safety and effectiveness of Avonex in combination with oral methotrexate, intravenous methylprednisolone, or both.

Geisinger Medical Center, Danville
Information: (570) 214-9321

This randomized, double-blind, placebo-controlled study of patients with relapsing-remitting MS is testing the safety and effectiveness of Avonex in combination with oral methotrexate, intravenous methylprednisolone, or both.

Greenstein Neurology Associates, Philadelphia
Information: (215) 985-2267

This randomized, double-blind, placebo-controlled study of patients with relapsing-remitting MS is testing the safety and effectiveness of Avonex in combination with oral methotrexate, intravenous methylprednisolone, or both.

Lehigh Valley Hospital, Allentown
Information: (610) 402-9001

This open-label study is designed to determine the safety and effectiveness of Avonex and Imuran in patients with relapsing-remitting MS.

Lehigh Valley Neurosciences and Pain Research Center, Allentown
Information: (800) 669-0281
http://www.pseudobulbar.com

This double-blind, placebo-controlled study will determine the safety and effectiveness of AVP-923 (an orally administered combination of dextromethorphan and quinidine sulfate). This drug is designed to improve the symptom of emotional lability (uncontrollable laughing or crying).

MS Neurosciences Research MS Center, Allentown
Information: (610) 402-9008

This open-label study of patients with relapsing-remitting MS is designed to compare low-dose Campath versus high-dose Campath versus high-dose Rebif.

Neurological Associates of Delaware Valley, Upland
Information: (800) 669-0281
http://www.pseudobulbar.com

This double-blind, placebo-controlled study will determine the safety and effectiveness of AVP-923 (an orally administered combination of dextromethorphan and quinidine sulfate). This drug is designed to improve the symptom of emotional lability (uncontrollable laughing or crying).

Neuroscience Research/MS Center, Allentown
Information: (610) 402-9005

This randomized, double-blind, placebo-controlled study of patients with relapsing-remitting MS is testing the safety and effectiveness of Avonex in combination with oral methotrexate, intravenous methylprednisolone, or both.

Thomas Jefferson University, Philadelphia
Information: (215) 955-7310

This randomized, double-blind, placebo-controlled study of patients with relapsing-remitting MS is testing the safety and effectiveness of Avonex in combination with oral methotrexate, intravenous methylprednisolone, or both.

University of Pennsylvania MS Center, Philadelphia
Information: (800) 972-2505

This randomized, double-blind, placebo-controlled study of patients with relapsing-remitting and secondary progressive MS is designed to evaluate the safety, tolerability, and effectiveness of NBI-5788 (an altered peptide ligand; a modified portion of a myelin protein that induces an immune response).

University of Pennsylvania, Philadelphia
Information: (215) 662-4893

This randomized, double-blind, placebo-controlled study of patients with relapsing-remitting MS is testing the safety and effectiveness of Avonex in combination with oral methotrexate, intravenous methylprednisolone, or both.

University of Pennsylvania, Philadelphia
Information: (215) 662-4893

This double-blind, placebo-controlled study is designed to determine the safety and efficacy of inosine (a dietary supplement in oral capsule form) on the number of newly active lesions in patients with relapsing-remitting MS.

University of Pittsburgh, Pittsburgh
Information: (412) 692-4918

This randomized, double-blind, placebo-controlled study of patients with relapsing-remitting MS is testing

the safety and effectiveness of Avonex in combination with oral methotrexate, intravenous methylprednisolone, or both.

Westmoreland Neurology, Greensburg and sites nationwide
Information: (800) 669-0281
http://www.pseudobulbar.com

This double-blind, placebo-controlled study will determine the safety and effectiveness of AVP-923 (an orally administered combination of dextromethorphan and quinidine sulfate). This drug is designed to improve the symptom of emotional lability (uncontrollable laughing or crying).

TENNESSEE
Knoxville Neurology Associates
Information: (865) 549-4812

This open-label study of patients with relapsing-remitting MS is designed to compare low-dose Campath versus high-dose Campath versus high-dose Rebif.

Vanderbilt University, Nashville
Information: (615) 963-4442

This randomized, double-blind, placebo-controlled study of patients with relapsing-remitting MS is testing the safety and effectiveness of Avonex in combination with oral methotrexate, intravenous methylprednisolone, or both.

TEXAS
Baylor College of Medicine, Houston
Information: (713) 798-7707

This open-label study of patients with relapsing-remitting MS is designed to compare low-dose Campath versus high-dose Campath versus high-dose Rebif.

Central Texas Neurology Consultants, Round Rock
Information: (512) 218-1222

This open-label study of patients with relapsing-remitting MS is designed to compare low-dose Campath versus high-dose Campath versus high-dose Rebif.

Central Texas Neurology Consultants, Round Rock
Information: (512) 218-1222

This randomized, double-blind, placebo-controlled study of patients with relapsing-remitting MS is testing the safety and effectiveness of Avonex in combination with oral methotrexate, intravenous methylprednisolone, or both.

Dallas Neurological Associates
Information: (972) 783-8900

This open-label study of patients with relapsing-remitting MS is designed to compare low-dose Campath versus high-dose Campath versus high-dose Rebif.

Integra Clinical Research, LLC, San Antonio
Information: (210) 692-1245

This open-label study of patients with relapsing-remitting MS is designed to compare low-dose Campath versus high-dose Campath versus high-dose Rebif.

Integra Clinical Research, LLC, San Antonio
Information: (800) 972-2505

This randomized, double-blind, placebo-controlled study of patients with relapsing-remitting and secondary progressive MS is designed to evaluate the safety, tolerability, and effectiveness of NBI-5788 (an altered peptide ligand; a modified portion of a myelin protein that induces an immune response).

Neurology Center of San Antonio
Information: (210) 225-5334

This open-label study of patients with relapsing-remitting MS is designed to compare low-dose Campath versus high-dose Campath versus high-dose Rebif.

North Texas Neurology, Wichita Falls
Information: (800) 972-2505

This randomized, double-blind, placebo-controlled study of patients with relapsing-remitting and secondary progressive MS is designed to evaluate the safety, tolerability, and effectiveness of NBI-5788 (an altered peptide ligand; a modified portion of a myelin protein that induces an immune response).

Texas Neurology, PA, Dallas
Information: (800) 972-2505

This randomized, double-blind, placebo-controlled study of patients with relapsing-remitting and secondary progressive MS is designed to evaluate the safety, tolerability, and effectiveness of NBI-5788 (an altered peptide ligand; a modified portion of a myelin protein that induces an immune response).

VERMONT

FACH-UHC Department of Neurological Services, Burlington
Information: (800) 669-0281
http://www.pseudobulbar.com

This double-blind, placebo-controlled study will determine the safety and effectiveness of AVP-923 (an orally administered combination of dextromethorphan and quinidine sulfate). This drug is designed to improve the symptom of emotional lability (uncontrollable laughing or crying).

Neurological Consultants, PC, Bennington
Information: (802) 447-2598, ext. 122

This randomized, double-blind, placebo-controlled study of patients with relapsing-remitting MS is testing the safety and effectiveness of Avonex in combination with oral methotrexate, intravenous methylprednisolone, or both.

VIRGINIA

Hunter Holmes McGuire VA Medical Center, Richmond
Information: (804) 675-5000, ext. 4873

This randomized, double-blind, placebo-controlled study of patients with relapsing-remitting MS is testing the safety and effectiveness of Avonex in combination with oral methotrexate, intravenous methylprednisolone, or both.

Neuroscience Consultants, PLC, Reston
Information: E-mail: sparlow@nscplc.com

This randomized, double-blind, placebo-controlled study of patients with relapsing-remitting MS is testing the safety and effectiveness of Avonex in combination with oral methotrexate, intravenous methylprednisolone, or both.

University of Virginia Health Sciences, Charlottesville
Information: (434) 243-5457

This randomized, double-blind, placebo-controlled study of patients with relapsing-remitting MS is testing the safety and effectiveness of Avonex in combination with oral methotrexate, intravenous methylprednisolone, or both.

VA Commonwealth University/Medical College of Virginia, Richmond
Information: (804) 828-0078

This randomized, double-blind, placebo-controlled study of patients with relapsing-remitting MS is testing the safety and effectiveness of Avonex in combination with oral methotrexate, intravenous methylprednisolone, or both.

WASHINGTON

Neurology and Neurosurgery Associates of Tacoma
Information: (800) 669-0281
http://www.pseudobulbar.com

This double-blind, placebo-controlled study will determine the safety and effectiveness of AVP-923 (an orally administered combination of dextromethorphan and quinidine sulfate). This drug is designed to improve the symptom of emotional lability (uncontrollable laughing or crying).

Swedish Medical Center, Seattle
Information: (800) 669-0281
http://www.pseudobulbar.com

This double-blind, placebo-controlled study will determine the safety and effectiveness of AVP-923 (an orally administered combination of dextromethorphan and quinidine sulfate). This drug is designed to improve the symptom of emotional lability (uncontrollable laughing or crying).

Virginia Mason Medical Center, Seattle
Information: (206) 223-6835

This randomized, double-blind, placebo-controlled study of patients with relapsing-remitting MS is testing the safety and effectiveness of Avonex in combination with oral methotrexate, intravenous methylprednisolone, or both.

APPENDIX IV
STATE CHAPTERS OF THE NATIONAL MULTIPLE SCLEROSIS SOCIETY

ALABAMA

3840 Ridgeway Drive
Birmingham, AL 35209
(205) 879-8881
(800) FIGHT-MS
http://www.nationalmssociety.org/alc
E-mail: alc@nmss.org

This chapter serves more than 4,000 people with multiple sclerosis within the state of Alabama.

ALASKA

511 West 41st Avenue
Suite 101
Anchorage, AK 99503
(907) 563-1115
(800) FIGHT-MS
http://www.nationalmssociety.org/aka
E-mail: aka@nmss.org

ARIZONA

315 South 48th Street
Suite 101
Tempe, AZ 85281
(480) 968-2488
(800) FIGHT-MS
http://www.nationalmssociety.org/aza
E-mail: info@dsw.nmss.org

The Arizona Chapter of the National Multiple Sclerosis Society, founded in 1956, is a not-for-profit agency serving more than 4,700 people with MS and their families in Arizona. The Arizona Chapter offers education, information and referrals, counseling, assistance with employment concerns, social activities and more. The major fund-raising campaigns are the MS Walks, the MS Bike Tours, and Dinner of Champions.

Over 1,000 volunteers give their expertise and time to the Arizona Chapter by serving on the board, leading support groups, raising funds, and many other tasks.

ARKANSAS

Evergreen Place
1100 North University
Suite 255
Little Rock, AR 72207
(501) 663-6767
(800) FIGHT-MS
http://www.nationalmssociety.org/arr
E-mail: arr@nmss.org

Mid-South
4219 Hillsboro Road
Suite 306
Nashville, TN 37215
(615) 269-9055
(800) FIGHT-MS
http://www.msmidsouth.org
E-mail: tns@nmss.org

The Mid-South Chapter offers a wide range of programs to help people cope with the everyday demands of living with a chronic illness. The society serves people with MS, their families, and health care professionals through education, advocacy, information, peer support, therapeutic recreation, and many other programs.

CALIFORNIA

Channel Islands
14 West Valerio Street
Santa Barbara, CA 93101
(805) 682-8783
(800) FIGHT-MS

http://www.nmssci.org/
E-mail: joan.young@cat.nmss.org

The Channel Islands Chapter serves more than 3,000 people affected by MS by providing comprehensive support services and educational programs and by funding national research into the cause, treatments, and cure for this chronic neurological disease.

Great Basin Sierra
255 West Moana
Suite #107
Reno, NV 89509-4942
(775) 329-7180
(800) FIGHT-MS
http://www.nationalmssociety.org/nvn
E-mail: nvn@nvn.nmss.org

Northern California Chapter Headquarters
150 Grand
Oakland, CA 94612
(510) 268-0572
(800) FIGHT-MS
http://www.msconnection.org
E-mail: info@msconnection.org

Orange County
17500 Redhill Avenue
Suite 240
Irvine, CA 92614
(949) 752-1680
(800) FIGHT-MS
http://www.nmssoc.org/
E-mail: msinfo@cao.nmss.org

San Diego
8840 Complex Drive
Suite 130
San Diego, CA 92123
(858) 974-8640
(800) FIGHT-MS
http://www.mssd.org
E-mail: mssd@mssd.org

Silicon Valley
2589 Scott Boulevard
Santa Clara, CA 95050
(408) 988-7557
(800) FIGHT-MS
http://www.nationalmssociety.org/cau
E-mail: cau@nmss.org

Southern California
2440 South Sepulveda Boulevard
Suite 115
Los Angeles, CA 90064
(310) 479-4456
(800) FIGHT-MS
http://www.nationalmssociety.org/cal
E-mail: ms@cal.nmss.org

COLORADO

700 Broadway
Suite 808
Denver, CO 80203-3442
(303) 831-0700
(800) FIGHT-MS
http://www.fightmscolorado.org
E-mail: general.information@coc.nmss.org

CONNECTICUT

Greater Connecticut
705 North Mountain Road
Newington, CT 06111
(860) 953-0601
(800) FIGHT-MS
http://www.ctnmss.org
E-mail: lgerrol@ctnmss.org

A nonprofit agency serving more than 4,000 people with MS and their families in Hartford, New Haven, New London, Tolland, Middlesex, and Windham Counties. The Greater Connecticut Chapter offers education, information and referrals, counseling, assistance with employment concerns, social activities, and more.

Western Connecticut
One Selleck Street
Suite 500
Norwalk, CT 06855
(203) 838-1033
(800) FIGHT-MS
http://www.msswct.org
E-mail: lparizeau@msswct.org

The Western Connecticut Chapter was established in 1947 and currently counts 1,150 persons with MS in the state. The chapter delivers programs and services to people with MS and their families by supporting research into the cause and cure of MS.

DELAWARE

Two Mill Road
Suite 106
Wilmington, DE 19806
(302) 655-5610
(800) FIGHT-MS
http://www.msdelaware.org
E-mail: kate.cowperthwait@ded.nmss.org

DISTRICT OF COLUMBIA

National Capital
2021 K Street, NW
Suite 715
Washington, DC 20006-1035
(202) 296-5363
(800) FIGHT-MS
http://www.MSandYOU.org
E-mail: information@msandyou.org

The National Capital Chapter provides programs and services to people in the District of Columbia; Prince George's and Montgomery Counties in Maryland; and Alexandria, Arlington, Fairfax, Fauquier, Loudoun, and Prince William Counties in Virginia. The chapter serves about 6,000 people with MS. When taken together with their families and caregivers, approximately 18,000 people are affected by MS in the Washington, DC, metro area.

FLORIDA

Mid-Florida
3659 Maguire Boulevard
Suite 110
Orlando, FL 32803
(407) 896-3873
(800) FIGHT-MS
http://www.nationalmssociety.org/flc
E-mail: info@flc.nmss.org

North Florida
4237 Salisbury Road
Suite 406
Jacksonville, FL 32216
(904) 332-6810
(800) FIGHT-MS
http://www.nationalmssociety.org/FLN
E-mail: msnorfla@fln.nmss.org

The North Florida Chapter serves more than 18,000 people affected by MS, including family members, in a 34-county area. The chapter provides educational programs, wellness programs, a lending library, Kids Camp, advocacy efforts, teleconferences, and monthly newsletters. Key events are the PGA Tour MS 150 Bike Tour each September, the MS Walks in the spring, the Dinner of Champions, and an annual golf classic.

South Florida
3201 West Commercial Boulevard
Suite 127
Fort Lauderdale, FL 33309
(954) 731-4224
(800) FIGHT-MS
http://www.nmssfls.org
E-mail: fls@nmss.org

GEORGIA

455 Abernathy Road NE
Suite 210
Atlanta, GA 30328
(404) 256-9700
(800) FIGHT-MS
http://www.nationalmssociety.org/gaa
E-mail: mailbox@nmssga.org

HAWAII

418 Kuwili Street
#105
Honolulu, HI 96817
(808) 532-0811
(800) FIGHT-MS
http://www.nationalmssociety.org/hih
E-mail: hih@nmss.org

IDAHO

Idaho Division
1674 Hill Road
Suite 18
Boise, ID 83702
(208) 388-1998 (option 2)
(800) FIGHT-MS
http://www.nationalmssociety.org/idi
E-mail: idi@nmss.org

Inland Northwest
818 East Sharp
Spokane, WA 99202
(509) 482-2022
(800) FIGHT-MS

http://www.nationalmssociety.org/wai/home
E-mail: wai@nmss.org

Chartered in 1954, the Inland Northwest Chapter provides services and programs to 2,000 people with MS and their families within a 25-county territory—15 counties in eastern Washington and 10 counties in northern Idaho. The Inland Northwest Chapter area has the second highest rate of MS in the world.

ILLINOIS

Gateway Area
1867 Lackland Hill Parkway
Saint Louis, MO 63146
(314) 781-9020
(800) FIGHT-MS
http://www.gatewaymssociety.org
E-mail: info@gatewaymssociety.org

Greater Illinois
910 West Van Buren
Fourth Floor
Chicago, IL 60607
(312) 421-4500
(800) FIGHT-MS
http://www.msillinois.org
E-mail: cgic@ild.nmss.org

INDIANA

Indiana State
7301 Georgetown Road
Suite 112
Indianapolis, IN 46268
(317) 870-2500
(800) FIGHT-MS
http://www.msindiana.org
E-mail: astevenson@msindiana.org

The Indiana State Chapter of the National Multiple Sclerosis Society provides its clients with help through a variety of programs for families living with MS and through national research to find a cure. The Indiana State Chapter serves the residents of the state of Indiana and has more than 6,300 registered clients.

Southeast Indiana/Kentucky
11700 Commonwealth Drive
Suite 500
Louisville, KY 40299
(502) 451-0014
(800) FIGHT-MS

http://www.kynmss.org
E-mail: doug.dressman@kyw.nmss.org

Providing services to 109 Kentucky counties as well as Clark and Floyd Counties in Southern Indiana, the Kentucky–Southeast Indiana Chapter of the National Multiple Sclerosis Society offers a variety of services to both individuals and families who are coping with the changes in lifestyles mandated by this disease. Chapter program staff work with a network of volunteers to provide opportunities to 4,000 clients.

IOWA

1300 50th Street
Suite 106
West Des Moines, IA 50266-5499
(515) 270-6337
(800) FIGHT-MS
http://www.ianmss.org
E-mail: info@iac.nmss.org

KANSAS

Eastern Kansas/Western Missouri
P.O. Box 2292
Mission, KS 66201
(913) 432-3926
(800) FIGHT-MS
http://www.msmidamerica.org
E-mail: info@nmsskc.org

The Mid-America Chapter, originally the Kansas City Chapter, began in 1955 with one staff member working out of his home. By 1982, the chapter had grown large enough to move to its current address and established the Ozark and St. Joseph branches. By 1985, the name was changed to the Mid-America Chapter, and in 1990, the Mid-America Chapter merged with the Eastern Kansas Chapter. The chapter and its branches currently serve 105 counties in eastern Kansas and western Missouri and annually raises more than $2.5 million for the fight against MS.

South Central and Western Kansas
250 South Laura
Wichita, KS 67211
(316) 264-7043
(800) FIGHT-MS
http://www.nationalmssociety.org/kss
E-mail: kss@nmss.org

KENTUCKY

Kentucky/Southeast Indiana
11700 Commonwealth Drive
Suite 500
Louisville, KY 40299
(502) 451-0014
(800) FIGHT-MS
http://www.kynmss.org
E-mail: doug.dressman@kyw.nmss.org

Providing services to 109 Kentucky counties as well as Clark and Floyd Counties in Southern Indiana, the Kentucky–Southeast Indiana Chapter of the National Multiple Sclerosis Society offers a variety of services to both individuals and families who are coping with the changes in lifestyles mandated by this disease. Chapter program staff work with a network of volunteers to provide much-needed opportunities to the 4,000 clients serviced in the chapter's area.

Ohio Valley
4460 Lake Forest Drive
Suite 236
Cincinnati, OH 45242
(513) 769-4400
(800) FIGHT-MS
http://www.nationalmssociety.org/ohg
E-mail: melissa.roby@ohg.nmss.org

The Ohio Valley Chapter of the National Multiple Sclerosis Society is committed to empowering people with MS, family, friends, and professionals to maximize their understanding and knowledge regarding this often-frustrating disease. The chapter currently serves about 5,163 people with MS and their families in a 27-county area, which includes southwestern Ohio as well as three counties in northern Kentucky.

West Virginia
#2 Players Club Drive
Suite 104
Charleston, WV 25311
(304) 343-5152
(800) FIGHT-MS
http://www.nationalmssociety.org/wvt
E-mail: programs@charterinternet.com

LOUISIANA

3129 Edenborn Avenue
Metairie, LA 70002
(504) 832-4013

(800) FIGHT-MS
http://www.nationalmssociety.org/LAM/home
E-mail: louisianachapter@nmss.org

The Louisiana Chapter serves more than 3,000 individuals and their families living in the 64-parish territory of the state. Local programs such as information and referral services, a quarterly newsletter, support and self-help groups, caregiver groups, teleconferences, newly diagnosed programs, a lending library, free literature, educational seminars, equipment loan and assistance, and more are offered.

MAINE

Maine Chapter
P.O. Box 8730
77 Preble Street
Portland, ME 04104
(207) 761-5815
(800) FIGHT-MS
http://www.msmaine.org
E-mail: info@msmaine.org

MARYLAND

Maryland State
10946 Beaver Dam Road
Suite E
Hunt Valley, MD 21030
(410) 527-1770
(800) FIGHT-MS
http://www.nmss-md.org
E-mail: info@nmss-md.org

The Maryland Chapter of the National Multiple Sclerosis Society, founded in 1956, is a nonprofit agency serving more than 4,500 people with MS and their families in Maryland, except Prince George's and Montgomery Counties. The Maryland Chapter offers education, information and referral, counseling, assistance with employment concerns, and social activities. Major fund-raising campaigns include the MS Walk, the MS150 Bike Tour, and Dinner of Champions.

National Capital
2021 K Street, NW
Suite 715
Washington, DC 20006-1035
(202) 296-5363
(800) FIGHT-MS
http://www.MSandYOU.org
E-mail: information@msandyou.org

The National Capital Chapter provides programs and services to people in the District of Columbia, Prince George's and Montgomery Counties in Maryland, and Alexandria, Arlington, Fairfax, Fauquier, Loudoun, and Prince William Counties in Virginia. The chapter serves about 6,000 people with MS. When taken together with their families and caregivers, about 18,000 people in the Washington, D.C. metro area are affected by MS.

MASSACHUSETTS

101A First Avenue
Suite 6
Waltham, MA 02451-1115
(781) 890-4990
(800) FIGHT-MS
http://www.msnewengland.org/
E-mail: communications@mam.nmss.org

For 54 years, the Central New England Chapter has worked to improve quality of life for nearly 13,000 families affected by multiple sclerosis in New Hampshire and Massachusetts; 86 percent of chapter resources are spent on local, community-based programs that increase knowledge about the disease and available treatments, that improve health through exercise and support systems, that build independence through disability access training and employment counseling, and that support vital MS research making progress toward the cause, a cure, and better treatments.

MICHIGAN

21311 Civic Center Drive
Southfield, MI 48076
(248) 350-0020
(800) FIGHT-MS
http://www.nmssmi.org
E-mail: info@mig.nmss.org

MINNESOTA

200 12th Avenue South
Minneapolis, MN 55415
(612) 335-7900
(800) FIGHT-MS
http://www.mssociety.org/
E-mail: info@mssociety.org

The Minnesota Chapter represents an estimated 7,500 people with MS in Minnesota and western Wisconsin.

The chapter provides research dollars, innovative special events, hundreds of programs, services, and advocacy efforts, which promote greater independence and seek to enhance the lives of people who have MS.

MISSISSIPPI

Mississippi State
145 Executive Drive
Suite 1
Madison, MS 39110
(601) 856-7575
(800) FIGHT-MS
http://www.nationalmssociety.org/msm
E-mail: msm@nmss.org

Mid-South
4219 Hillsboro Road
Suite 306
Nashville, TN 37215
(615) 269-9055
(800) FIGHT-MS
http://www.msmidsouth.org
E-mail: tns@nmss.org

The Mid-South Chapter offers a wide range of programs to help people cope with the everyday demands of living with a chronic illness, serving people with MS, their families, and health care professionals through education, advocacy, information, peer support, therapeutic recreation, and many other programs. The Mid-South Chapter provides information based on professional advice, published experience, and expert opinion, but it does not give therapeutic recommendations, nor does it endorse products, services, or manufacturers.

MISSOURI

1867 Lackland Hill Parkway
Saint Louis, MO 63146
(314) 781-9020
(800) FIGHT-MS
http://www.gatewaymssociety.org
E-mail: info@gatewaymssociety.org

MONTANA

1629 Avenue D
Suite 2-C
Billings, MT 59102
(406) 252-9500

(800) FIGHT-MS
http://www.nationalmssociety.org/mtt
E-mail: mtt@nmss.org

For more than 50 years, the Montana Division of the National Multiple Sclerosis Society has been committed to expanding knowledge and awareness of MS, to enhancing access to MS specialty medical care, and to empowering people with MS to live as independently as possible. The goals are achieved through national and local programs and activities that educate people with MS and their families, professional, public officials, and the general public about MS. The chapter provides support programs that help people with MS and their families cope with the changes and challenges that MS presents, helps people gain access to community and public policy, and fills gaps in community resources.

NEBRASKA

Community Health Plaza
7101 Newport Avenue
Suite 304
Omaha, NE 68152
(402) 572-3190
(800) FIGHT-MS
http://www.nationalmssociety.org/nen
E-mail: nen@nmss.org

The Nebraska Chapter of the National Multiple Sclerosis Society serves more than 5,000 people in Nebraska and Pottawattamie County, Iowa. The chapter supports research into the cure, prevention, and treatment of MS, and it provides programs and services to help improve the quality of life for those with MS. It also provides programs, services, and activities in areas such as knowledge, health, and independence to empower those affected by multiple sclerosis. Major fund-raising campaigns are the MS Walk, the MS150 Bike Tour, Celebrate Cycling (one-day bike ride), and Dinner of Champions.

NEVADA

Great Basin Sierra
255 West Moana
Suite #107
Reno, NV 89509-4942
(775) 329-7180
(800) FIGHT-MS
http://www.nationalmssociety.org/nvn
E-mail: nvn@nvn.nmss.org

The Great Basin Sierra Chapter of the National Multiple Sclerosis Society was founded in 1960 as part of a nationwide network of organizations developed to support the overall mission: to end the devastating effects of multiple sclerosis. The chapter offers education, information and referrals, counseling, and social activities. The major fund-raising campaigns are the MS Walk and the MS 150 Bike Tour.

Nevada State
6000 South Eastern Avenue
#5C
Las Vegas, NV 89119-5151
(702) 736-7272
(800) FIGHT-MS
http://www.nationalmssociety.org/nvl
E-mail: nvl@nmss.org

NEW HAMPSHIRE

101A First Avenue
Suite 6
Waltham, MA 02451-1115
(781) 890-4990
(800) FIGHT-MS
http://www.msnewengland.org/
E-mail: communications@mam.nmss.org

For 54 years, the Central New England Chapter has worked to improve the quality of life for nearly 13,000 families affected by multiple sclerosis in New Hampshire and Massachusetts; 86 percent of chapter resources are spent on local, community-based programs that increase knowledge about the disease and available treatments, that improve health through exercise and support systems, that build independence through disability access training and employment counseling, and that support vital MS research making progress toward the cause, a cure, and better treatments.

NEW JERSEY

Greater Delaware Valley
1 Reed Street
Suite 200
Philadelphia, PA 19147
(215) 271-1500
(800) FIGHT-MS
http://www.pae.nmss.org
E-mail: pae@nmss.org

The Greater Delaware Valley Chapter is one of 83 chapters and branches of the National Multiple Sclerosis Society and serves a number of communities in New Jersey, including Atlantic, Burlington, Camden, Cape May, Cumberland, Gloucester, and Salem.

Greater North Jersey
1 Kalisa Way
Suite 205
Paramus, New Jersey, NJ 07652
(201) 967-5599
(800) FIGHT-MS
http://www.njbnmss.org
E-mail: chapter@njb.nmss.org

The Greater North Jersey Chapter, located in Paramus, New Jersey, serves northern New Jersey in Bergen, Essex, Hudson, Morris, Passaic, Sussex, Union, and Warren Counties. It provides over 100 programs and services to 4,500 people with MS and their families and caregivers, all of whom are dealing daily with the physical and emotional challenges of the disease. It also supports the national research effort to find the cause, treatments, and cure for MS.

Mid-Jersey
246 Monmouth Road
Oakhurst, NJ 07755
(732) 660-1005
(800) FIGHT-MS
E-mail: gail.svenciunas@njm.nmss.org

The Mid-Jersey Chapter was established in 1975 to serve the central Jersey area. The chapter services individuals and families with MS living in Monmouth, Ocean, Somerset, Middlesex, Hunterdon, and Mercer Counties.

NEW MEXICO

Panhandle Division
6222 Canyon Drive
Amarillo, TX 79109
(806) 468-7500
(800) FIGHT-MS
http://www.nationalmssociety.org/txp
E-mail: txp@nmss.org

The Panhandle Division is located in Amarillo, Texas, the heart of the Texas Panhandle. It is currently serving the 700 people with MS in the Texas and Oklahoma Panhandles and the four easternmost counties of New Mexico.

Rio Grande Division
2021 Girard SE
Suite 201
Albuquerque, NM 87106
(505) 244-0625
(800) FIGHT-MS
http://www.nationalmssociety.org/nmx
E-mail: nmx@nmss.org

For more than 50 years, the Rio Grande Division of the National Multiple Sclerosis Society has been committed to expanding knowledge and awareness of multiple sclerosis, to enhance access to MS specialty medical care, and to empower people with MS to live as independently as possible. The goals are achieved through national and local programs and activities.

NEW YORK

Long Island
200 Parkway Drive South
Hauppauge, NY 11788
(631) 864-8337
(800) FIGHT-MS
http://www.nationalmssociety.org/nyh
E-mail: pmastrota@nmssli.org

In the 1950s, grassroots efforts on Long Island resulted in the establishment of offices in both Nassau and Suffolk counties. In 1986, in order to provide more comprehensive coverage and services, these two divisions merged and gave rise to the Long Island Chapter. Today the Long Island Chapter serves the needs of more than 38,000 people with MS and their families and is dedicated to ending the devastating effects of MS and promoting access to a multitude of programs and services to help individuals lead useful and fulfilling lives.

New York City
30 West 26th Street
9th Floor
New York, NY 10010
(212) 463-7787
(800) FIGHT-MS
http://www.msnyc.org
E-mail: info@msnyc.org

The chapter provides its clients with many programs and services such as education, information and referrals, counseling, assistance with employment concerns, self-help and support groups, social activities, and much more.

Southern New York

2 Gannett Drive
Suite LC
White Plains, NY 10604
(914) 694-1655
(800) FIGHT-MS
http://www.nationalmssociety.org/nyv
E-mail: nyv@nmss.org

The chapter provides its clients with many programs and services such as education, information and referrals, counseling, assistance with employment concerns, self-help and support groups, social activities, and much more.

Upstate New York

1650 South Avenue
Suite 100
Rochester, NY 14620-3901
(585) 271-0801
(800) FIGHT-MS
E-mail: chapter@msupstatcny.org

The chapter provides its clients with many programs and services such as education, information and referrals, counseling, assistance with employment concerns, self-help and support groups, social activities, and much more.

Western New York/Northwestern Pennsylvania

4245 Union Road
Suite 108
Buffalo, NY 14225
(716) 634-2261
(800) FIGHT-MS
E-mail: nyw@nmss.org

Founded on November 23, 1954, the chapter is a nonprofit agency serving nearly 3,300 people with MS and their families within 11 counties located throughout western New York and northwestern Pennsylvania. They include Allegany, Cattaraugus, Chautauqua, Erie, Genesee, Niagara, Orleans, and Wyoming Counties in western New York and Erie, McKean, and Warren counties in northwestern Pennsylvania. The chapter provides its clients with many programs and services such as education, information and referrals, counseling, assistance with

employment concerns, self-help and support groups, social activities, and much more. Three major events the chapter hosts are the MS Walk, the MS Bike Tour—A Tour of Chautauqua, and the Dinner of Champions.

NORTH CAROLINA

Central North Carolina

2211 West Meadowview Road
Suite 30
Greensboro, NC 27407
(336) 299-4136
(800) FIGHT-MS
http://www.nationalmssociety.org/ncc
E-mail: ncc@nmss.org

The chapter is committed to expanding knowledge of MS, enhancing access to MS specialty medical care, and empowering people with MS to live as independently as possible within the limits of their disabilities, and to the maximum of their capabilities, within the least-restrictive environment.

Eastern North Carolina

3101 Industrial Drive
Suite 210
Raleigh, NC 27609
(919) 834-0678
(800) FIGHT-MS
http://www.nationalmssociety.org/nct
E-mail: nct@nmss.org

Mid-Atlantic

9844 C Southern Pines Boulevard
Charlotte, NC 28273
(704) 525-2955
(800) FIGHT-MS
http://www.nationalmssociety.org/ncp
E-mail: ncp@nmss.org

The Mid-Atlantic Chapter of the National Multiple Sclerosis Society, established in 1955, contributes funds for the society's national research program and provides programs to people with MS throughout 33 counties of western North Carolina. Chapter programs help improve the quality of life of people living with MS and their families by improving knowledge about the disease, emotional health, physical health, and independence. The chapter provides the latest information on all aspects of MS including current research, community resources, and government programs.

NORTH DAKOTA

3800 West Technology Circle
Suite 201
Sioux Falls, SD 57106
(605) 336-7017
(800) FIGHT-MS
http://www.msdakotachapter.org
E-mail: mona.schrader@ndn.nmss.org

OHIO

Northwestern Ohio

401 Tomahawk Drive
Maumee, OH 43537
(419) 897-9533
(800) FIGHT-MS
http://www.nationalmssociety.org/oho
E-mail: nwohio@amplex.net

The Northwestern Ohio Chapter has been serving people with MS and their families for more than 36 years. Today the service area includes 26 counties, with approximately 3,000 people registered.

Ohio Buckeye Chapter

1422 Euclid Avenue
Suite 333
Cleveland, OH 44115
(800) 667-7131
(800) FIGHT-MS
http://www.msohiobuckeye.org
E-mail: oha@nmss.org

The Ohio Buckeye Chapter serves 8,000 people living with MS in 36 eastern and central Ohio counties through offices in Akron, Cleveland, Columbus, and Youngstown. The chapter was founded on September 24, 1953. The Ohio Buckeye Chapter offers education, information and referrals, counseling, assistance with employment concerns, equipment loan programs, social activities, and much more.

Ohio Valley

4460 Lake Forest Drive
Suite 236
Cincinnati, OH 45242
(513) 769-4400
(800) FIGHT-MS
http://www.nationalmssociety.org/ohg
E-mail: melissa.roby@ohg.nmss.org

The Ohio Valley Chapter of the National Multiple Sclerosis Society is committed to empowering people with MS, family, friends, and professionals to maximize their understanding and knowledge regarding this often-frustrating disease. The chapter currently serves about 5,163 people with MS and their families in a 27-county area, which includes southwestern Ohio as well as three counties in northern Kentucky.

OKLAHOMA

Oklahoma State

4606 East 67th Street
Building 7
Suite 103
Tulsa, OK 74136
(918) 488-0882
(800) 777-7814
http://www.nationalmssociety.org/oke
E-mail: paula.cortner@oke.nmss.org

The Oklahoma Chapter, established in 1954, funds research programs and provides services to the more than 21,000 Oklahomans affected in a 74-county service area covering most of Oklahoma. The three panhandle counties are covered by the Panhandle Division.

Panhandle Division

6222 Canyon Drive
Amarillo, TX 79109
(806) 468-7500
(800) FIGHT-MS
http://www.nationalmssociety.org/txp
E-mail: txp@nmss.org

The Panhandle Division is located in Amarillo, Texas, the heart of the Texas Panhandle. It is currently serving the 700 people with MS in the Texas and Oklahoma Panhandles and the four easternmost counties of New Mexico.

OREGON

1650 NW Naito Parkway
Suite 190
Portland, OR 97209
(503) 223-9511
(800) FIGHT-MS
http://www.orcnmss.org
E-mail: info@orcnmss.org

The Oregon Chapter of the National Multiple Sclerosis Society is aggressively pursuing the mission to end the devastating effects of MS by providing programs designed to enhance the quality of life for people with MS and their families throughout Oregon and Clark

County, Washington, and by raising funds to support these programs and national research efforts aimed at solving the puzzle of MS. The Oregon Chapter is 36 years old and is currently serving over 5,800 people with MS, plus family members, friends, and health care professionals.

PENNSYLVANIA

Allegheny District
1040 Fifth Avenue
2nd Floor
Pittsburgh, PA 15219
(412) 261-6347
(800) FIGHT-MS
http://www.nmss-pgh.org
E-mail: pax@nmss.org

The Allegheny District Chapter of the National Multiple Sclerosis Society, founded in 1957, is a not-for-profit agency serving more than 4,900 people with MS and their families in 23 counties of western Pennsylvania. The Allegheny District Chapter offers self-help groups, equipment assistance, respite for caregivers, exercise and wellness classes, and more. Major fund-raising campaigns are the MS Walk, the MS 150 Bike Tour, the MS Read-a-Thon, and the Coors Light U.G.L.Y Bartender Contest.

Central Pennsylvania
2209 Forest Hills Drive
Suite 18
Harrisburg, PA 17112
(717) 652-2108
(800) FIGHT-MS
http://www.pac.nmss.org
E-mail: pac@nmss.org

The National Multiple Sclerosis Society, Central Pennsylvania Chapter, those with MS, serves their family, and their friends through education, information and referrals, counseling, assistance with employment concerns, social activities, and more. Members receive chapter newsletters. The quarterly *MSConnection* include research updates invitations to educational seminars calendars for special events, self-help groups, physical activities and social opportunities, and programs specialized for family members; and other valuable information.

Greater Delaware Valley
1 Reed Street
Suite 200

Philadelphia, PA 19147
(215) 271-1500
(800) FIGHT-MS
http://www.pae.nmss.org
E-mail: pae@nmss.org

The Greater Delaware Valley Chapter is one of 83 chapters and branches of the National Multiple Sclerosis Society in the United States. It serve Berks, Bucks, Carbon, Chester, Delaware, Lehigh, Monroe, Montgomery, Northampton, Philadelphia, and Schuylkill Counties.

Northwestern Pennsylvania/Western New York
4245 Union Road
Suite 108
Buffalo, NY 14225
(716) 634-2261
(800) FIGHT-MS
E-mail: nyw@nmss.org

Founded on November 23, 1954, the Western New York/Northwestern Pennsylvania Chapter is a nonprofit agency serving nearly 3,300 people with MS and their families in northwestern Pennsylvania, including Erie, McKean, and Warren. The chapter provides its clients with many programs and services such as education, information and referrals, counseling, assistance with employment concerns, self-help and support groups, social activities, and much more. Three major events the chapter hosts are the MS Walk, the MS Bike Tour—A Tour of Chautauqua, and the Dinner of Champions.

RHODE ISLAND
205 Hallene Road
Suite 209
Warwick, RI 02886
(401) 738-8383
(800) FIGHT-MS
http://www.nationalmssociety.org/rir
E-mail: sean.mcauliffe@rir.nmss.org

SOUTH CAROLINA

Mid-Atlantic
9844 C Southern Pines Boulevard
Charlotte, NC 28273
(704) 525-2955
(800) FIGHT-MS
http://www.nationalmssociety.org/ncp
E-mail: ncp@nmss.org

The Mid-Atlantic Chapter of the National Multiple Sclerosis Society, established in 1955, contributes funds for the society's national research program and provides programs to people with MS throughout all of South Carolina. Chapter programs help improve the quality of life of people living with MS and their families by improving knowledge about the disease, emotional health, physical health, and independence. The chapter provides the latest information on all aspects of MS including current research, community resources, and government programs.

South Carolina, Regional
2711 Middleburg Drive
Suite 105
Columbia, SC 29204
(803) 799-7848
(800) FIGHT-MS

SOUTH DAKOTA
3800 West Technology Circle
Suite 201
Sioux Falls, SD 57106
(605) 336-7017
(800) FIGHT-MS
http://www.msdakotachapter.org
E-mail: mona.schrader@ndn.nmss.org

The Dakota Chapter is dedicated to offering programs that will support knowledge of MS, family support and MS, employment, emotional, physical accessibility, and independence in MS.

TENNESSEE
4219 Hillsboro Road
Suite 306
Nashville, TN 37215
(615) 269-9055
(800) FIGHT-MS
http://www.msmidsouth.org
E-mail: tns@nmss.org

The Mid-South Chapter offers a wide range of programs to help people cope with the everyday demands of living with a chronic illness. It serves people with MS, their families, and health care professionals through education, advocacy, information, peer support, therapeutic recreation, and many other programs.

TEXAS
Lone Star
8111 North Stadium Drive
Suite 100
Houston, TX 77054
(713) 526-8967
(800) FIGHT-MS
http://www.nationalmssociety.org/txh
E-mail: txh@nmss.org

The chapter staff and volunteers are committed to helping end the devastating effects of MS and providing educational and wellness programs, social activities, recreational camps, information and referral services, advocacy efforts, self-help groups, and direct assistance to people living with MS, their family, friends, and the professionals who serve them. Members of the Lone Star Chapter receive invitations to programs; the quarterly chapter newsletter *MS Connection,* and the quarterly national magazine *InsideMS.* These publications are packed with information about living well with MS, research updates, information from health care professionals, and a calendar of events. This chapter serves 141 counties in Texas with offices in Austin, Corpus Christi, Dallas, Houston, and San Antonio.

North Central Texas
4086 Sandshell Drive
Fort Worth, TX 76137
(817) 306-7003
(800) FIGHT-MS
http://www.nctms.org
E-mail: nms@nctms.org

The North Central Texas Chapter of the National Multiple Sclerosis Society, founded in 1984, is a not-for-profit agency serving more than 7,500 people with MS and their families in North-Central Texas. The chapter offers education, information and referrals, counseling, assistance with employment concerns, social activities, and more.

Panhandle Division
6222 Canyon Drive
Amarillo, TX 79109
(806) 468-7500
(800) FIGHT-MS
http://www.nationalmssociety.org/txp
E-mail: txp@nmss.org

The Panhandle Division is located in Amarillo, Texas, the heart of the Texas Panhandle. It is currently serving the 700 people with MS in the Texas and Oklahoma Panhandles and the four easternmost counties of New Mexico.

West Texas Division
1031 Andrews Hwy

Suite 201
Midland, TX 79701
(432) 522-2077
(800) FIGHT-MS
http://www.nationalmssociety.org/txq
E-mail: txq@nts-online.net

For more than 50 years, the West Texas Division of the National Multiple Sclerosis Society has been committed to expanding knowledge and awareness of MS, enhancing access to MS specialty medical care, and empowering people with MS to live as independently as possible. The goals are achieved through national and local programs and activities that inform and educate people with MS and their families, professionals, public officials, and the general public about MS; provide support programs that help people with MS and their families cope with changes and challenges; help people gain access to community and public policy beneficial to people with MS; and fill gaps in community resources.

UTAH

2995 South West Temple
Suite C
Salt Lake City, UT 84115
(801) 493-0113
(800) FIGHT-MS
http://www.fightmsutah.org
E-mail: info@fightmsutah.org

The Utah State Chapter provides valuable support, resources, and services for Utah residents with MS, their families, and friends. Although membership with the Utah State Chapter is not required to receive informative materials about MS, membership does offer many advantages. Members receive two chapter newsletters: the quarterly *MSConnection* and bimonthly *Program Connection,* including research updates; invitations to educational seminars; calendars for special events, self-help groups, physical therapy opportunities, and care partner meetings; and other information. Members also receive *InsideMS,* a national quarterly magazine. In addition, the Utah State Chapter offers many support programs, special events, informational seminars, and other services to members.

VERMONT

75 Talcott Road
Williston, VT 05495
(802) 862-0912
(800) FIGHT-MS

http://www.nationalmssociety.org/vtn
E-mail: vtn@nmss.org

For more than 50 years, the Vermont Division of the National Multiple Sclerosis Society has been committed to expanding knowledge and awareness of MS, to enhance access to MS specialty medical care, and to empower people with MS to live as independently as possible. The goals are achieved through national and local programs and activities that inform and educate people with MS and their families, professionals, public officials, and the general public about MS. The chapter also provides support programs that help people with MS and their families cope with the changes and challenges that MS presents, helps people gain access to community and public policy beneficial to people with MS, and fills gaps in community resources.

VIRGINIA

Blue Ridge
1 Morton Drive
Suite 106
Charlottesville, VA 22903
(434) 971-8010
(800) FIGHT-MS
http://www.nationalmssociety.org/vab
E-mail: vab@nmss.org

Central Virginia
2104 West Laburnum Avenue
Suite 102
Richmond, VA 23227
(804)353-5008
(800) FIGHT-MS
http://www.nmss-centralva.org
E-mail: melina.davis-martin@var.nmss.org

Hampton Roads
405 South Parliament Drive
Suite 105
Virginia Beach, VA 23462
(757) 490-9627
(800) FIGHT-MS
http://www.fightms.com
E-mail: info@fightms.com

The Hampton Roads Chapter of the National Multiple Sclerosis Society serves more than 2,600 people in the greater Hampton Roads area including the Southside, the Peninsula, the northern Neck, the eastern Shore, and three counties in North Carolina. The chapter supports research into the cure, prevention, and treatment of MS and provides programs and services to help improve the quality of life for those with MS.

National Capital
2021 K Street, NW
Suite 715
Washington, DC 20006-1035
(202) 296-5363
(800) FIGHT-MS
http://www.MSandYOU.org
E-mail: information@msandyou.org

The National Capital Chapter provides programs and services to people in the District of Columbia; Prince George's and Montgomery Counties in Maryland; and Alexandria, Arlington, Fairfax, Fauquier, Loudoun, and Prince William Counties in Virginia. The chapter serves approximately 6,000 people with MS. When taken together with their families and caregivers, the chapter has identified that approximately 18,000 people are affected by MS in the Washington, DC, metro area.

WASHINGTON

Greater Washington
192 Nickerson Street
Suite 100
Seattle, WA 98109
(206) 284-4236
(800) FIGHT-MS
http://www.nationalmssociety.org/was
E-mail: greaterwainfo@nmsswas.org

The Greater Washington Chapter serves 23 counties in western and central Washington and provides support to more than 50,000 people, including 7,000 with MS and nearly 40,000 others whose lives are directly impacted (ranging from spouses, children, and relatives to friends, coworkers, and caregivers). The chapter programs include information and referrals, educational seminars, self-help groups, and financial assistance for counseling, durable medical equipment, and fitness scholarships. The chapter also funds national research efforts to discover the cause and cure for MS.

Inland Northwest
818 East Sharp
Spokane, WA 99202
(509) 482-2022

(800) FIGHT-MS
http://www.nationalmssociety.org/wai/home
E-mail: wai@nmss.org

The Inland Northwest Chapter of the National Multiple Sclerosis Society is one of a 70-plus-chapter network across the United States that advances the society's mission. Chartered in 1954, the Inland Northwest Chapter provides services and programs to 2,000 people with MS and their families within the chapter's 25-county territory. The Inland Northwest Chapter serves 15 counties in eastern Washington and 10 counties in northern Idaho. The Inland Northwest Chapter area has the second highest rate of MS in the world.

WEST VIRGINIA

2 Players Club Drive
Suite 104
Charleston, WV 25311
(304) 343-5152
(800) FIGHT-MS
http://www.nationalmssociety.org/wvt
E-mail: programs@charterinternet.com

For more than 50 years, the West Virginia Division of the National Multiple Sclerosis Society has been committed to expanding knowledge and awareness of MS, to enhancing access to MS specialty medical care, and to empowering people with MS to live as independently as possible.

Wisconsin
Minnesota State
200 12th Avenue South
Minneapolis, MN 55415
(612) 335-7900
(800) FIGHT-MS
http://www.mssociety.org
E-mail: info@mssociety.org

The Minnesota Chapter represents an estimated 7,500 people with MS in Minnesota and western Wisconsin. The chapter provides research dollars, innovative special events, and hundreds of programs, services, and advocacy efforts that promote greater independence and seek to enhance the lives of people who have MS.

Wisconsin Chapter
1120 James Drive
Suite A
Hartland, WI 53029

(262) 369-4400
(800) FIGHT-MS
http://www.wisms.org
E-mail: info@wisms.org

WYOMING

400 East 1st Street
Suite 203

Casper, WY 82601
(307) 234-2340
(Casper)
(307) 433-8664
(Cheyenne)
(800) FIGHT-MS
http://www.nationalmssociety.org/wyy
E-mail: nicholle.bridgmon@nmss.org

APPENDIX V
INTERNATIONAL MULTIPLE SCLEROSIS SOCIETIES

Multiple Sclerosis International Federation (MSIF)

3rd Floor Skyline House
200 Union Street
London
SE1 OLX
44 (020) 7620 1911
http://www.msif.org
E-mail: info@msif.org

The Multiple Sclerosis International Federation was established in 1967 as an international body linking the activities of national MS societies around the world. Current information is available in several languages at the MSIF web site.

ARGENTINA

Esclerosis Múltiple Argentina

Uriarte 1465
(1414) Buenos Aires
Tel: (54) 1 831 6617
Fax: (54) 1 831 6786
http://www.ema.org.ar
E-mail: info@ema.org.ar

This nonprofit society was established in 1986 in Buenos Aires to collaborate in finding a cure for multiple sclerosis (MS) and to help people with MS and their families to improve their quality of life. About 10,000 people in Argentina have MS; the society has about 950 members.

AUSTRALIA

National MS Society of Australia

c/o Studdy MS Center
Joseph Street,
Lidcombe, NSW 2141
(61) 02 9646 0600
http://www.msaustralia.org.au
E-mail: info@mssociety.com.au

This nonprofit society was established in 1975 in North Sydney to provide information exchange between state multiple sclerosis (MS) societies, coordinate funding of research projects, and develop a national communications program. About 20,000 people in Australia have MS; the society includes members from seven states.

AUSTRIA

Österreichische Multiple Sklerose Gesellschaft

Universitätsklink für Neurologie
Währinger-Gürtel 18-20
A-1090 Wien
(43) 1-40400-3123
http://www.ms-ges.or.at
E-mail: oemsges@akh-wien.ac.at

This nonprofit society was established in 1965 in Vienna to support people with multiple sclerosis (MS), distribute information about MS, and support scientific research. About 8,000 people in Austria have MS; the society has about 3,500 members.

BELGIUM

Ligue Nationale Belge de la Sclérose en Plaques/Nationale Belgische Multiple Sclerose Liga

Avenue Eugene Plasky
173/bte 11, B-1030 Bruxelles
(32) 2 736 1638
http://www.ms-sep.be
E-mail: ms.sep@ms-sep.be

This nonprofit society was established in 1958 in Brussels to empower people with multiple sclerosis (MS), provide information, defend the rights and interests of MS patients, provide financial support to people with MS, and support medical and social research. About 12,000 people in Belgium have MS; the society has about 5,500 members.

BRAZIL

Associação Brasileira de Esclerose Múltipla

Avenida Indianópolis, 2752
Indianópolis, São Paulo, SP
04062-003
(55) 11 5587 6050
http://www.abem.org.br
E-mail: abem@abem.org.br

This nonprofit society was established in 1984 to provide information about multiple sclerosis (MS), support people with MS and their families, and offer a full range of services. About 25,000 people in Brazil have MS; the society has about 21,000 members.

CANADA

MS Society of Canada/Société Canadienne de la Sclérose en Plaques

175 Bloor Street East
Suite 700 North Tower
Toronto, Ontario M4W 3R8
(1) 416 922 6065
http://www.mssociety.ca
http://www.scleroseenplaques.ca
E-mail: info@mssociety.ca

This nonprofit society was founded in 1948 in Toronto to help find a cure for multiple sclerosis (MS); fund research into the cause, prevention, treatment and management of MS; provide services for patients and family members; educate the public; and work to change government policies, private industry practices, and public attitudes about MS. About 50,000 Canadians have MS, and society has about 28,500 members.

CHILE

Corporación Chilena contra la Esclerosis Múltiple

Los Cerezos 278
Ñuñoa, Santiago
(56) 2 276 5556
E-mail: lmikin@redbanc.cl

This nonprofit organization was founded in 1991 to develop a better quality of life for people with multiple sclerosis by providing information, psychological support, and social support. About 2,000 Chileans have MS; the society has about 330 members.

CYPRUS

Cyprus Multiple Sclerosis Association

67-69 Ayiou Nicolaou Street, 2408
Engomi, Nicosia
(357) 22 590949
E-mail: multips@logos.cy.net

This nonprofit association was founded in 1986 in Nicosia to support the 350 Cypriots with multiple sclerosis. There are about 200 members in this society.

CZECH REPUBLIC

Unie Roska Ceská MS Spolecnots

P.O. Box 38
120 00 Praha 2
(420) 2 4172 8619
http://www.roska-czmss.cz/
E-mail: roska@roska-czmss.cz

A nonprofit society founded in 1992 to help people with multiple sclerosis (MS) become fully integrated into society. About 10,000 people in the Czech Republic have MS, and about 2,500 are members of the CzMSS.

DENMARK

Danish MS Society

Scleroseforeningen
Mosedalvej 15
DK-2500 Valby
(45) 36 46 36 46
http://www.scleroseforeningen.dk
E-mail: info@scleroseforeningen.dk

This nonprofit society was founded in 1957 to support research and to provide information about multiple sclerosis (MS). About 7,000 Danes have MS; about 5,000 belong to the society.

FINLAND

Suomen MS-Liitto Finlands MS-Förbund

Seppalantie 90, PL 15
FIN–21251 Masku
(358) 2 439 2111
http://www.ms-liitto.fi
E-mail: ms-liitto@ms-liitto.fi

This nonprofit society was founded in 1972 to support people with multiple sclerosis (MS) and guide and supervise the activities of the affiliated MS societies. About 6,000 Finns have MS, and the society has about 10,000 members.

FRANCE

Ligue Française Contre la Sclérose en Plaques
40 Rue Duranton
75015 Paris
(33) 1 53 98 98 80
http://www.lfsep.com
E-mail: info@lfsep.asso.fr

This nonprofit society was founded in 1986 in Paris to provide information, fund research, and help people with multiple sclerosis (MS). About 60,000 people in France have MS; the society has about 2,600 members.

GERMANY

Deutsche Multiple Sklerose Gesellschaft
Bundesverband e.V.
Küsterstrasse 8
D-30519 Hannover
(49) 511 9 68 34 0
http://www.dmsg.de
E-mail: dmsg@dmsg.de

This nonprofit society was founded in 1953 in Hannover to support and sponsor research into multiple sclerosis (MS), improve outpatient aftercare, represent patient interests in the legislature, and provide more information about MS. The society also funds and sponsors nursing institutions and clinics, and it supports self-help groups, seminars, public education, advice centers, driving services, outpatient care services, living care projects, rehabilitation, and acute clinics. About 122,000 Germans have MS; the society has about 43,125 members.

GREAT BRITAIN

See UNITED KINGDOM

GREECE

Greek Multiple Sclerosis Society
2-4 Faethonos Str
Thessaloniki 54351
(30) 23109 49909
E-mail: mssoc@hol.gr

This nonprofit society was founded in 1992 to support people with multiple sclerosis (MS) and to promote research into treatments and a possible cure. Between 6,000 and 10,000 Greeks have MS; the society has about 3,500 members.

HUNGARY

Hungarian Multiple Sclerosis Society
Székesfehérvár
Jancsár u. U 9, 8000 Hungary
(36) 22 314 198
http://www.sm.alba.hu/
E-mail: info@sm.alba.hu

This nonprofit society was founded in 1985 to coordinate the work of the Hungarian multiple sclerosis (MS) organizations, to provide information for the media about MS, and to protect the interests of people with MS. The society also informs people with MS through the MS journal *ESEMÉNYEK*. An estimated 12,000 Hungarians have MS; the society has about 24 members.

ICELAND

MS Felag Islands
Slettluvegur 5
103 Reykjavík
(354) 568 8620
http://www.msfelag.is
E-mail: msfelag@msfelag.is

This nonprofit society was founded in 1968 in Reykjavík to promote the welfare of people with multiple sclerosis, facilitate their equal participation in the fabric of the country, and encourage their rehabilitation. About 100 people out of every 100,000 have MS in Iceland.

INDIA

Multiple Sclerosis Society of India
No. 4 Ground Floor, Shree Laxmi
Sadan, 49/50
Gokhale Road (North)
Dadar (West)
Mumbai–400 028
(91) 22 444 2067
http://www.mssi.info
E-mail: mssindia@bom8.vsnl.net.in

This nonprofit society was established in 1985 to promote the welfare of people with multiple sclerosis (MS), to provide information about MS, and to promote activities intended to help people with MS. About 50,000 Indians have MS; about 1,000 members belong to the society.

IRAN

Iranian MS Society
58 Shirazi Avenue
Vessal
Terhan
(98) 216 490945
http://www.irmss.org
E-mail: info@irmss.org

This nonprofit society was established in 2000 in Tehran to support patients with multiple sclerosis (MS), gather information and compile statistics, provide information, and support research into MS. About 15,000 Iranians have MS, and about 4,000 are members of the society.

IRELAND

MS Society of Ireland Limited
4th Floor, Dartmouth House
Grand Parade, Dublin 6
(353) 1 269 4599
http://www.ms-society.ie
E-mail: info@ms-society.ie

This nonprofit society was founded in 1963 in Dublin to help people with multiple sclerosis (MS) regain control over their lives and their environment, live with dignity, and participate in the community; it also helps people with MS. In addition, the society promotes scientific research into the cause, cure, and management of MS, provides information about MS, and develops an effective and caring organization to serve the needs of people with MS. More than 6,000 Irish citizens have MS; the society includes 3,000 members.

ISRAEL

Israel MS Society
75 Yehuda Halevi Street
Tel Aviv, 65796
(972) 3 560 9222
http://www.mssociety.org.il
E-mail: agudaims@netvision.net.il

This nonprofit society was founded in 1976 in Tel Aviv to help people with MS and their families. About 5,000 Israelis have MS; the society includes about 2,200 members.

ITALY

Associazione Italiana Sclerosi Multipla
Vico Chiuso Paggi, 3-16128
Genova
(39) 010 27 131
http://www.aism.it
E-mail: aism@aism.it

This nonprofit society was founded in 1968 in Genoa to identify the cause and a cure for the disease, to help people with multiple sclerosis (MS) and their families, and to provide information about MS. About 50,000 Italians have MS; the society includes about 20,000 members.

JAPAN

Japan Multiple Sclerosis Society
4-1-2 Kotobuki
Taito-Ku
Tokyo
(81) 3 3847 3561
E-mail: jmss@tk.sanyeicorp.co.jp

This nonprofit society was founded in 1977 in Tokyo to further research into multiple sclerosis (MS) and related diseases and to provide services for patients. About 5,000 Japanese have MS; the society includes about 29 members.

KOREA

Korean MS Society
421 Koryo Academitel
437-3 Ahyoun-dong
Mapo-Gu
Seoul 121-011
(82) 2 362 7774
http://www.kmss.or.kr/
E-mail: kmss@kmss.or.kr

LATVIA

Latvijas Multiplas Sklerozes Asociacija
Melidaiela 10, Riga, LV-1015
(371) 7 351 792
http://www.lmsa.lv
E-mail: lmsa@e-apollo.lv

This nonprofit society was founded in 1995 in Riga. About 2,500 Latvians have MS; the society includes about 1,368 members.

LUXEMBOURG

Ligue Luxembourgeoise de la Sclérose en Plaques
Boîte Postale 1444
L-1014 Luxembourg

(352) 40 08 44

E-mail: mslux@pt.lu

This nonprofit society was founded in 1980 to improve the quality of life of people with multiple sclerosis (MS) and to help improve their integration into society. The society also tries to promote contact among people with MS, to help them find suitable housing, to create a suitable social services, and to provide information about MS. The society also supports scientific research into MS. About 400 people in Luxembourg have MS; the society has about 1,550 members.

MALTA

Multiple Sclerosis Society of Malta

P.O. Box 209

Valetta

(356) 418 066

http://www.msmalta.org.mt/

E-mail: lagius@onvol.net

This nonprofit society was founded in 1997 to provide updated medical information about multiple sclerosis (MS), to provide those with MS with an environment where they can meet and share experiences, and to provide medical and other services to people with MS. About 80 Maltese have MS; the society includes about 120 members.

MEXICO

Esclerosis Múltiple México

Callejón del Río 33 Bis

Col. del Carmen Coyoacan

México, D.F.

(52) 55 5659 2419

E-mail: emmex_ac@hotmail.com

NETHERLANDS

Multiple Sclerose Vereniging Nederland

Laan van Meerdervoort 51, Postbus

30470, 2500 GL Den Haag

(31) 70 374 7777

http://www.msweb.nl

E-mail: info@msvn.nl

This nonprofit society was founded in 1963 to protect the interests of people with multiple sclerosis (MS) and people with similar diseases. The society also tries to maintain adequate provisions for people with MS

in order to help them maintain their independence. About 16,000 Dutch people have MS; the society has about 12,000 members.

NEW ZEALAND

MS Society of New Zealand, Inc.

P.O. Box 2627

Wellington

(64) 4 499 4677

http://www.msnz.org

E-mail: info@msnz.org

This nonprofit society was founded in 1967 in Wellington to provide ongoing support, education, and advocacy for people with multiple sclerosis (MS) and their support networks. It also educates the general public, employers, and health professionals about MS. The society supports (both financially and through lobbying) ongoing medical research into MS. About 2,500 New Zealanders have MS; 18 regional societies belong to the national organization.

NORWAY

Multipel Sklerose Forbundet I

Norge Sørkedalsveien 3

0369 Oslo

(47) 2296 3580

http://www.ms.no

E-mail: post@ms.no

This nonprofit society was founded in 1966 in Oslo to provide information to newly diagnosed people with multiple sclerosis (MS) and to provide both financial help and information to people with MS. The society can arrange courses for people with MS and their families, and it provides information to local communities and the government. About 8,000 Norwegians have MS; the society has about 6,923 members.

POLAND

Polskie Towarzystwo Stwardnienia Rozsianego

c/o Hotel Marriott, Al Jerozolimskie

65/79, 00-697 Warszawa

(48) 22 630 7220

http://ptsr.idn.org.pl/

E-mail: ptsr-rg@idn.org.pl

This nonprofit society was founded in 1990 in Warsaw to distribute information about mutliple sclerosis (MS). About 60,000 Poles have MS; the society has about 6,000 members.

PORTUGAL

Sociedade Portuguesa de Esclerose Múltipla
Rua Zofimo Pedroso, 66
1950-291, Lisboa
(351) 21 839 4720
http://www.spem.org
E-mail: spem@spem.org

This nonprofit society was founded in 1984 in Lisbon to provide information to people with multiple sclerosis (MS), to provide referrals to professionals and facilities, and to provide home care for people with MS. The society also offers summer vacations, legal and psychological advice, and leisure activities. About 5,000 Portuguese have MS; the society has about 1,370 members.

ROMANIA

Uniunea Nationala a organizatiilor de Multipla Scleroza din România
2/B Str Buzaului, CP11 OP7
Oradea 3700 Romania
(40) 5941 7136
http://www.smromania.ro
E-mail: unoms@roetco.ro

This nonprofit society was established to help people with multiple sclerosis (MS) and their families. The society also tries to strengthen existing regional MS foundations and, through its development plan, help to establish new foundations in regions not yet covered. It provides information and, where possible, social and medical support through the regional groups. With its newly formed medical advisory board, the society informs national and local health agencies so the state can provide the most effective treatment, therapy, and care possible for people with MS. The practical philosophy of this society is a commitment to keep families together where possible by supporting the person with MS so that he or she can continue to live as independently as possible in the community, rather than be sent to institutions. About 20,000 people in Romania have MS.

SLOVAKIA

Slovensky Zväz Sclerosis Multiplex
Culenova 12
917 01 Trnava
(421) 33 551 3009
http://web.stonline.sk/szsm/
E-mail: msinslovakia@pobox.sk

This nonprofit society was founded in 1990 to support and encourage people with multiple sclerosis (MS) and support the formation of regional societies. About 5,500 people in Slovakia have MS; the society has about 1,286 members.

SLOVENIA

Zdruzenje Multiple Skleroze Slovenije
Maroltova 14, 1000 Ljubljana
(386) 1 568 72 99
http://www.zdruzenje-ms.si/
E-mail: info@zdruzenje-ms.si

This nonprofit society was founded in 1973 to provide rehabilitation for people with multiple sclerosis (MS) at its MS center in Toplosica. The society also tries to help people with MS remain in the workforce and to help people maintain, for as long as possible, an independent life. About 2,400 people in Slovenia have MS; the society has about 1,750 members.

SPAIN

Associación Española de Esclerosis Múltiple
c/o Modesto Lafuente
8 1st Centro Derecha
28010 Madrid
(34) 91 448 1261
http://www.aedem.org/aedem/home.htm
E-mail: aedem26884@teleline.es

This nonprofit society was founded in 1984 in Madrid to provide a link between people with multiple sclerosis (MS) and people with similar diseases and also to disseminate information about the treatment of MS. The society also provides information to people with MS and to their families to help achieve the social integration of people with MS and promotes the scientific investigation of MS. About 30,000 people in Spain have MS; the society has about 7,600 members.

SWEDEN

Neurologiskt Handikappades Riksforbund
Box 3284, 103 65
Stockholm
(46) 8 677 7010
http://www.nhr.se
E-mail: nhr@nhr.se

This nonprofit association was founded in 1957 in Stockholm to provide service and fellowship for individuals interested in neurological problems such as multiple sclerosis (MS). About 15,000 Swedes have MS; the association has about 15,000 members.

SWITZERLAND

Schweizerische Multiple Sklerose Gesellschaft
Josefstrasse 129,
Postfach, CH-8031
Zürich
(41) 43 444 43 43
http://www.multiplesklerose.ch
E-mail: info@multiplesklerose.ch

This nonprofit society was founded in 1959 to provide services that help people with multiple sclerosis (MS) lead an autonomous life. The society also supports research and provides information to the public and people with MS about the disease. About 10,000 Swiss have MS; the society has about 17,762 members.

TURKEY

Türkiye Multipl Skleroz Derncgi
Buyukdere Caddesi, Hukukcular
Sitesi No 24/21, Mecidiyekoy
Istanbul
(90) 212 275 2296
E-mail: cokyuk@ixir.com

This nonprofit society was founded in 1989 in Istanbul to bring people with MS and their families together, to support them, and to keep them up-to-date with clinical research. About 30,000 people in Turkey have MS; the society has about 750 members.

UNITED KINGDOM

MS Society of Great Britain and Northern Ireland
MS National Centre
372 Edgware Road
London, NW2 6ND
(44) 020 8438 0700
http://www.mssociety.org.uk
E-mail: info@mssociety.org.uk

This nonprofit society was established in 1953 in London to support people affected by multiple sclerosis (MS) and to encourage people affected by MS to attain their full potential as members of society by improving their quality of life. The society also promotes research into MS and allied conditions. About 85,000 people in the U.K. have MS; the society has about 45,000 members.

ZIMBABWE

MS Society of Zimbabwe
P.O. Box BE 1234, Beldevere
Harare
(263) 4 740 472
E-mail: therobs@mweb.co.zw

This nonprofit society was established in 1973 in Harare to aid and alleviate the suffering of those who have multiple sclerosis (MS) to help any person with MS requiring financial assistance or care, and to cooperate closely with the MS societies in other countries, bringing to Zimbabwe the benefits of all the latest advances in the care and treatment of MS. About 35 people in Zimbabwe have MS; the society has about 70 members.

GLOSSARY

antagonist   A chemical that blocks the action of a neurotransmitter receptor. Antagonists inhibit the effects of agonists.

anterior   In medicine, a directional term meaning "toward the front."

brain stem   Brain area composed of midbrain, pons, and medulla; contains reticular activating system and other key centers.

central nervous system (CNS)   One of the two major divisions of the nervous system. Composed of the brain and spinal cord, the CNS is the control network for the entire body.

cerebral cortex   The outer layer of the brain, consisting of nerve cells and the pathways that connect them. The cerebral cortex is the part of the brain in which thought processes (including learning, language, and reasoning) take place.

chromosome   An H-shaped structure inside the cell nucleus made up of tightly coiled strands of genes. Each chromosome is numbered (in humans, from 1 to 46), and contains DNA, sequences of which make up genes.

cognition   The process of recognizing, interpreting, judging, reasoning and knowing. Perception is considered a part of cognition by some psychologists, but not by others.

cognitive   The process of knowing in the broadest sense, including perception, memory, and judgment.

cognitive abilities   Mental abilities such as judgment, memory, learning, comprehension, and reasoning.

cognitive deficit   A perceptual, memory, or conceptual problem that interferes with learning.

cognitive retraining   Developing or relearning the processes involved in thinking.

coping skills   The ability to deal with problems and difficulties by attempting to overcome them or accept them.

dendrites   Branched extensions of the nerve cell body that receive signals from other nerve cells. Each nerve cell usually has many dendrites.

emotional lability   Exhibiting rapid and drastic changes in emotions (such as laughing, crying, anger) without apparent reason.

frustration tolerance   The ability to deal with frustrating events in daily life without becoming angry or aggressive.

gene   The biological unit of heredity. Each gene is located at a specific spot on a particular chromosome, and is made up of a string of chemicals arranged in a certain sequence along the DNA molecule.

genome   All the genes of an organism.

hippocampus   An area buried deep in the forebrain that helps regulate emotion and is important for learning and memory.

hypothalamus   A brain structure composed of many nuclei with different functions, including regulation of activities of internal organs, monitoring information from the autonomic nervous system and controlling the pituitary gland.

limbic system   A group of brain structures including the amygdala, hippocampus, septum and basal ganglia, that regulate emotions, memory and certain aspects of movement.

nervous system   The brain, spinal cord, nerves, ganglia, and parts of the receptor organs that receive and interpret stimuli and transmit impulses.

neurotransmitter   A chemical the nervous system uses to carry messages from one neuron to another.

prefrontal area   Brain location of processes of foresight, abstract thinking, and judgment.

receptor   A site on a nerve cell that receives a specific neurotransmitter; the message receiver.

synapse   The tiny gap between two nerve cells; messages are transmitted across this gap from one nerve cell to another, usually by a neurotransmitter.

tactile   The ability to receive and interpret stimuli through contact with the skin.

temporal lobe   The section of the cerebral hemisphere primarily concerned with hearing and emotions.

ventricles   Four natural cavities in the brain which are filled with cerebrospinal fluid.

BIBLIOGRAPHY

Aarli, J. A. "Role of Cytokines in Neurological Disorders." *Current Medicinal Chemistry* 10, no. 19 (2003): 1,931–1,937.

Aboul-Enein, F., H. Rauschka, et al. "Preferential Loss of Myelin-Associated Glycoprotein Reflects Hypoxia-like White Matter Damage in Stroke and Inflammatory Brain Diseases." *Journal of Neuropathology and Experimental Neurology* 62, no. 1 (2003): 25–33.

Achiron, A. and Y. Barak. "Cognitive Impairment in Probable Multiple Sclerosis." *Journal of Neurology and Neurosurgical Psychiatry* 74, no. 4 (2003): 443–446.

Ackerman, K. D., A. Stover, et al. "Relationship of Cardiovascular Reactivity, Stressful Life Events, and Multiple Sclerosis Disease Activity." *Brain Behavior and Immunity* 17, no. 3 (2003): 141–151.

Aktas, O. and F. Zipp. "Regulation of Self-Reactive T Cells by Human Immunoglobulins—Implications for Multiple Sclerosis Therapy." *Current Pharmaceutical Design* 9, no. 3 (2003): 245–256.

Alpini, D., L. Pugnetti, D. Caputo, et al. "Vestibular Evoked Myogenic Potentials in Multiple Sclerosis: Clinical and Imaging Correlations." *Multiple Sclerosis* 10, no. 3 (June 2004): 316–321.

Alter, A., M. Duddy, S. Hebert, et al. "Determinants of Human B Cell Migration Across Brain Endothelial Cells." *Journal of Immunology* 170 (2003): 4,497–4,505.

Angelov, D. N., S. Waibel, et al. "Therapeutic Vaccine for Acute and Chronic Motor Neuron Diseases: Implications for Amyotrophic Lateral Sclerosis." *Proceedings of the National Academy of Sciences U.S.A.* 100, no. 8 (2003): 4,790–4,795.

Anlar, B. "Infection and multiple sclerosis." *Journal of Neurology and Neurosurgical Psychiatry* 74, no. 5 (2003): 692–693.

Anlar, O., M. Kisli, et al. "Visual Evoked Potentials in Multiple Sclerosis Before and After Two Years of Interferon Therapy." *International Journal of Neuroscience* 113, no. 4 (2003): 483–489.

Antel, J. P. and A. Bar-Or. "Do Myelin-Directed Antibodies Predict Multiple Sclerosis?" *New England Journal of Medicine* 349, no. 2 (2003): 107–109.

Antel, J. P. and T. Owens. "Immune Regulation and CNS Autoimmune Disease." *Journal of Neuroimmunology* 100 (1999): 181–189.

Araki, I., M. Matsui, et al. "Relationship of Bladder Dysfunction to Lesion Site in Multiple Sclerosis." *Journal of Urology* 169, no. 4 (2003): 1,384–1,347.

Arbour, N., A. Holz, et al. "A New Approach for Evaluating Antigen-Specific T Cell Responses to Myelin Antigens During the Course of Multiple Sclerosis." *Journal of Neuroimmunology* 137, no. 1/2 (2003): 197–209.

Arevalo-Martin, A., J. M. Vela, et al. "Therapeutic Action of Cannabinoids in a Murine Model of Multiple Sclerosis." *Journal of Neuroscience* 23, no. 7 (2003): 2,511–2,516.

Ascherio A., K. L. Munger, E. T. Lennette, et al. "Epstein-Barr Virus Antibodies and Risk of Multiple Sclerosis: A Prospective Study." *Journal of the American Medical Association* 286, no. 24 (December 2001): 3,083–3,088.

Ascherio A. and M. Munch. "Epstein-Barr Virus and Multiple Sclerosis." *Epidemiology* 11, no. 2 (March 2000): 220–224.

Ashton, E. A., C. Takahashi, et al. "Accuracy and Reproducibility of Manual and Semiautomated Quantification of MS Lesions by MRI." *Journal of Magnetic Resonance Imaging* 17, no. 3 (2003): 300–308.

Avasarala, J. R., A. H. Cross, et al. "Comparative Assessment of Yale Single Question and Beck

Depression Inventory Scale in Screening for Depression in Multiple Sclerosis." *Multiple Sclerosis* 9, no. 3 (2003): 307–310.

Babcock, A. and T. Owens. "Chemokines in Experimental Autoimmune Encephalomyelitis and Multiple Sclerosis." *Advances in Experimental Medical Biology* 520 (2003): 120–132.

Baker, D. and D. J. Hankey. "Gene Therapy in Autoimmune, Demyelinating Disease of the Central Nervous System." *Gene Therapy* 10, no. 10 (2003): 844–853.

Baker, D., P. Adamson, et al. "Potential of Statins for the Treatment of Multiple Sclerosis." *Lancet* 2, no. 1 (2003): 9–10.

Baker, D. and G. Pryce. "The Therapeutic Potential of Cannabis in Multiple Sclerosis." *Expert Opinions in Investigational Drugs* 12, no. 4 (2003): 561–567.

Baker, D., G. Pryce, et al. "The Therapeutic Potential of Cannabis." *Lancet* 2, no. 5 (2003): 291–298.

Bakshi, R. "Fatigue Associated with Multiple Sclerosis: Diagnosis, Impact and Management." *Multiple Sclerosis* 9, no. 3 (2003): 219–227.

Balassy, C., G. Bernert, C. Wober-Bingol, et al. "Long-Term MRI Observations of Childhood-Onset Relapsing/Remitting Multiple Sclerosis." *Neuropediatrics* 32, no. 1 (February 2001): 28–37.

Balcer, L. J., M. L. Baier, J. A. Cohen, et al. "Contrast Letter Acuity as a Visual Component for the Multiple Sclerosis Functional Composite." *Neurology* 61 (2003): 1,367–1,373.

Ballabh, P., A. Braun, and M. Nedergaard. "The Blood-Brain Barrier: An Overview: Structure, Regulation, and Clinical Implications." *Neurobiological Disease* 16, no. 1 (June 2004): 1–13.

Barkhof, F., M. Rocca, et al. "Validation of Diagnostic Magnetic Resonance Imaging Criteria for Multiple Sclerosis and Response to Interferon Beta1a." *Annals of Neurology* 53, no. 6 (2003): 718–724.

Barnes, M. P., R. M. Kent, et al. "Spasticity in Multiple Sclerosis." *Neurorehabilitation Neural Repair* 17, no. 1 (2003): 66–70.

Bashir, K. and R. A. Kaslow. "*Chlamydia pneumoniae* and Multiple Sclerosis: The Latest Etiologic Candidate." *Epidemiology* 14, no. 2 (2003): 133–134.

Batocchi, A. P., M. Rotondi, et al. "Leptin as a Marker of Multiple Sclerosis Activity in Patients Treated with Interferon-Beta." *Journal of Neuroimmunology* 139, no. 1/2 (2003): 150–154.

Baumhackl, U., C. Franta, et al. "A Controlled Trial of Tick-borne Encephalitis Vaccination in Patients with Multiple Sclerosis." *Vaccine* 21, suppl. 1 (2003): S56–61.

Beatty, W. W., D. M. Orbelo, et al. "Comprehension of Affective Prosody in Multiple Sclerosis." *Multiple Sclerosis* 9, no. 2 (2003): 148–153.

Beck, R., H. Wiendl, et al. "Human Herpesvirus 6 in Serum and Spinal Fluid of Patients with Multiple Sclerosis?" *Archives of Neurology* 60, no. 4 (2003): 639; author reply 639–640.

Belopitova, L., P. V. Guergueltcheva, and V. Bojinova. "Definite and Suspected Multiple Sclerosis in Children: Long-Term Follow-Up and Magnetic Resonance Imaging Findings." *Journal of Child Neurology* 16, no. 5 (May 2001): 317–324.

Benedict, R. H., D. A. Carone, and R. Bakshi. "Correlating Brain Atrophy with Cognitive Dysfunction, Mood Disturbances, and Personality Disorder in Multiple Sclerosis." *Journal of Neuroimaging* 14, no. 3 suppl. (July 2004): 36–45.

Benedict, R. H., F. Munschauer, et al. "Screening for Multiple Sclerosis Cognitive Impairment Using a Self-Administered 15-Item Questionnaire." *Multiple Sclerosis* 9, no. 1 (2003): 95–101.

Benito-Leon, J. and P. Martinez-Martin. "Health-Related Quality of Life in Multiple Sclerosis." *Neurologia* 18, no. 4 (2003): 210–217.

Benjamins, J. A., L. Nedelkoska, et al. "Protection of Mature Oligodendrocytes by Inhibitors of Caspases and Calpains." *Neurochemical Research* 28, no. 1 (2003): 143–152.

Berger, T., P. Rubner, et al. "Antimyelin Antibodies as a Predictor of Clinically Definite Multiple Sclerosis After a First Demyelinating Event." *New England Journal of Medicine* 349, no. 2 (2003): 139–145.

Bermel, R. A., J. Sharma, et al. "A Semiautomated Measure of Whole-Brain Atrophy in Multiple Sclerosis." *Journal of Neurological Science* 208, no. 1/2 (2003): 57–65.

Bielekova, B., N. Richert, T. Howard, et al. "Humanized Anti-CD25 (Daclizumab) Inhibits Disease Activity in Multiple Sclerosis Patients Failing to Respond to Interferon {Beta}." *Proceedings of the National Academy of Sciences U.S.A.* 101 (May 2004): 8,705–8,708.

Bjartmar, C. and B. D. Trapp. "Axonal and Neuronal Degeneration in Multiple Sclerosis: Mechanisms and Functional Consequences." *Current Opinions in Neurology* 14 (2001): 271–278.

———. "Axonal Degeneration and Progressive Neurologic Disability in Multiple Sclerosis." *Neurotoxicity Research* 5, no. 1/2 (2003): 157–164.

Bjartmar, C., J. R. Wujek, et al. "Axonal Loss in the Pathology of MS: Consequences for Understanding the Progressive Phase of the Disease." *Journal of Neurological Science* 206, no. 2 (2003): 165–171.

Blackstone, Margaret. *Multiple Sclerosis: An Essential Guide for the Newly Diagnosed.* New York, N.Y.: Marlowe & Co., 2003.

Bobholz, J. A. and S. M. Rao. "Cognitive Dysfunction in Multiple Sclerosis: A Review of Recent Developments." *Current Opinions in Neurology* 16, no. 3 (2003): 283–288.

Boggild, M. and H. Ford. "Multiple Sclerosis." *Clinical Evidence* 7 (2002): 1,195–1,207.

Bolviken, B., E. G. Celius, et al. "Radon: A Possible Risk Factor in Multiple Sclerosis." *Neuroepidemiology* 22, no. 1 (2003): 87–94.

Bowling, A. C. and T. M. Stewart. "Current Complementary and Alternative Therapies for Multiple Sclerosis." *Current Treatment Options in Neurology* 5, no. 1 (2003): 55–68.

Brass, S. D., S. Narayanan, J. P. Antel, et al. "Axonal Damage in Multiple Sclerosis Patients with High Versus Low Expanded Disability Status Scale Score." *Canadian Journal of Neurological Science* 31, no. 2 (May 2004): 225–228.

Brescia Morra, V., G. Coppola, G. Orefice, et. al. "Interferon-ß Treatment Decreases Cholesterol Plasma Levels in Multiple Sclerosis Patients." *Neurology* 62 (2004): 829–830.

Brostrom, S., J. L. Frederiksen, et al. "Motor Evoked Potentials from the Pelvic Floor in Patients with Multiple Sclerosis." *Journal of Neurological Neurosurgical Psychiatry* 74, no. 4 (2003): 498–500.

Brown, J. S. "Correlation of Mollicutes and Their Viruses with Multiple Sclerosis and Other Demyelinating Diseases." *Medical Hypotheses* 60, no. 2 (2003): 298–303.

Bruce, J. M. and P. A. Arnett. "Self-reported Everyday Memory and Depression in Patients with Multiple Sclerosis." *Journal of Clinical and Experimental Neuropsychology* 26, no. 2 (April 2004): 200–214.

Bruck, W., T. Kuhlmann, et al. "Remyelination in Multiple Sclerosis." *Journal of Neurological Science* 206, no. 2 (2003): 181–185.

Bruno, R., L. Sabater, M. Sospedra, et al. "Multiple Sclerosis Candidate Autoantigens Except Myelin Oligodendrocyte Glycoprotein Are Transcribed in Human thymus." *European Journal of Immunology* 32, no. 10 (October 2002): 2,737–2,747.

Buchanan, R. J., S. Wang, et al. "Analyses of Nursing Home Residents with Multiple Sclerosis and Depression Using the Minimum Data Set." *Multiple Sclerosis* 9, no. 2 (2003): 171–188.

Buljevac, D., H. Z. Flach, W. C. Hop, et al. "Prospective Study on the Relationship Between Infections and Multiple Sclerosis Exacerbations." *Brain* 125 (2002): 952–964.

Carroll, David L. and Jon Dudley Dorman. *Living Well with MS.* New York, N.Y.: HarperCollins, 1993.

Chaudhuri, A. and P. O. Behan. "Mitoxantrone Trial in Multiple Sclerosis." *Lancet* 361, no. 9,363 (2003): 1,133–1,134; author reply 1134.

Chaudhuri, A., P. O. Behan, D. H. Miller, et al. "Natalizumab for Relapsing Multiple Sclerosis." *New England Journal of Medicine* 348 (2003): 1,598–1,599.

Chelmicka-Schorr, E. and B. G. Arnason. "Nervous System-Immune System Interactions and Their Role in Multiple Sclerosis." *Annals of Neurology* 36, Suppl. (1994): s29–s32.

Chitnis, T. and S. J. Khoury. "20. Immunologic Neuromuscular Disorders." *Journal of Allergy and Clinical Immunology* 111, no. 2 suppl. (Oct. 2003): S659–S668.

Ciccarelli, O., D. J. Werring, et al. "A Study of the Mechanisms of Normal-Appearing White Matter Damage in Multiple Sclerosis Using Diffusion Tensor Imaging—Evidence of Wallerian Degeneration." *Journal of Neurology* 250, no. 3 (2003): 287–292.

Clark, A. J., M. A. Ware, E. Yazer, et al. "Patterns of Cannabis Use Among Patients with Multiple Sclerosis." *Neurology* 62, no. 11 (June 8, 2004): 2,098–2,100.

Colman, D., C. Lubetzki, et al. "Multiple Paths Towards Repair in Multiple Sclerosis." *Trends in Neuroscience* 26, no. 2 (2003): 59–61.

Confavreux, C., S. Vukusic, et al. "Early Clinical Predictors and Progression of Irreversible Disability in Multiple Sclerosis: An Amnesic Process." *Brain* 126, Pt. 4 (2003): 770–782.

Comi, G., M. Filippi, J. S. Wolinsky. "European Canadian Glatiramer Acetate. European/Canadian Multicenter, Double-Blind, Randomized, Placebo-Controlled Study of the Effects of Glatiramer Acetate on Magnetic Resonance Imaging—Measured Disease Activity and Burden in Patients with Relapsing Multiple Sclerosis." *Annals of Neurology* 49, no. 3 (2001): 290–297.

Comi, G., M. Filippi, F. Barkhof, et al. "Effect of Early Interferon Treatment on Conversion to Definite Multiple Sclerosis: A Randomised Study." *Lancet* 357, no. 9,268 (2001): 1,576–1,582.

Confavreux, C. "Rate of Pregnancy-Related Relapse in Multiple Sclerosis." *New England Journal of Medicine* 339, no. 5 (1998): 285–291.

Confavreux, C., et al. "Relapses and Progression of Disability in Multiple Sclerosis." *New England Journal of Medicine* 343, no. 20 (2000): 1,430–1,438.

Damasio, A. R. "Aphasia." *New England Journal of Medicine.* 326 (1992): 531–539.

Dan, B., F. Christiaens, C. Christophe, et al. "Trans-Cranial Magnetic Stimulation and Other Evoked Potentials in Pediatric Multiple Sclerosis." *Pediatric Neurology* 22, no. 2 (February 2000): 136–138.

Davey, R., and A. Al-Din. "Secondary Trigeminal Autonomic Cephalgia Associated with Multiple Sclerosis." *Cephalalgia* 24, no. 7 (July 2004): 605–607.

Devere, T. R., J. L. Trotter, and A. H. Cross. "Acute Aphasia in Multiple Sclerosis." *Archives of Neurology* 57 (2000): 1,207–1,209.

Ebers, G. for The PRISMS (Prevention of Relapses and Disability by Interferon beta-1a Subcutaneously in Multiple Sclerosis) Study Group. "Randomised Double-Blind Placebo-Controlled Study of Interferon Beta-1a in Relapsing/Remitting Multiple Sclerosis." *Lancet* 352 (1998): 1,498–1,504.

Edan, G., D. Miller, M. Clanet, et al. "Therapeutic Effect of Mitoxantrone Combined with Methylprednisolone in Multiple Sclerosis: A Randomised Multicentre Study of Active Disease Using MRI and Clinical Criteria." *Journal of Neurology and Neurosurgical Psychiatry* 62 (1997): 112–118.

Feinstein, A., P. Roy, N. Lobaugh, et al. "Structural Brain Abnormalities in Multiple Sclerosis Patients with Major Depression." *Neurology* 62 (2004): 586–590.

Filippi, M., M. Rovaris, and M. A. Rocca. "Imaging Primary Progressive Multiple Sclerosis: The Contribution of Structural, Metabolic, and Functional MRI Techniques." *Multiple Sclerosis* 10, suppl. 1 (June 2004): S36–S44; discussion S44–S45.

Filippi, M., M. Rovaris, M. A. Rocca, et al. "Glatiramer Acetate Reduces the Proportion of New MS Lesions Evolving into 'Black Holes.' " *Neurology* 57 (2001): 731–733.

Francis, G. "Secondary Progressive Efficacy Clinical Trial of Recombinant Interferon-beta-1a in MS (SPECTRIMS) Study Group. Randomized Controlled Trial of Interferon-Beta-1a in Secondary Progressive MS: Clinical Results." *Neurology* 56 (2001): 1,496–1,504.

Frank, J. A., N. Richert, C. Bash, et al. "Interferon-β-1b Slows Progression of Atrophy in RRMS: Three-year Follow-up in NAb– and NAb+ Patients." *Neurology* 62 (2004): 719–725.

Fredrikson, S. and S. Kam-Hansen. "The 150-year anniversary of Multiple Sclerosis: Does Its Early History Give an Etiological Clue?" *Perspectives in Biology and Medicine* 32 (1989): 237–243.

Friedman, J., H. Brem, and R. Mayeux. "Global Aphasia in Multiple Sclerosis." *Annals of Neurology* 13 (1993): 222–223.

Ge, Y., O. Gonen, and M. Inglese. "Neuronal Cell Injury Precedes Brain Atrophy in Multiple Sclerosis." *Neurology* 62 (2004): 624–627.

Gilroy, J. "Multiple Sclerosis," in *Basic Neurology,* 3rd ed., New York, N.Y.: McGraw-Hill, 2000, pp. 199–223.

Goodin, D. S., B. G. Arnason, P. K. Coyle, et al. "The Use of Mitoxantrone (Novantrone) for the Treatment of Multiple Sclerosis: Report of the Therapeutics and Technology Assessment Subcommittee of the American Academy of Neurology." *Neurology* 61 (2003): 1,332–1,338.

Goodin, D. S., E. M. Frohman, and G. P. Garmany, Jr., et al. "Disease Modifying Therapies in Multiple Sclerosis: Subcommittee of the American Academy of Neurology and the MS Council for Clinical Practice Guidelines." *Neurology* 58 (2002): 169–178.

Goodin, D. S., G. C. Ebers, K. P. Johnson, et al. "The Relationship of MS to Physical Trauma and Psychological Stress: Report of the Therapeutics and Technology Assessment Subcommittee of the American Academy of Neurology." *Neurology* 52 (1999): 1,737–1,745.

Haahr, S., N. Koch-Henriksen, A. Moller-Larsen, et al. "Increased Risk of Multiple Sclerosis After Late Epstein-Barr Virus Infection: A Historical Prospective Study." *Multiple Sclerosis* 1, no. 2 (June 1995): 73–77.

Hafler, D. A. "Multiple Sclerosis." *Journal of Clinical Investigation.* 113 (2004): 788–794.

Hahn, Cecil D., M. Manohar, Susan Shroff, et al. "MRI Criteria for Multiple Sclerosis: Evaluation in a Pediatric Cohort." *Neurology* 62 (2004): 806–808.

Hernan, M. A., S. M. Zhang, L. Lipworth, et al. "Multiple Sclerosis and Age at Infection with Common Viruses." *Epidemiology* 12, no. 3 (May 2001): 301–306.

Hilton, D. A., S. Love, A. Fletcher, et al. "Absence of Epstein-Barr Virus RNA in Multiple Sclerosis as Assessed by In Situ Hybridization." *Journal of Neurology and Neurosurgical Psychiatry* 57, no. 8 (August 1994): 975–976.

Hogancamp, W. E. "The Epidemiology of Multiple Sclerosis." *Mayo Clinic Proceedings* 72 (1997): 871–878.

Nancy J. Holland and Robin Frames. "Bowel Problems: The Basic Facts 2003," Available online. URL: http://www.nationalmssociety.org/Brochures-BowelProblems1.asp Downloaded on September 28, 2004.

Hollsberg, P., H. J. Hansen, and S. Haahr. "Altered CD8+ T Cell Responses to Selected Epstein-Barr Virus Immunodominant Epitopes in Patients with Multiple Sclerosis." *Clinical Experimental Immunology* 132, no. 1 (April 2003): 137–143.

Hughes, R. A. C., for The PRISMS (Prevention of Relapses and Disability by Interferon-β-1a Sub-cutaneously in Multiple Sclerosis) Study Group, and The University of British Columbia MS/MRI Analysis Group. PRISMS-4. "Long-Term Effi-cacy of Interferon in Relapsing MS." *Neurology* 56 (2001): 1,628–1,636.

Hunter, S. F., et al. "Rational Clinical Immunother-apy for Multiple Sclerosis." *Mayo Clinic Proceedings* 72 (1997): 765–780.

Jacobs, L. D., D. L. Cookfair, R. A. Rudick, et al. "Intramuscular Interferon Beta-1a for Disease Progression in Relapsing Multiple Sclerosis. The Multiple Sclerosis Collaborative Research Group (MSCRG)." *Annals of Neurology* 39 (1996): 285–294.

Jacobs, L. D., R. W. Beck, J. H. Simon, et al. "Intra-muscular Interferon Beta-1a Therapy Initiated During a First Demyelinating Event in Multiple Sclerosis. CHAMPS Study Group." *New England Journal of Medicine* 343 (2000): 898–904.

Jafarian-Tehrani, M. and E. M. Sternberg. "Animal Models of Neuroimmune Interactions in Inflammatory Diseases." *Journal of Neuroim-munology* 100 (1999): 13–20.

Johnson, K. P., B. R. Brooks, J. A. Cohen, et al. "Extended Use of Glatiramer Acetate (Copaxone) Is Well Tolerated and Maintains Its Clinical Effect on Multiple Sclerosis Relapse Rate and Degree of Disability. Copolymer 1 Multiple Sclerosis Study Group." *Neurology* 50 (1998): 701–708.

Kantarci, O. H., D. D. Hebrink, and S. J. Achen-bach. "Association of APOE Polymorphisms with Disease Severity in MS Is Limited to Women." *Neurology* 62 (2004): 811–814.

Kappos, L. "Effect of Drugs in Secondary Disease Progression in Patients with Multiple Sclerosis." *Multiple Sclerosis* 10, suppl. 1 (June 2004): S46–S54; discussion S54–S55.

Kolesnikova, T. V., C. S. Stipp, R. M. Rao, et al. "EWI-2 Modulates Lymphocyte Integrin α4β1 Functions." *Blood* 103 (2004): 3,013–3,019.

Kreitman, R. R. and F. Blanchette. "On the Hori-zon: Possible Neuroprotective Role for Glati-ramer Acetate." *Multiple Sclerosis* 10, suppl. 1 (June 2004): S81–S86; discussion S86–S89.

Kroencke, D. C. and D. R. Denney. "Stress and Coping in Multiple Sclerosis: Exacerbation, Remission and Chronic Subgroups." *Multiple Sclerosis* 5 (1999): 89–93.

Lacour, A., J. de Seze, E. Revenco, et. al. "Acute Aphasia in Multiple Sclerosis: A Multicenter Study of 22 Patients." *Neurology* 62 (2004): 974–977.

Lang, H. L., H. Jacobsen, S. Ikemizu, et al. "A Functional and Structural Basis for TCR Cross-Reactivity in Multiple Sclerosis." *Natural Immunology* 3, no. 10 (October 2002): 940–943.

Laplaud, D. A., C. Ruiz, S. Wiertlewski, et al. "Blood T-Cell Receptor {Beta} Chain Transcriptome in Multiple Sclerosis. Characterization of the T Cells with Altered CDR3 Length Distribution." *Brain* 127 (2004): 981–995.

Larsen, P. D., L. C. Bloomer, and P. F. Bray. "Epstein-Barr Nuclear Antigen and Viral Capsid Antigen Antibody Titers in Multiple Sclerosis." *Neurology* 35, no. 3 (March 1985): 435–438.

Levin, L. I., K. L. Munger, M. V. Rubertone, et al. "Multiple Sclerosis and Epstein-Barr Virus." *Journal of the American Medical Association* 289, no. 12 (March 26, 2003): 1,533– 1,536.

Li, D. K., and D. W. Paty. "Magnetic Resonance Imaging Results of the PRISMS Trial: A Randomized, Double-Blind, Placebo-Controlled Study of Interferon-Beta1a in Relapsing-Remitting Multiple Sclerosis." *Annals of Neurology* 46 (1999): 197–206.

Li, J., C. Johansen, and E. H. Brønnum-Hansen. "The Risk of Multiple Sclerosis in Bereaved Parents: A Nationwide Cohort Study in Denmark." *Neurology* 62 (2004): 726–729.

Lim, E. T., D. Grant, M. Pashenkov, et al. "Cerebrospinal Fluid Levels of Brain Specific Proteins in Optic Neuritis." *Multiple Sclerosis* 10, no. 3 (June 2004): 261–265.

Lin, X., C. R. Tench, N. Evangelou, et al. "Measurement of Spinal Cord Atrophy in Multiple Sclerosis." *Journal of Neuroimaging* 14, no. 3 suppl. (July 2004): 20–26.

Lublin, Fred D., Monika Baier, and Gary Cutter. "Effect of Relapses on Development of Residual Deficit in Multiple Sclerosis." *Neurology* 61 (2003): 1,528–1,532.

Lucchinetti, C., and W. Bruck. "The Pathology of Primary Progressive Multiple Sclerosis." *Multiple Sclerosis* 10, suppl. 1 (June 2004): S23–S30.

Maggs, F. G. and J. Palace. "The Pathogenesis of Multiple Sclerosis: Is It Really a Primary Inflammatory Process?" *Multiple Sclerosis* 10, no. 3 (June 2004): 326–329.

Malmeström, C., S. Haghighi, L. Rosengren, et al. "Neurofilament Light Protein and Glial Fibrillary Acidic Protein as Biological Markers in MS." *Neurology* 61 (2003): 1,720–1,725.

Mansson, E., and J. Lexell. "Performance of Activities of Daily Living in Multiple Sclerosis." *Disability Rehabilitation* 26, no. 10 (May 20, 2004): 576–585.

Marrie, R. A., C. Wolfson, M. C. Sturkenboom, et al. "Multiple Sclerosis and Antecedent Infections: A Case-Control Study." *Neurology* 54, no. 12 (June 2000): 2,307–2,310.

Martínez, A., A. Rubio, and E. Urcelay. "TNF-376A Marks Susceptibility to MS in the Spanish Population: A Replication Study." *Neurology* 62 (2004): 809–810.

Mayr, W. T., S. J. Pittock, R. L. McClelland, et al. "Incidence and Prevalence of Multiple Sclerosis in Olmsted County, Minnesota, 1985–2000." *Neurology* 61 (2003): 1,373–1,377.

McDonald, W. I. "The Dynamics of Multiple Sclerosis." *Journal of Neurology* 240 (1993): 28–36.

McDonald, W. I., A. Compston, G. Edan, et al. "Recommended Diagnostic Criteria for Multiple Sclerosis: Guidelines from the International Panel on the Diagnosis of Multiple Sclerosis." *Annals of Neurology* 50 (2001): 121–127.

McDonald, W. I., et al. "Recommended Diagnostic Criteria for Multiple Sclerosis: Guidelines from the International Panel on the Diagnosis of Multiple Sclerosis." *Annals of Neurology* 50 (2001): 121–127.

Medaer, R. "Does the History of Multiple Sclerosis Go Back as Far as the 14th Century?" *Acta Neurologica Scandinavica* 60 (1979): 189–192.

Meesters, Y. "Light Treatment and Multiple Sclerosis." *Multiple Sclerosis* 10, no. 3 (June 2004): 336.

Mestas, J. and C. C. W. Hughes. "Of Mice and Not Men: Differences Between Mouse and Human Immunology." *Journal of Immunology* 172 (2004): 2,731–2,738.

Miller, David H., Omar A. Khan, and William A. Sheremata. "A Controlled Trial of Natalizumab for Relapsing Multiple Sclerosis." *New England Journal of Medicine* 348, no. 1 (January 2, 2003): 15–23.

Mohr, D. C., D. E. Goodkin, P. Bacchetti, et al. "Psychological Stress and the Subsequent Appearance of New Brain: MRI Lesions in MS." *Neurology* 55 (2000): 55–61.

Morgan, J. C., D. C. Hess, and K. D. Sethi. "Botulinum Toxin Treatment of Painful Tonic Spasms in Multiple Sclerosis." *Neurology* 62, no. 11 (June 8, 2004): 2,143; author reply 2,143.

Morre, S. A., J. van Beek, C. J. De Groot, et al. "Is Epstein-Barr Virus Present in the CNS of Patients with MS?" *Neurology* 56, no. 5 (March 13, 2001): 692.

MS Disease Management Advisory Task Force. "National Multiple Sclerosis Society (NMSS) Disease Management Consensus Statement," Available online. URL: http://www.nationalmssociety.org/Sourcebook-Early.asp Downloaded on 2/1/05.

Myers, L. W. "Treatment of Multiple Sclerosis with ACTH and Corticosteroids," in Rudick, R. A. and D. E. Goodkin, eds. *Treatment of Multiple Sclerosis: Trial Design, Results, and Future Perspectives.* New York, N.Y.: Springer Verlag, 1992, pp. 146–147.

Noseworthy, J. H., et al. "Multiple Sclerosis." *New England Journal of Medicine* 343, no. 13 (2000): 938–952.

O'Connor, Paul. *Multiple Sclerosis: The Facts You Need.* Buffalo, N.Y.: Firefly Books, 1998.

O'Connor, P. W., A. Goodman, A. J. Willmer-Hulme, et al. "Randomized Multicenter Trial of Natalizumab in Acute MS Relapses: Clinical and MRI Effects." *Neurology* 62, no. 11 (2004): 2,038–2,043.

Oken, B. S., S. Kishiyama, D. Zajdel, et al. "Randomized Controlled Trial of Yoga and Exercise in Multiple Sclerosis." *Neurology* 62, no. 11 (June 8, 2004): 2,058–2,064.

Olson, J. K., T. N. Eagar, and S. D. Miller. "Functional Activation of Myelin-Specific T Cells by Virus-Induced Molecular Mimicry." *Journal of Immunology* 169, no. 5 (2002): 2,719–2,726.

Operskalski, E. A., B. R. Visscher, R. M. Malmgren, et al. "A Case-Controlled Study of Multiple Sclerosis." *Neurology* 39, no. 6 (June 1989): 825–829.

Pachner, Andrew R. "An Improved ELISA for Screening for Neutralizing Anti-IFN-β Antibodies in MS Patients." *Neurology* 61 (2003): 1,444–1,446.

Patten, S. B., C. A. Beck, J. V. A. Williams, et al. "Major Depression in Multiple Sclerosis: A Population-Based Perspective." *Neurology* 61 (2003): 1,524–1,527.

Pengiran Tengah, C. D., R. J. Lock, D. J. Unsworth, et al. "Multiple Sclerosis and Occult Gluten Sensitivity." *Neurology* 62, no. 12 (June 22, 2004): 2,326–2,327.

Peterson, J. W., L. Bö, S. Mörk, et al. "Transected Neurites, Apoptotic Neurons, and Reduced Inflammation in Cortical Multiple Sclerosis Lesions." *Annals of Neurology* 50 (2001): 389–400.

Phillips, J. T., G. Rice, E. Frohman, et al. "A Multicenter, Open-Label, Phase II Study of the Immunogenicity and Safety of a New Prefilled Syringe (Liquid) Formulation of Avonex in Patients with Multiple Sclerosis." *Clinical Therapeutics* 26, no. 4 (April 2004): 511–521.

Pittock, S. J., W. T. Mayr, R. L. McClelland, et al. "Disability Profile of MS Did Not Change Over 10 Years in a Population-Based Prevalence Cohort." *Neurology* 62 (2004): 601–606.

Rabins, P. V., B. R. Brooks, P. O'Donnell, et al. "Structural Brain Correlates of Emotional Disorder in Multiple Sclerosis." *Brain* 109 (1986): 585–597.

Racke, M. K., K. Hawker, and E. M. Frohman. "Fatigue in Multiple Sclerosis: Is the Picture Getting Simpler or More Complex?" *Archives of Neurology* 61, no. 2 (February 2004): 201–207.

Rosner, Louis J. and Shelley Ross. *Multiple Sclerosis: New Hope and Practical Advice for People with MS and Their Families.* New York, N.Y.: Simon & Schuster, 1992.

Rudick, R. A. "Impact of Disease-Modifying Therapies on Brain and Spinal Cord Atrophy in Multiple Sclerosis." *Journal of Neuroimaging* 14, no. 3 suppl. (July 2004): 54–64.

Rudick, R. A., E. Fisher, J. C. Lee, et al. "Use of the Brain Parenchymal Fraction to Measure Whole Brain Atrophy in Relapsing-Remitting MS. Multiple Sclerosis Collaborative Research Group." *Neurology* 53 (1999): 1,698–1,704.

Schwartz, C. E., et al. "Utilization of Unconventional Treatments by Persons with MS: Is It Alternative or Complementary." *Neurology* 52 (1999): 626–629.

Schwartz, C. E., F. W. Foley, S. M. Rao, et al. "Stress and Course of Disease in Multiple Sclerosis." *Behavioral Medicine* 25 (1999): 110–116.

Shirodaria, P. V., M. Haire, E. Fleming, et al. "Viral Antibody Titers: Comparison in Patients with

Multiple Sclerosis and Rheumatoid Arthritis." *Archives of Neurology* 44, no. 12 (December 1987): 1,237–1,241.

Sirven, J. I., and A. T. Berg. "Marijuana as a Treatment for Epilepsy and Multiple Sclerosis? A 'Grass Roots' Movement." *Neurology* 62, no. 11 (June 8, 2004): 1,924–1,925.

Sormani, M. P., M. Rovaris, P. Valsasina, et al. "Measurement Error of Two Different Techniques for Brain Atrophy Assessment in Multiple Sclerosis." *Neurology* 62 (2004): 1,432–1,434.

Sternberg, E. M. "Neuroendocrine Regulation of Autoimmune/Inflammatory Disease." *Journal of Endocrinology* 169 (2001): 429–435.

Stuve, O., M. Kita, D. Pelletier, et al. "Mitoxantrone as a Potential Therapy for Primary Progressive Multiple Sclerosis." *Multiple Sclerosis* 10, suppl. 1 (June 2004): S58–S61.

Sullivan, G. W., D. D. Lee, W. G. Ross, et al. "Activation of A2A Adenosine Receptors Inhibits Expression of α4/β1 Integrin (Very Late Antigen-4) on Stimulated Human Neutrophils." *Journal of Leukocyte Biology* 75 (2004): 127–134.

Sun, X., M. Tanaka, S. Kondo, et al. "Clinical Significance of Reduced Cerebral Metabolism in Multiple Sclerosis: A Combined PET and MRI Study." *Annals of Nuclear Medicine* 12, no. 2 (1998): 89–94.

Sundstrom, P., P. Juto, G. Wadell, et al. "An Altered Immune Response to Epstein-Barr Virus in Multiple Sclerosis: A Prospective Study." *Neurology* 62, no. 12 (June 22, 2004): 2,277–2,282.

The IFNB Multiple Sclerosis Study Group. "Interferon Beta-1b Is Effective in Relapsing-Remitting Multiple Sclerosis. I. Clinical Results of a Multicenter, Randomized, Double-Blind, Placebo-Controlled Trial," *Neurology* 43 (1993): 655–661.

The IFNB Multiple Sclerosis Study Group and The University of British Columbia MS/MRI Analysis Group. "Interferon Beta-1b in the Treatment of Multiple Sclerosis: Final Outcome of the Randomized Controlled Trial," *Neurology* 45 (1995): 1,277–1,285.

Torelli, P. and G. C. Manzoni. "Risk Factors of Multiple Sclerosis." *Neurological Science* 25, no. 2 (June 2004): 116–117.

Tremlett, Helen L., Eric M. Yoshida, and Joel Oger. "Liver Injury Associated with the β-Interferons

for MS: A Comparison Between the Three Products." *Neurology* 62 (2004): 628–631.

Van Kaer, L. "Natural Killer T Cells as Targets for Immunotherapy of Autoimmune Diseases." *Immunology and Cell Biology* 82, no. 3 (June 2004): 315–322.

van Oosten, B. W., J. Killestein, E. M. Mathus-Vliegen, et al. "Multiple Sclerosis Following Treatment with a Cannabinoid Receptor-1 Antagonist." *Multiple Sclerosis* 10, no. 3 (June 2004): 330–331.

van Veen, T., L. van Winsen, J. B. A. Crusius, et al. "B-Crystallin Genotype Has Impact on the Multiple Sclerosis Phenotype." *Neurology* 61 (2003): 1,245–1,249.

Victor, M. and A. H. Ropper. "Multiple Sclerosis and Allied Demyelinative Diseases." *Adams and Victor's Principles of Neurology,* 7th ed. New York, N.Y.: McGraw-Hill, 2001.

von Andrian, U. H. and B. Engelhardt. "{Alpha}4 Integrins as Therapeutic Targets in Autoimmune Disease." *New England Journal of Medicine* 348 (2003): 68–72.

Waegemans, T. "Auto-Antibodies in Multiple Sclerosis: An Hypothesis." *Biomedical Pharmacotherapy.* 58, no. 5 (June 2004): 282–285.

Walther, E. U. and R. Hohlfield. "Multiple Sclerosis: Side Effects of Interferon Beta Therapy and Their Management." *Neurology* 53 (1999): 1,622–1,627.

Wandinger, K., W. Jabs, A. Siekhaus, et al. "Association Between Clinical Disease Activity and Epstein-Barr Virus Reactivation in MS." *Neurology* 55, no. 2 (July 25, 2000): 178–184.

Warner, H. B. and R. I. Carp. "Multiple Sclerosis and Epstein-Barr Virus." *Lancet* 2, no. 8,258 (December 1981): 1,290.

Wolinsky, J. S. and PROMiSe Trial Study Group. "The PROMiSe Trial: Baseline Data Review and Progress Report." *Multiple Sclerosis* 10, suppl. 1 (June 2004): S65–S71; discussion S71–S72.

Zifko, U. A. "Management of Fatigue in Patients with Multiple Sclerosis." *Drugs* 64, no. 12 (2004): 1,295–1,304.

Zivadinov, R. and R. Bakshi. "Central Nervous System Atrophy and Clinical Status in Multiple Sclerosis." *Journal of Neuroimaging* 14, no. 3, suppl. (July 2004): 27–35.

INDEX